THE AMA AND U.S. HEALTH POLICY
SINCE 1940

THE AMA AND U.S. HEALTH POLICY

SINCE 1940

Frank D. Campion

CHICAGO REVIEW PRESS, CHICAGO

Copyright © 1984 by American Medical Association
All rights reserved
Published by Chicago Review Press, Chicago

Library of Congress Cataloging in Publication Data

Campion, Frank D., 1921-
  The AMA and U.S. health policy since 1940.

  Bibliography: p.
  Includes index.
  1. American Medical Association—History—20th century. 2. Medical
policy—United States—History—20th century. 3. Medical care—United
States—History—20th century. I. Title. II. Title: The A.M.A. and US health policy
since 1940. [DNLM: 1. Health Policy—history—United States. 2. Societies,
Medical history—United States. WB 1 AA1 C19a]
R15.A55C36   1984   610'.6'073   84-7817

Manufactured in the United States of America
First Printing
First Edition

ISBN 0-914091-57-3

Contents

Preface

The oldest and most reliable way to write a history is to set down the significant facts in chronological sequence. "Begin at the beginning," as the King says in *Alice's Adventures in Wonderland*, "and go on till you come to the end; then stop." That advice is hard to follow in the case of an organization as big, as complex, and as heterogeneous as the American Medical Association (AMA). The major difficulty is one of pace, for some parts of the essential material consist of well-contained, suddenly occurring episodes, while other parts—no less important—consist of long-established, continuing operations. Moreover, some of the most important issues that weave through this period have a way of appearing, disappearing, and then reappearing, a phenomenon that would require the author of an orthodox chronology to take his reader back and forth endlessly to pick up various threads in the story. Organizing the history of the AMA into an orderly and readable form has not been a simple assignment.

The same challenge evidently faced Morris Fishbein, M.D., the editor of the *Journal of the American Medical Association* from 1924 to 1949, when he wrote his 1,242-page *A History of the American Medical Association*, published in 1947 during the 100th anniversary of the founding of the association. Fishbein solved his organizational problems by dividing his history into several sections, many of them written by others. Walter L. Bierring, M.D., for example, an AMA president himself in 1934, contributed biographies of the 100 other men who had been elected President of the AMA.* Fishbein

---

*The only man to serve more than one year was Nathan S. Davis, M.D., (1817-1904). More responsible than any other person for the founding of the AMA, he served two years as president during the Civil War and became the first editor of *JAMA* in 1883.

wrote a section consisting of portraits of those who had received the AMA's Distinguished Service Medal. Various others helped by writing chapter-long histories of each AMA council, each AMA publication, and each AMA administrative department.

The core of the book was, however, Fishbein's 515-page chronicle. For the most part, this was a year-by-year record of events with emphasis on the actions of the House of Delegates taken at the annual meetings. Fishbein made only occasional efforts to interpret the broad trends and identify the continuities that can give isolated actions the perspective of history. He also wrote for a reader already familiar with the AMA or interested in it.

This book, which picks up at the approximate time when Fishbein left off, aims at a wider audience and takes a different approach. It is designed to be read easily by a reader with virtually no knowledge of medicine, the AMA, or United States health policy. For that reason, time is devoted at the beginning of the book to the economic, political, and scientific setting (Part I) and to the structural workings of the AMA as an organization (Part II). Most physician readers will find that they can skim chapters 2, 3, and 4; those who have been active in AMA affairs can probably move quickly through chapters 5, 6, 7, and 8. The central element of this book—the essential history—is to be found in Part III. Events here are arranged in generally chronological order, though an exact time sequence has sometimes been sacrificed so that a thematic structure could be followed. However satisfactory in other respects, that format imposed restrictions, necessitating Part IV so that suitable emphasis could be given to some of the AMA's long-standing but less dramatic operations.

In developing material for this book, the author has relied on the craft of the journalist and the resources of the historian. Much of the information herein is, of course, a matter of record. The actions of the AMA House of Delegates are recorded in the published *Proceedings* of each meeting; those of the Board of Trustees are to be found in the minutes for its meetings, which were available to the author. The mere report of an action does not, however, always reveal its full dimensions. The AMA's publications, especially the weekly *Journal of the American Medical Association* and the *American Medical News* (the weekly AMA newspaper), have often helped to identify the underlying causes or motivations for some action. The transcripts of the dialogue in the house have proven invaluable in appreciating the intensity that surrounded many issues. In further efforts to put flesh on the bones, the author has interviewed people close to the major events—present employees of the AMA, retired employees, present and former officers of the association, and people entirely outside of the organization who, for various reasons, were close to events. Virtually all of the major interviews were taped and the recordings deposited with the AMA archive library.

This is, of course, an authorized history, approved for publication by the AMA Board of Trustees. At the time of writing, and for more than ten years before that, the author was a full-time employee of the AMA. He was, however, allowed wide latitude; he was not directed as to the sort of history that was wanted nor told what to include or omit. The same book would very likely have resulted had the author undertaken it on his own, independently of the AMA's sponsorship. Whatever lack of objectivity or whatever shortcomings may appear are therefore the responsibility of the author. Total objectivity is, of course, beyond human achievement. About all that can be said on the matter here is that the author set out to write a full and fair-minded account of events for a sponsor who asked only for a history that was complete and balanced.

During the first 100 years of the AMA's existence, the principal changes tended to spring from internally generated initiatives for reform in American medicine. But during the forty or so years on which this book concentrates—roughly from the outbreak of World War II into the early 1980s—external phenomena such as wondrous advances in science, profound shifts in economic policy, and a new concept of the governmental function presented challenges of a different sort and required a new brand of leadership. The United States health care system, American medicine, and the American Medical Association have all changed more in the last four decades than in the century that preceded them.

Acknowledgements

This history has benefited from the generous help of many people, several of them members of the staff of the American Medical Association. I am particularly indebted to Eleanor Barry, who as a member of the executive secretarial staff attended, took notes, and prepared the minutes of virtually every meeting of the Board of Trustees during the key periods of this history. One of those remarkable persons who unfailingly knows where things are and what happened when, she was invaluable in challenging assumptions, unearthing relevant source material, and documenting facts. Equally cordial thanks are due Linda Abbott, who typed the manuscript, to Dolores Anderson who did the word-processing, and to several people in the AMA library: Terry Austin, director of special collections, Mary Jo Dwyer, Jackie Kuhl, Micaela Sullivan, and especially Marguerite Fallucco, in charge of the archives, and George Kruto, who did the indexing. The credit for the graphic design of this book belongs to Herbert L. Hinkelman and David LaHoda of the creative services department; Joseph F. Fletcher took many of the photographs and supervised the photocopying of others. Elizabeth K. White edited the the manuscript.

I wish to express my thanks also to other members of the AMA staff (plus several elected officers, many members, and others outside of the AMA) who reviewed parts of this book dealing with their areas of special knowledge and experience. I want to say a final word about Leo E. Brown, for many years the director of communications for the AMA and later a special assistant to the AMA's chief executive officer. It was his memo, written shortly before his retirement, that originally set this work in motion.

Part I

The Environment

Chapter One

The Elements of Change

The American medical care system—that populous and protean agglomeration of physicians, nurses, technicians, administrators, clinics, hospitals, insurance companies, and government agencies—has evolved in the way many of our other national institutions have evolved. Responsive to changing perceptions of need, it has been shaped by our history, our traditions, and our culture as well as by our economic and political choices. During the last forty years, with rising insistence, many forces have pushed and pulled at the system and brought about substantial change. One of the principal participants in that process of change is the subject of this book, the American Medical Association (AMA).

At the time this history begins, roughly 1940, the American medical care system had developed around both private and public institutions. Some of these were federal, state, county, and municipal; others were religious, fraternal, proprietary (privately owned), and community. But with the government then financing only 20 percent of the total national health bill, the system was overwhelmingly private. Odin W. Anderson, Ph.D., the University of Chicago sociologist, points out that the United States system of medical care grew up in a climate of laissez-faire economics and in the presence of the largest, most affluent middle class the world has ever known. He writes:

> The American hospitals were subsidized without interest or thought of repayment by the newly rich, and by contributions from the not-so-rich, in community after community across the nation...In exchange for the privilege of hospital appointments, the physicians were expected to provide care to indigent patients without charge. Thus the American health service delivery system became largely a private system, both as to ownership of facilities and the provision of

skills—the voluntary hospital and the physician in private practice. No other country has been able to support as expensive and as socially necessary a service from a large middle income group, because the mass purchasing power was not present elsewhere.[1]

Economist Victor R. Fuchs, Ph.D., emphasizes an additional factor in our history that helped cast our medical system in a pluralistic mold. Citing the "distrust of government on the part of many Americans who came to this country to escape oppressive rule," he attributes the largely private nature of our system to "the heterogeneity of the population in terms of race, religion and ethnicity" and the consequent desire of separate groups to have their own medical care institutions.[2]

Another salient characteristic of the American medical care system in the early 1940s was its commitment to quality. This stemmed from a decision made early in the century by the AMA that standards of American medical education should be second to none, that they should, specifically, at least match the standards then existing in England, France, and Germany.[3]

At the turn of the twentieth century, the United States had more medical schools than the rest of the countries of the world put together. A few American schools were first-rate, among them Harvard, Rush, Western Reserve, the University of California and, notably, Johns Hopkins. But others, a decided majority, were a disgrace; many were little more than cram schools or diploma mills run for the benefit of their proprietors.

No one knew better how shameful the conditions were than the five physicians appointed by the Board of Trustees of the AMA in 1904 to serve as its newly created Council on Medical Education. Four of them held professorial rank at well established medical schools: Harvard, the University of Pennsylvania, Vanderbilt, and Rush; the fifth was dean of the University of Michigan Medical School. As one important step in a long series of actions to upgrade American medical education, the council in 1905 announced minimum and ideal standards for medical education. These embraced higher entrance requirements, longer academic training in medical school, more clinical work with patients, and the satisfactory completion of a state licensing exam. The ideal standard, which included a year's internship in a hospital, gave educators a target to shoot for, and they proceeded to do so in surprisingly large numbers.

Those who did not respond to the Council on Medical Education's carrot soon felt the stick. Reviewing the pass/fail statistics of recent medical school graduates taking state licensing board examinations, the council concluded that performance on the exams constituted a measure of the quality of medical education in the schools from which the candidates came. Accordingly, in 1905 the *Journal of the American Medical Association* (*JAMA*) began publishing statistical tables listing the nation's medical colleges, the number of graduates from each taking the previous year's state licensing board examinations, and the number and the percentage of those failing. Thus the schools found themselves rated, and rated *publicly*, for all to see, in the pages of *JAMA*.[4]

To give the drive for reform an even sharper edge the next year, Arthur Dean Bevan, M.D., the chairman of the Council on Medical Education, singled out "five especially rotten spots which are responsible for most of the bad medical instruction." Illinois, Kentucky, Maryland, Missouri, and Tennessee, he said, had among them fifty-four medical schools of which "not more than six can be considered acceptable."[5]

By 1907 the council could take an even tougher stand because its ratings of medical schools were now based on the evidence gained from site visits. During the 1906-1907 school year either a member of the council or the council's full-time secretary, Nathan P. Colwell, M.D., visited each of the 162 United States medical schools then operating. The visitors from the AMA graded the schools on such things as admission requirements, laboratory equipment, library facilities, number of full-time instructors, character of the curriculum, and clinical instruction facilities. Chairman Bevan's report, given at the third annual AMA conference on medical education and published in *JAMA*, came down hard on some schools that the inspecting teams found "no better equipped to teach medicine than a Turkish-bath establishment or a barber shop." The survey gave eighty-two schools a Class A rating (acceptable), forty-six a Class B rating (doubtful), and thirty-two a Class C rating (unacceptable).[6] Though the individual medical schools were not named publicly, they were notified of their ratings by letter. But that was enough. Years later, Bevan, who headed the council from its start in 1904 until 1928, recalled that from that point onward, "A great wave of improvement in medical education swept over the country."[7]

The council, however, was not yet fully satisfied that maximum pressure had been applied. In 1908 the AMA approached the prestigious Carnegie Foundation for the Advancement of Teaching to present the evidence it had accumulated and to ask if the foundation would make the status of medical education the subject of a special report. "If we could obtain the publication and approval of our work by the [foundation]," Bevan later reported, "it would assist materially in securing the results we were attempting to bring about." The president of the Carnegie Foundation enthusiastically agreed to the AMA proposal and engaged a distinguished educator, Abraham Flexner, M.A., to conduct the continuing investigation.[8]

During the 1909-10 school year, Flexner and Colwell, the Council on Medical Education's secretary, together inspected the medical schools of the United States and, at the request of the Canadians themselves, those of Canada. Published in the spring of 1910, the Flexner report accomplished several things. Far more harsh in its criticisms than the previous AMA inspection reports had been, it dramatized the issue and won wide public support. Confirming what the AMA had been uncovering, it served also to remove the suspicion of self-serving motives on the part of the AMA in unmasking the disreputable schools.

History tends to credit the Flexner report alone for the turnabout in American medical education, and, indeed, much credit is properly directed to the report. It should be emphasized, however, as Bevan reported to the AMA House of Delegates in 1919, that "the great changes in medical education had their beginning in, and are mainly due to, the efforts of the organized profession, the American Medical Association, to put its own house in order."[9]

A chart included in Bevan's 1919 report confirms the degree of progress already made before the Flexner report was issued. In 1906, for example, the United States had 162 medical schools, only six of which required a student to have any college level preparation before admission. In 1910, the year the Flexner report was released, there were thirty-one fewer schools, and, of the 131 that survived, thirty-five were requiring at least one year of college for admission. Thus, the upgrading of American medical education was clearly underway when the Flexner report appeared.

By the 1940s the AMA's concern with medical education (which continues undiminished) had led to impressive results. To be sure, the number of schools had dropped to seventy-seven in 1945. But it was the second- and third-rate schools that were gone, largely the proprietary (for-profit) schools. Those that survived were bigger and better equipped schools than those of 1905, stronger financially and stronger academically. As a consequence, the overall quality of American medicine was beginning to match or surpass the levels of medicine in the more advanced nations of Europe.

By 1945, the essentially private character of the American medical care system had come under fire. During the Great Depression of the 1930s, at least two of the supporting elements that had given the system its uniqueness had suffered severe blows. The affluent middle class had temporarily lost its affluence, and laissez-faire economic theory, largely abandoned in Europe, had sunk from favor.

It is difficult now to appreciate the extent and the suddenness of the political change that the United States underwent during the 1930s. To correct the frightening economic collapse—unemployment rates soared to 25 percent—President Roosevelt ushered in the New Deal. Citing as authority a phrase in the preamble to the Constitution—"to promote the general welfare," the administration began to transform the role of government. In *The Powers That Be*, Pulitzer Prize-winning author David Halberstam ably describes the atmosphere of tumultuous change that Roosevelt and the New Deal brought to Washington:

> There was so much energy, so much action...the rhythms of the times, the great inventions, the changing shape of society, were working to centralize power.... The speed of decision was becoming faster and faster, and, as it did, local governments simply could not keep up with the growing power and affluence of the federal government. The federal government's taxing power increased as its mandate increased, and as its taxing power increased, so did its real power.[10]

Not surprisingly, plans were drawn for the federal government to develop a new role in medical care. Late in 1934, as the newly created federal Committee on Economic Security drafted what would become the Social Security Act, the AMA became more and more fearful of what the forthcoming bill might propose.

On this issue, medicine's most effective advocate was Harvey Cushing, M.D., who held no office in the AMA but, as a noted brain surgeon, author, and teacher, was easily one of the most respected men in American medicine. Appointed to an advisory committee on medical matters to the Committee on Economic Security, Cushing urged his strong negative feelings on Frances Perkins, the Secretary of Labor and the person appointed by President Roosevelt to oversee the development of the new legislation. "Most of the agitation regarding the high cost of medical care," he wrote the Secretary, "has been voiced by public health officials and members of foundations, most of whom do not have a medical degree, much less any first-hand experience with what the practice of medicine and the relation of doctor to the patient means."[11]

Shortly thereafter, the AMA registered its reservations. Unaware of what the bill actually contained but afraid nevertheless, the AMA became so aroused that it summoned a special session of its House of Delegates in Chicago, February 15-16, 1935. This was only the second time in its history that it had done so. Declaring itself opposed to "all forms of compulsory sickness insurance," the AMA was as alarmed over what the government might do to medicine as businessmen were regarding the government's new economic and regulatory programs.

What did not come out at the time was Cushing's use of a special line of communication to the White House. Cushing's daughter Betsey was the wife of the President's oldest son, James, and Cushing used them to place his arguments directly before the President. Wilbur J. Cohen was fresh out of the University of Wisconsin then and, as a staff employee of the Committee on Economic Security, just beginning his long career in government. Cohen, who rose to become Secretary of the U.S. Department of Health, Education, and Welfare in 1968 and, in the early 1980s, was professor of public affairs at the University of Texas, does not believe that anything close to what would be regarded today as national health insurance was ever contemplated in the Social Security Act of 1935. Grants to the states to expand their public health programs were included, but not much more. "The feeling that some sort of massive health plan would be enacted was broken quite early," Cohen says. He doubts that the young Roosevelts had a difficult selling job. "President Roosevelt," he says, "already had so damn much in the social security bill—social security and unemployment insurance—that he was opposed to any additional health insurance provisions in it."[12]

As it turned out, the medical provisions in the Social Security Act, as submitted to Congress, as passed and signed into law in late 1935, were modest. They included some provisions for child and maternal health and assistance for the blind and for crippled children—measures that the AMA could and did accept.

President Roosevelt never did press long and hard for a specific health insurance bill. In 1939, when Democratic Senator Robert F. Wagner of New York proposed legislation that would have authorized federal grants to the states to develop health insurance programs and step up existing medical services, the President first gave his support but later withdrew it.[13] A more conservative political tide was then running, and in Congress a group of southern Democrats and northern Republicans had forged a powerful legislative bloc.

Without question, though, Roosevelt believed in wider federal participation in the medical care of the people. In 1944, for example, when the sacrifices of the war were being felt more sharply and the electorate was asking with greater insistence, "What are we fighting for?" Roosevelt offered what was called a Second Bill of Rights as a statement of the sort of new social benefits that victory would bring. The President's rationale stemmed from his belief that "necessitous men are not free men." That is, men who lacked the necessities of life could be forced into trading their freedom to obtain them. To guarantee freedom, therefore, it was necessary to guarantee new "rights"—the rights to a job, to an education, to food, and to medical care. It was the proper role of government, Roosevelt argued, to underwrite such underpinnings of freedom.[14]

That position was far from being public policy in 1945. In fact, the electorate turned sufficiently conservative to elect a Republican Congress in 1946, the first since 1932. Yet despite the end of the Depression and the death of Roosevelt, the New Deal had not run out of steam. The liberal wing of the Democratic party continued to press for more social legislation, for an expanded federal role in health care, for the continuation of New Deal politics. And for postwar liberals, the great unenacted social reform was national health insurance.

How medical care should be financed was a controversial and unresolved issue in 1945. Traditionally, in all but charity cases, the patient or his family paid physician and hospital bills. Group health insurance had started, but only a small percentage of the population was enrolled. Moreover, compared to today, few people felt an overwhelming demand for either health insurance or medical services; medical care was not then perceived to be all that effective. Before World War II, even the best of medical care possessed nothing like the capabilities it developed afterwards; treatment was not especially expensive (comparatively), and people did not seek it with the frequency they do now. But with the availability of antibiotics, new technological advances, and a return to prosperity, the demand for access to medical care gradually grew more insistent. In time, as the effectiveness of medical treatment continued to improve, society would reach a point where it asserted a *moral* claim on medical care.

Near the end of the war, the United States medical care system began to reap the benefits of what can only be described as a prolonged explosion of new knowledge in the biomedical sciences. Up to the entry of the United States into World War II, scientific research in this country was regarded as the almost exclusive province of industry, academia, and private philanthropic institutions. Research was not perceived to be a function of government. But the war changed that. In 1941, an Office of Scientific Research and Development was established, and its director, Vannevar Bush, Sc.D., a former vice president and dean of engineering at the Massachusetts Institute of Technology, brilliantly organized and mobilized national scientific resources to serve the military. This centralized effort underlay the success of such programs as the atomic bomb, the perfection of radar, and the mass production of sulfa drugs and penicillin.

When the war ended, it seemed logical to apply the same sort of organized effort to peaceful ends. In collaboration with a number of scientific leaders, Bush drew up a report on the desirability of federal financial support for research, including medical research. At its 1945 annual meeting, the AMA House of Delegates expressed its support for the Bush report, though with some reservations.[15] These were articulated a few months later by AMA President Roger I. Lee, M.D., who said "...I'm sure the intent is benevolent. But I believe that dangers to the profession lurk there just the same as in the more obvious attempts of governmental intervention...."[16] The Bush report gained acceptance quickly and soon became translated into law. The federal dollars followed, in amounts that quickly swelled.

The pace of discovery and invention leapt forward. From 1945 through 1982, ninety-two individuals from all over the world received the Nobel Prize for medicine and physiology. Of those scientists, forty-nine were American. No other nation could claim even half that number. Riding a crest of federal dollars, the United States swept on to a clear, international pre-eminence in the biological sciences.

And as physicians learned how to prevent, cure, and manage more and more of mankind's afflictions, society began to place a new and different value on medical services.

Chapter Two

"Overnight, We Became Optimists..."

By the standards of today, the pre-World War II physician had few weapons to help him in the fight against disease. Thanks to Louis Pasteur, Paul Ehrlich, Robert Koch and the other early microbe hunters, he did have effective vaccines to protect his patients against the historical scourges: smallpox, cholera, typhoid, typhus, and the plague. And he had antitoxins for tetanus, rabies, and diphtheria. Vitamins could correct conditions like scurvy, beriberi, and pellagra. There was liver extract for pernicious anemia. The hormone insulin allowed him to manage the patient with diabetes. For the relief of pain, the doctor could prescribe aspirin and the derivatives of opium. Available too were drugs from other botanical sources, such as digitalis for the flagging heart and quinine for malaria. But the physician's powers were restricted. Except for a handful of drugs—quinine was one; salvarsan (arsphenamine), for syphilis, was another—he had no medicines that attacked the real source of disease. What few therapeutics there were could only relieve symptoms.[1]

But suddenly, almost on the eve of the war, that all began to change. Slowly at first, then with an increasing tempo, a whole succession of therapeutic discoveries occurred, transforming medicine as profoundly as the jet would transform air travel or the atomic bomb would transform military thinking. Lives—at least a million by one estimate[2]—were saved and suffering was reduced, often quickly, painlessly, and, in the context of preceding years, miraculously.

They were indeed miracle drugs, for they were drugs with anti-biological properties, drugs that could enter the human body and destroy disease-causing organisms. "These events," writes Lewis

Thomas, M.D., a distinguished medical educator, essayist, and president of Memorial Sloan-Kettering Cancer Center, "were simply overwhelming when they occurred. I was a medical student at the time of sulfanilamide and penicillin, and I remember the earliest reaction of flat disbelief concerning such things. We had given up on therapy a century earlier...We were educated to be skeptical about the treatment of disease.

"Overnight, we became optimists, enthusiasts. The realization that disease could be turned around by treatment...was a totally new idea just forty years ago."[3]

The first of the miracle drugs emerged in 1935 from the laboratory of a biochemist named Gerhard Domagk, a scientist on the staff of the German chemical cartel, I.G. Farbenindustrie. Domagk was working on dyes, a subject fascinating to business because of their wide use in the textile industry but fascinating to biomedical science for quite another reason. Ever since the nineteenth century it had been known that dyes, many of them at least, had the chemical property of being able to home in selectively on cellular targets. Applied to a specimen on a microscopic slide, for example, a dye might seek out and color the cells of only one type of bacterium, leaving the surrounding cells of other bacteria unaffected. The property was useful in microscopy. But it also exemplified Paul Ehrlich's idea of the "magic bullet,"—chemically constructed medicines with a special affinity for certain cells, an ability to bond with them and thus neutralize them or destroy their power while at the same time leaving other cells alone. This concept of Ehrlich's is the basis of modern chemotherapy, the use of drugs to destroy cancer cells.

In the course of his work, Domagk found that a deep red dye called prontosil not only had such selective affinity, but also, when injected into mice, could cure a streptococcal infection. At about this time it happened that Domagk's own young daughter was severely ill, suffering from a severe streptococcal disease that was not responding to conventional treatment. In desperation, Domagk administered the dye to his own child. The results were stunning. The girl's recovery was so quick and so complete that a new, widespread, scientific interest focused on the dye. One question that intrigued researchers was why prontosil seemed to be more effective in the human body than it was in the test tube. Soon it was found that the body metabolized prontosil into sulfanilamide. That was the active, disease-fighting substance.[4]

Then came the process that was to follow the discovery of virtually all antibiotics: efforts to make slight variations in the molecular structure of the original drug in order to create new compounds that might be stronger, have less harmful side effects, or be more useful in the treatment of still other diseases. Since 1940, through the process of molecular tinkering and trials of the resulting variants, some thirty-three sulfonamides have been introduced in the United States alone. Like the original sulfonamide, most of these drugs are used to control infectious disease. But there are additional sulfa drugs, some of which exploit the side effects of the early drugs. These are useful for such diverse purposes as eliminating excess fluids and preventing seizures. Discovery, it is clear, begets discovery.

Electrifying as the potential of sulfanilamide was, penicillin was the drug that burst open the doorways to the development of whole new families of drugs—the antibiotics. In 1928 the British physician Alexander Fleming left an agar plate containing a culture of *Staphylococcus aureus* (the bacterium that causes boils) open to the air in the research laboratory of the London hospital where he worked. The spore of a somewhat rare airborne fungus settled on the culture and sprouted a mold. When, after some time, Fleming returned to the neglected dish, he observed a curious thing: around the mold, like the circular band on a target, was a no-man's-land clear of the *Staphylococci*. It was an event of truly cosmic serendipity. It was the first recognition of something that was to be seen again and again, on countless culture plates, in countless laboratories: a visible "ring of inhibition" signaling the presence of a mold capable of destroying the micro-organisms planted in the agar on the dish.

Fleming, who was later knighted for his work and awarded the Nobel Prize, identified the fungus (*Penicillium notatum*), extracted the substance its mold produced, and established its germicidal properties. However, Fleming's hospital lacked the facilities and resources for further developmental work, and he went on to other things. But with the outbreak of World War II, two other scientists (who were to share Fleming's Nobel Prize) revived and extended the early research. By 1941 penicillin was serving military needs; by 1944 it was being mass-produced, satisfying both civilian and military requirements.

Like prospectors in the Klondike, pharmacologists then began to scour the earth in search of other fungi that might have the antibiotic power of penicillin.[5] Louis Pasteur, it was recalled, once examined the soil of graveyards, expecting to find the presence of the microbial organisms that had caused the death of recent arrivals. Surprised when he could not find them, he concluded that nature played host to a merciless, never-ending, underground war—microbe against microbe. What made fungi such a target of the pharmacological search was a trait peculiar to this form of vegetable life. Most plants contain chlorophyll, the substance that enables them to create carbohydrates through the process of photosynthesis. Fungi, however, have no chlorophyll. They have no element of green in them; they grow in the dark. They are predators that subsist by devouring other things. Thus their therapeutic power; they eat microbes.

To widen the search, pharmaceutical companies asked their stockholders to send in distant soil samples. World-traveling pilots, missionaries, and explorers were similarly approached. And not without result. Soil from Venezuela yielded a fungus from which one useful antibiotic was developed. In more mundane fashion, another drug company did the same thing with a soil sample taken from the grounds behind one of its midwestern factories.

A parade of new antibiotics followed the development of penicillin: the streptomycins, which were the first drugs really effective against tuberculosis; the broad spectrum tetracyclines, which are effective against a wide range of infections; and countless others, nearly 200 in all.

The development of these antibiotics, with frequent tests along the way for safety and genuine effectiveness, generally followed a three-step sequence: (1) the discovery of a fungus with antimicrobial properties, revealed by the ring of inhibition on a culture plate; (2) chemical elucidation, i.e., discovery, of the molecular architecture of the antimicrobial ingredient; and (3) chemical synthesis of the material; that is, its manufacture from non-biological sources. Between a naturally produced drug and a synthesized drug there is no practical difference. A *Staphylococcus* cell cannot distinguish between a natural penicillin molecule—one created, say, from a mold growing on Fleming's agar dish—and a penicillin molecule manufactured from chemical materials in a pharmaceutical plant in New Jersey.

Though powerless against viruses, such as those that cause influenza and the common cold, antibiotics have been developed that are effective against nearly all forms of bacteria. At present, roughly

20 percent of the prescriptions written in the United States call for antibiotics, and no other class of drugs has had such a worldwide impact on death rates.

All that is not to say, however, that antibiotics constitute the sum of biomedical progress in the last forty years. The development of the steroids is nearly as important. These medicines cannot kill bacteria, as the antibiotics do; their effect is symptomatic. But they can and do save lives.

Steroids (the best known is cortisone, and that name is often used as a generic term to describe this whole class of drugs) are hormones. Biologically, they act as the naturally generated hormones act—as messengers and signalers within the human body. Probably the best known natural hormone is epinephrine, or adrenaline. It is the substance that goes through your body when you feel that "all your juices are flowing." In fact, the word hormone comes from the Greek word that means, "I excite."

What hormones do—what steroids do—is to trigger a wide variety of remote reactions within the human system. For example, one particular steroid, the birth control pill, "instructs" the female ovaries not to send a human egg into the fallopian tubes where it can be fertilized.

Most steroids are used, however, not for birth control but for their anti-inflammatory properties. Steroids set off reactions that, in effect, make peace between body enemies (antigens) and body defenders (antibodies). When first introduced in 1949, steroids promised to be the answer to rheumatoid arthritis. They were so effective in soothing inflamed joints that people who had been bedridden for years could stand and walk. But it was soon found that taken over long periods of time, which would be the case with arthritis, steroids gradually caused harmful side effects.

Though still used in the treatment of arthritis, the steroids have a wide range of application elsewhere.[6] Sometimes called the dermatologist's delight, steroids can relieve itches, rashes, and other skin outbreaks that are seldom fatal by themselves but can be so persistent and annoying as to make the sufferer wish they were. But steroids are also effective with far more serious ailments. They can head off allergic reactions that can sometimes prove fatal; they can interrupt the once lethal course of ulcerative colitis. Used now in the treatment of some 150 different diseases, steroids are the great palliatives, the great soothers of the human body. As antibiotics scored dramatic breakthroughs in making diseases less frequently fatal, steroids have proved to be almost as dramatic in making diseases more frequently bearable.

Drugs of an entirely different sort are now making inroads on what may well be the nation's most threatening disease: hypertension. Hypertension, or high blood pressure (the terms are interchangeable), accounts for about 60,000 deaths each year by itself. But its real danger lies elsewhere, as the forerunner and cause of heart attacks and strokes, which are the number one and number three causes of death in the United States. Hypertension can do damage in many places throughout the body. It can ruin the eyes and seriously harm the kidneys. But it exacts its worst toll from the vascular system. It can cause arteries to burst in the brain and, by increasing fatty deposits on arterial walls, it can force the heart to pump against greater and greater resistance. That in turn creates overwork for the heart—enlargement, muscle damage and, finally, failure. Someone whose blood pressure is 160/90 runs three to seven times the risk of a heart attack or stroke as someone whose blood pressure is close to a more normal reading of 120/80.

Lowering a person's blood pressure is a complex medical procedure. To understand it in the simplest terms, think of the human circulatory system as being like the system of hot water pipes that heats an office building. One way to relieve excess pressure in such a closed circuit of piping is to reduce the volume of fluid in it. There are drugs that can accomplish that. The other way to relieve pressure is to expand the capacity of the circuit itself, by widening the diameter of some of the pipes for example. And there are drugs that, in effect, do that.

The volume-reducing drugs are the diuretics, the most common type being the thiazides. As blood filters through the kidneys, both waste products and some water are removed, but much of the water is returned to the bloodstream. What thiazides (and other diuretics) do is cause the kidneys to return a smaller than normal portion of water. Thus, urination is increased, the volume of fluid in the circulatory system is reduced, and blood pressure is lowered.

Other drugs lower the pressure in the vascular system by enlarging the human "pipes." What these drugs do, more exactly, is diminish or slow the constricting power of the arterioles, which are small blood vessels connecting the arteries with the capillaries.

Some of these drugs dilate the vessels directly. Others, like reserpine (which derives from *Rauwolfia serpentina*, a plant used for centuries by Asian herb doctors), deplete the transmitter substance that carries the signal to constrict from the sympathetic nervous system to the arterioles.

The attention that has been focused on hypertension is well-deserved. An estimated 20 percent of the adult population of the United States has high blood pressure. And while one out of seven adult white males is thought to be hypertensive, the estimate for black adult males is one in four. Various programs have increased both physician and patient awareness, and these efforts, together with the new medicines, seem to be having an impact. In the last ten years the mortality rate for heart disease, the leading cause of death in the United States, has dropped by 22 percent. In the case of stroke, the third leading killer in the United States, the decline has been even more abrupt: 30 percent.[7] Though they are not the only factors contributing to those improvements, both increased awareness and better treatment of hypertension have to be playing significant roles.

Another important category of new drugs is the psychotherapeutics, drugs that can calm the psychotic and restore him or her to rationality. Historically, the treatment of psychoses has been discouraging. Insulin coma and electric shock were used with results that were far from satisfactory. Depressants of the central nervous system such as barbiturates were tried, but they had to be administered in such heavy dosages as to leave the patient stupified. For the psychotic patient, confinement in county and state mental hospitals seemed to be the best that society could do.

But in the early 1950s researchers in France who were testing a phenothiazine compound (thought originally to be helpful in malaria) observed some remarkable behavior in the mice they were using. These had been psychologically conditioned, much in the manner of Pavlov's dog, to climb a pole in their cage in response to the sound of a buzzer. The conditioning had been done by sending a sharp jolt of electricity through the floor of their cage at the moment the buzzer sounded.

Having been conditioned, the mice then received doses of phenothiazine. Now when subjected to the electrical charge, the mice would still scamper up the pole. But no longer would they do so merely in response to the buzzer. It was apparent that the phenothiazine acted selectively: it could depress the nervous system of the mice sufficiently to quiet the conditioned reflexes while leaving the psychomotor reactions unimpaired.

On the strength of this finding, the drug was tried on an institutionalized psychotic with such astounding results that he was discharged three weeks later, his behavior adjudged to be nearly normal.[8] Derivatives (or elaborations, in the language of the pharmacologist) of phenothiazine have come into wide use in the United States since 1955, resulting in a startling but welcome drop in the resident population of state and county mental institutions from something near 600,000 to under 200,000 in 1975. Thus large numbers of patients suffering severe emotional disturbances are managed on an outpatient basis, a treatment that is far less costly and far more humane.

Dramatic discoveries have come so frequently and have produced such wide improvement in the treatment of so many different diseases that the public often seems to expect a similar miracle to cure cancer. People ask: Why won't cancer yield to the sort of urgent, massive, multi-million-dollar effort that produced the first atomic bomb or sent the first man to the moon? Advocates of various federal cancer programs have pleaded their case in just those terms. But what is ignored here is something basic. Physicists had answers to the theoretical questions on atomic energy well before the Manhattan Project began, just as engineers possessed the theoretical knowledge needed to get to the moon years before the first astronaut was launched into orbit.

That is not true of cancer research. Despite the money expended, despite the intensity of human effort, even despite the considerable advances made, we do not yet possess the equivalent theoretical knowledge that preceded the other achievements. As a matter of fact, cancer is not really a single disease; it is several, each with a distinctive behavior, each with a distinctive reaction to treatment. Furthermore, developing an anticancer drug is uniquely difficult. Drugs such as antibiotics really assist the body's own capacity to fight invasive bacteria; they are not required to achieve a kill rate of 100 percent to be effective. But in the case of anticancer drugs the demands are that stringent, for against cancer, natural body defenses appear to be powerless. An effective anticancer drug must go it alone.

Historically, and even now, cancer treatment relies on surgery or irradiation or both. But drugs are playing a larger and larger role—

sometimes by themselves, more often in conjunction with surgery or irradiation. The basic action of a cancer drug is to destroy cells, interfere with their growth, or prevent their spread throughout the body. Cancer drugs are powerful, high-risk substances. They destroy tissue. But they are not indiscriminate destroyers, for they do more harm to the fast-growing cancer cells than to normal cells. Some anticancer drugs, like nitrogen mustard agents, inhibit the division process by which cells multiply. Other drugs enter malignant cells disguised—molecularly—as innocent vitamins or amino acids, but then turn on the host cell and poison it. The wide range of drugs used in cancer includes some classed as antibiotics and hormones.

The most dramatic accomplishment in the area of chemotherapy is the recently announced capacity of a four-drug combination called MOPP to cure Hodgkin's disease, a cancer of the lymph system. This disease was once considered incurable, but it has, in recent years, responded more and more favorably to drug treatment. Drugs have brought about higher cure rates and long-term remission rates in other leukemia-type cancers and lymphomas as well. One survey of acute leukemia victims in 100 hospitals found that between the 1940s and the late 1960s the percentage of patients surviving for one year or more rose from 5 percent to 37 percent. Once fatal, lymphatic leukemia in children, if detected and treated early, now has a 50 percent survival rate.

"There is probably more to be done in the area of neoplastic drugs than anywhere else," says John C. Ballin, Ph.D., director of the AMA Division of Drugs. "Researchers in the field have just begun to scratch the surface."

Relatively new on the frontiers of drug research is a class of substances called the beta blockers, whose actions proceed from a radically new hypothesis in pharmacology. These are the first drugs made that have a molecular configuration enabling them to bond with the so-called beta receptor sites of certain nerve cells and affect their biological behavior.

While several beta blocking drugs have been used abroad for some time, only one has been subject to widespread use here: propranolol. This drug consists of inactive molecules that link firmly with the message-sending sites of the nerve cells that tell the circulatory system to constrict, an action that increases blood pressure. By blocking the message-sending capability of these nerve cells, the constrictive action is modified. The vessels relax, and the patient's blood pressure stays down.

The whole human system is filled with a variety of special cells that send messages, receive messages, or manufacture cells that transmit messages. And each type of cell has a characteristic molecular structure. When chemical substances are developed that achieve a molecular fit with receptor sites on these cells, a binding process is made possible that in turn can stop or diminish the communication function. An example is a drug named cimetidine, introduced in 1978, which can stop the secretion of gastric acid, an excess of which is an important factor in duodenal ulcer disease. Cimetidine has not only relieved countless sufferers; it has eliminated a great deal of surgery. In many cases it is both a less risky and less costly way treat an ulcer.

In broad terms, the theories behind the continuing development of many drugs can be likened to the early affinity theories of Paul Ehrlich, with his vision of "charmed" chemical "bullets" able to bind themselves to the cells of selected bacteria and seal off their toxic actions.[9] "Underlying the work on the sulfas and the penicillins and the other antibiotics has been the process of discovering the relationship between chemical structure and biologic effect," notes William R. Barclay, M.D., former editor of *JAMA*. "You could call this a part of a continuum that begins with Ehrlich's concept of the magic bullet, proceeds throughout the development of new molecular structures and new antibiotics, and culminates—in a far, far more sophisticated way—in what science is now finding out about the chemistry of the human message system. Advances in recombinant DNA techniques, the recently demonstrated ability to implant human genetic material in the cells of bacteria and so produce human insulin, this sort of achievement lies at the endpoint of a remarkable scientific train."[10]

Chapter Three

The Breakthroughs in Surgery

Just as the first antibacterial medicines were beginning to work their early miracles in the early 1940s—and in large part because they were working those miracles—surgery embarked on a course of discovery that carried it well beyond its traditional horizons. Before the wide availability of antibiotics, the chance of postoperative infection was high. Except where injury was already done or the consequences of not operating were clearly fatal, surgeons had to weigh the risks of an operation against the possible benefits far more cautiously than they do now. "Surgery before World War II was all big surgery," recalls H. Thomas Ballantine, M.D., a pre-war surgical resident at the Massachusetts General Hospital, a neurosurgeon at the hospital after the war, and a recent AMA trustee. "It was difficult surgery...for the most part, gross surgery...the removal of tumors and the amputation of legs because of diabetic gangrene— ...things like that."[1]

But with antibiotics coming into use in the early 1940s, the inhibitions started to fade. And as the threat of infection dropped, the scope of surgery, which had remained constant for some years, abruptly began to broaden. Contributing an early and essential impetus to the new directions that surgery then took were advances in the field of anesthesia.

Down through time man has tried many ways to escape the pain of the surgeon's knife. Both the Greeks and the Romans describe the use of alcohol, derivatives from the poppy, and other herbal substances. Shakespeare mentions one of these, mandragora (from the mandrake root), and other "drowsy syrups." For its officers, the British Navy used to issue grog (rum) and laudanum (an opiate), and for seamen, soft lead bullets to bite. Because of pain, surgeons learned to practice their craft swiftly, par being somewhere between thirty seconds and three minutes for an early nineteenth century amputation. One practitioner of that day wrote admiringly of a colleague, "...the gleam of his knife was followed so instantaneously by the sound of sawing that the two actions appear almost simultaneous."[2]

Credit for the discovery of anesthesia is variously distributed among three nineteenth century Americans, one of whom was a physician, two of whom were dentists. The physician, Crawford W. Long, M.D., a Georgian, operated on an etherized patient as early as 1842, but he neglected, unfortunately, to describe his results in the medical literature until 1849. Horace Wells, invited to demonstrate his use of nitrous oxide (laughing gas) on a young dental patient at the Harvard Medical School in 1845, lost his opportunity when the youngster fled shrieking from the auditorium. So it is that the man in the painting in the National Library of Medicine is the other dentist, William T.G. Morton, who so successfully etherized a patient at the Massachusetts General Hospital in 1846 that a tumor was removed from the man's neck with no display of pain whatsoever.

Although the rival claims for the discovery of anesthesia were argued for years, the procedure itself was adopted overnight. Oliver Wendell Holmes, M.D., (the physician, poet, and essayist, not his son, the Supreme Court justice) gave the process its name, which is derived from the Greek and translated literally, means "without sensation."

For nearly a century afterwards, anesthesia underwent little change. Chloroform enjoyed a brief vogue, but only until harmful side effects were discovered. Nitrous oxide, still used in about 65 percent of present-day anesthesias, and ether, especially ether, remained the agents of choice. As technology, anesthesia ranked low, being looked upon by some as a rag-and-bottle science requiring nothing more than a nurse to drip fluid ether slowly onto gauze covering the patient's nose and mouth. That perception was far from universal; surgeons highly valued their trained nurse-anesthetists.

At the outbreak of World War II, new technology and new anesthetizing drugs were coming into use. Some, like sodium pentothol, could be injected intravenously; others were injected intraspinally; still others could be administered rectally. Open-drop ether anesthesia and the nurse-anesthetist were giving way more and more frequently to a physician trained in the recently recognized (1937) medical specialty of medical anesthesiology. Slowly, for there were only eighty-six active, board-certified anesthesiologists in the

United States in 1940,[3] a new concept took hold—that of a physician to put the patient to sleep and then assume responsibility for his physiological functions during and immediately after the operation. Not only does the anesthesiologist carefully track the level to which the patient is anesthetized; he monitors the workings of the bodily systems as well, especially the respiratory and circulatory systems. He or she frees the surgeon to concentrate on the operation, taking the responsibility for watching blood pressure and blood volume, for monitoring the levels of oxygen and carbon dioxide in the blood, and for seeing that the blood is maintained at the necessary level of mild alkalinity. From these signs, the anesthesiologist can tell whether the patient's vital organs are functioning as they should.

No one is precisely certain how anesthesia works, just as no one has solved all the mysteries of sleep. It is clear, however, that anesthesia slows the working of the brain in a progressive manner. First affected are the most neurologically refined areas—the seat of reason, intellect, and consciousness. Farther down is the part of the brain that controls breathing, and, below that, the area controlling the beat of the heart. Anesthesia seeks to keep the patient just below the edge of consciousness, in a sleep deep enough to dull sensation, but safely above the levels where breathing or circulation might be lost.

The other thing the anesthesiologist seeks to accomplish is a relaxed patient. Just because a person is unconscious does not mean that he or she is relaxed. Even after an incision is made, the muscles, especially the abdominal muscles, may remain so tense that the surgeon can proceed only with great difficulty.

Rather than put the patient into a deeper, more relaxing sleep, which might be dangerous, the anesthesiologist administers relaxants. Surprisingly, the earliest, most effective relaxant used was curare, the same lethal substance in which the Indians of the Amazon dip their arrows. Curare is rarely used today, although synthesized relaxants that do virtually the same thing are.

Curare "poisons" by relaxing muscles to the point of flaccidity. And among the muscles affected when it enters the bloodstream are the chest muscles. As they are relaxed to the point where they cease to function, death by asphyxiation quickly follows. Patients undergoing surgery—about 30 percent of them—are similarly relaxed and would die of asphyxiation except that a tube is inserted down the windpipe into the lungs through which the anesthesiologist introduces a mixture containing the needed oxygen. Use of this endotracheal tube and the relaxants make a number of other things possible. The surgeon has a perfectly quiet and relaxed muscular system to deal with: the anesthesiologist has a patient who is unconscious but not deeply unconscious.

Emboldened by the powers of the new antibiotics and encouraged further by the new anesthesia techniques, surgeons began to enter the chest with far greater confidence. The heart and the kidneys and the lungs had always been considered inviolable. Because of that, surgeons approached operations on them hesitantly. But in the late 1930s and early 1940s that began to change.[4] Operations on the lungs, once rare, became more common. Other surgery within the chest was undertaken: the "blue baby" operation, first performed in 1944, was the most widely acclaimed. What the surgeon did in that operation was to splice and reconnect vessels near the heart and lungs, rerouting a child's bloodstream so that its flow to the lungs was increased and its oxygen level raised. The operation compensated for congenital defects of the heart—the "leaks" between the chambers of the heart that allowed blood to be recirculated before it was oxygenated by the lungs.

At this level of sophistication, it was not a far step for surgeons to cross another barrier—surgery within the heart itself. This was not heart surgery as we know it now, accomplished with the heart at rest, its functions performed by a machine. This was closed heart surgery, surgery to widen the heart's valves within a live, pulsing heart upon whose function the life of the patient still depended. The first step in this operation called for a suture through a series of stitches in the exterior of the heart muscle to form something much like a purse string. Then, through a slit cut inside the sutured area, the surgeon inserted a finger into the interior of the heart, while an assistant quickly drew the purse string tight, thereby preventing the escape of blood. The surgeon then pushed his finger through the narrowed valve, or even cut it open wider with a small, retractable knife. Thus repairs were done on heart valves that were either malformed at birth, constricted by rheumatic fever, or calcified by age.

Though effective, closed heart surgery had obvious limitations. The surgeon could not see what he was doing; his actions were severely limited. Holes between the chambers of the heart—a nottoo-rare birth defect—could not be closed. Nor could artificial valves be installed.

Many parts of the body can survive a half an hour or more without freshly oxygenated blood, i.e. blood that has passed through the lungs to release carbon dioxide and take on oxygen. But not the brain. At 98.6° F, without fresh oxygen, only four minutes may elapse before brain cells perish irrevocably. If the body is chilled to 60°F, the metabolism is slowed. In this condition of artificial hibernation, the brain may survive up to eight minutes without fresh blood, but no more. Theoretically, that was the time limit for open heart surgery, unless there was something to perform the circulatory and respiratory functions.

That began to change on May 6, 1953, when surgeon John H. Gibbon, Jr., M.D., successfully diverted the bloodstream of an eighteen-year-old girl through a heart-lung machine he had developed, opened her still heart, sewed together a hole between the upper chambers, reconnected the blood vessels, and then restarted the regular functions of her heart and lungs.[5] For the first time, he had demonstrated that the human heart could be taken off-line, stopped, repaired, and returned to duty. His heart-lung machine worked smoothly throughout the twenty-six minutes it took to perform the heart surgery.

By today's standards, Gibbon's machine was crude. Unfairly, it was later blamed for failures that might have been charged elsewhere. But it blazed the trail. It performed the functions of the heart without squeezing and damaging the oxygen-bearing red blood cells. It performed the functions of the lungs without creating dangerous bubbles. By 1959 the death rate from congenital heart disease had started sharply down. Francis D. Moore, M.D., Moseley Professor of Surgery at the Harvard Medical School, wrote, "The techniques of open cardiac surgery, a vision in 1950, became practical in 1955 and routine by 1960."[6]

The wondrous capabilities of the heart-lung machine, so recently the stuff of science fiction, were matched at virtually the same time by surgery's newly found ability to transplant an organ from one human body to another. For many reasons, among them the existence of an artificial kidney machine and the progress in research on renal function, kidneys were the first organs to be transplanted. By the early 1950s physicians had worked out the hazardous surgical-anatomical problems. But the first successful transplant had to wait until 1954, when physicians found someone who needed a new kidney and also had a twin who could donate one. For a full nine years after this operation the host twin enjoyed fine health, dying eventually from causes having nothing to do with the function of his kidney.

What limited the success of early transplant attempts—and still does—is the body's rejection, through its immune system, of invasions by foreign tissue. In the case of twins, especially identical twins, the foreignness of the transplanted organ is minimal, and the rejection alarms tend to be weak. Properly reconnecting the arteries, veins, ducts, and so forth is not the governing factor for a successful transplant; suppressing the mechanism by which the body fends off invaders is.

The rejection problem has opened up a whole new field of tissue immunology. After antibiotics were discovered, the science of immunology seemed to go into a decline. But organ transplants have rekindled an enormous interest in the subject. Much has been learned about tissue typing (comparable to blood typing); there are immuno-suppressant drugs; techniques to create tolerance have been developed; and other ways have been found to weaken the immune system. As a result, rejection rates have improved. But during the 1970s the survival rate of kidney grafts from cadavers still hovered near 55 percent, though the survival rate for patients is higher than that. The five-year survival rate is closer to 70 percent for the 4,000 or so kidney transplants performed each year.[7] At present, relatively few transplants of other organs are being attempted.

Transplants, open heart surgery, the delicate vascular surgery now being done inside the abdomen, chest, and skull...these are the stuff of headlines. These are the visible forward steps that trigger the cover stories in *Time* or *Newsweek* and make the TV network news. What has to be emphasized is that the modern feats rest on a pyramid of earlier research and discovery. One expert cites no fewer than twenty-five separate bodies of medical knowledge that had to grow to a certain point before the first open heart operation could take place.

Dazzling progress can also depend on undramatized accomplishments. Modern surgery, for example, with its sometimes unforeseen needs for transfusions, could not function as well as it does without blood banks, and these, in turn, could not develop until reliable means of preserving whole blood were developed in the early 1940s. The use of a heart-lung machine, for example, requires a quantity of stored blood roughly equal to three times the blood volume of a normal sized adult. Intravenous feeding is hardly a subject to stir the creative juices of a Hollywood scriptwriter. Yet at least some difficult surgery would not be undertaken today without the knowledge that virtually every nutrient needed can be dripped into a patient's vein. Organizational accomplishments, too, evident in the transportation and communications systems of emergency services, can improve the surgeon's capabilities.

Medical technology also owes a great debt to the international chemical-electronic-industrial complex, which invented or did the basic development work on key instruments and materials. From chemistry came the materials that make possible the total replacement of an arthritic hip joint. Chemistry also developed materials that go far beyond the capabilities of glass or rubber, the plastics for angiographic catheters, for example, that can curl through the arteries and the aorta to release radio-opaque drugs that allow diagnostic observation of the coronary arteries. Tubes of knit Dacron, grafted to arteries, have brought a new reliability to surgery on aneurysms (sections of blood vessels that swell, weaken, and threaten to burst, like blisters on an old tire). Because of Dacron's remarkable tensile strength a surgeon may use sutures thinner than a human hair in the reattachment, say, of a severed hand or digit. These sutures come pre-attached to eyeless needles because an eye's additional width, a microscopic difference, could be enough to damage the delicate tissues involved. Special operating microscopes permit surgeons to stitch the tiny blood vessels back together. Fiber optics make possible some of the new endoscopic instruments that allow physicians to see around corners, to spot lesions or to examine tumors in the bronchial tree, the stomach, or the colon as readily as if they were located on the lip. New phosphorescent materials and new electronic cameras have led to the development of X-ray cinematography, which enables a cardiologist to watch malfunctions in a system of coronary arteries or an orthopedist to see the ends of fractured bones accurately fitting together, all at radiation levels low enough to be safe for patient and physician alike. Laser beams tack detached retinas back into place. Cryogenic probes freeze tiny bundles of nerves in the brain, guided to the exact spot through a complex, stereotaxic method that, in effect, plots the three-dimensional coordinates of the various parts of a brain. Nuclear science has given medicine radioisotope tracers and capabilities for powerful radiation treatment. Electronic developments have produced the pacemaker, a device that is surgically implanted and restores synchronization to out-of-phase heart muscles.

Then there is the computer. Not only has the computer revolutionized significant parts of the commercial world—banking, engineering, manufacturing, transportation, even sausage-making—

now it has given medicine the CAT scanner, a truly remarkable new diagnostic tool. CAT is an acronym; C for computerized; A for axial; and T for tomography. Tomography is an X-ray technique that can plot the outer dimensions of an organ within a cross-section of the body. A tomogram of your liver, for example, would show it to you as it would appear in outline from above as part of a thin horizontal slice of your torso. By taking tomograms of successive "slices" along an axis and then feeding the data through a computer, the CAT scanner can produce a detailed, rounded "picture" of your liver, or other soft-tissue parts of your body that up to now could never, in effect, be "photographed." A CAT scanner can be used to spot a tumor in the brain or locate injuries there, by bringing back data that heretofore could be obtained only through surgery or the use of dangerous dyes. Providing scans of the kidneys, the pancreas and other organs, the CAT scanner can reduce exploratory surgery of the chest and abdomen. "Sure, some people call it a doctor's toy," says Ballantine, a neurosurgeon. "But it is without question one of the most exciting inventions of the twentieth century. Now you can take a spine and look inside it and turn it around and look at it all up and down...why it's just unbelievable what it can do."

CAT scanners originally drew the fire of health planning agencies. They cost up to $750,000 installed, and there was initially little experience to indicate how many there should be in a given community. Accusations of "CAT fever" were leveled, implying an over-indulgence of the physician's love of gadgetry. Less controversial now, they are not as frequently denigrated as gadgets. The United States physicist who did the theoretical work on the CAT scanner and the British engineer who translated the theory into practical application shared the 1979 Nobel Prize for the medical/physiological discovery that "conferred the greatest benefit on mankind."

In extreme form, the CAT scanner represents a dilemma that faces medicine with growing frequency. New machines, new medicines, and new surgical procedures do save lives or prolong lives, or simply make the day-to-day living with a disease more bearable. But such things are expensive. And the question is asked, of course, "Is the cost justified?" It was, after all, United States government money (i.e., tax payers' money) that financed virtually all of the research that led to the heart-lung machine and organ transplants. What is the justification?

The massive *Study on Surgical Services for the United States* (SOSSUS), published by the American Surgical Association and the

American College of Surgeons in 1975, includes an earnest try at answering just that question. Among sixty-four leading contributions to surgical research developed between 1945 and 1970, the study participants judged that the benefits of fifteen could be analyzed from the standpoint of mortality; that is, their capability to prolong useful, productive life. Base-years antedating the new developments were selected, and death rates for 1970 projected. These rates showed what probably would have happened if the new procedures had not been developed. The projected death rates (after various adjustments) were then compared with the actual rates for 1970, resulting in the precise number of 78,538 lives saved that year by just the fifteen particular procedures. The procedures having the greatest impact included, in descending order: hemodialysis and kidney transplantation, vascular surgery, cardiac surgery, progress in burn treatment, and surgery for duodenal ulcer. In its dry, clinical language, the report adds, "If the number of lives saved were calculated for each year after a particular advance was introduced and these figures were added, the result would clearly prove to be very large."[8]

The study also attempted a financial judgment. This time sixteen new surgical developments were selected and the amount saved (mostly in terms of lost earnings) compared to the amount invested in surgical research for the year. Conclusion: the amount of money saved was sixty times larger than the amount currently invested in research. Such comparisons really satisfy few people, even though they are undoubtedly the best that can be made. They do indicate, however, that large investments in surgical research pay off, a proposition most people accept. They also indicate that we have not yet devised a meaningful yardstick of cost-effectiveness to apply to medical care. What, for example, should the price tag be on an extra month of life? On an extra year? On an extra five years?

Without question, though, as the SOSSUS chapter on surgical research says, "There has been no other period in surgical history in which the yield from scientific investigation was so bountiful and the resultant change in the practice of surgery so great."[9]

From across the Atlantic, from Sir George W. Pickering, Emeritus Regius Professor of Medicine at Oxford, comes this generous accolade: "Until [the twentieth century] ideas flowed to America from Europe, as Americans went to Europe to complete their scientific or professional training. Increasingly, since the turn of the century, ideas have come from the United States, and Europeans have gone there to perfect their education."[10]

Chapter Four

The Move to Specialization

As educational standards improved and scientific knowledge grew, it was inevitable that the medical profession would lay increasing emphasis on specialization. Although only 23.5 percent of American physicians were full-time specialists in 1940,[1] it was clear that change was coming. One early sign of the direction in which medicine was headed was the establishment during the 1930s of more than half of the approved medical specialty boards that exist today. Another was the AMA's survey in 1945 of physicians in the armed forces—about a third of the total physician population—revealing that an astonishing 63 percent of them planned to take specialized training upon their discharge.[2]

That news forewarned hospitals and training centers across the United States. The number of residency and fellowship training programs rapidly expanded, so that by 1946 *JAMA* was able to claim: "Never before in the history of medicine...has there even been an approximation of the demand for the advanced training of physicians. In 1941, before the war, there were 5,256 physicians in approved assistant residencies and fellowships...Today there are 8,930...an expansion of 70 percent."[3]

A tapering off was expected. Much of the demand was thought to be backlog—physicians who had forgone residency training for financial reasons in the late 1930s, physicians in the four successive classes of medical graduates that the armed forces had absorbed almost 100 percent, directly out of school. When this pent-up demand was met, it was thought, the pressure would ease. But that never occurred. By 1950 nearly 20,000 physicians were in residencies. By 1960 the figure had risen to over 30,000, and in 1980 it was nearly 70,000.[4] In the years since 1945, the ratio of generalists to specialists has been reversed,[5] and a 1978 study indicated that over 80 percent of recent medical school graduates had completed residency training and embarked on the process of specialty certification.*

It was a remarkable change. "Graduate medical education," concluded that 1978 study, "in essence has become a part of the formal education of physicians. This has happened without any legislative or legal requirements. It has resulted from a voluntary effort of the medical profession mainly through the policies and activities of specialty boards whose basic purpose is to assure the public that a physician has undergone a period of formal education in a specialty and has demonstrated an acceptable degree of professional competence according to standards set by the profession."[6]

The transformation has its critics. Many people, including many physicians, believe that along the road to specialization the profession has lost its human touch, that specialization serves physician needs more than patient needs. Others argue that specialization has caused medical care to become overly elaborate and, consequently, overly expensive. Those who support the concept of specialization respond that neither the remarkable advances in medical research nor the expanded ability to treat disease could have occurred without the stress on specialty training. It would be hard, moreover, to change the present system of specialization, for the American patient is accustomed to it, and it is often the patient who is the first to demand a specialist when something serious goes wrong.

Is the profession now over-specialized? That is an impossible judgment to make. But the pendulum seems to have swung back to more emphasis on the generalist. In 1973 the AMA House of Delegates adopted a report supporting the view that there was a shortage of physicians in primary care. Rather than trying to limit access to specialty education, the AMA started to promote—successfully, as it turned out—a goal to have at least 50 percent of all medical school graduates enter post-doctoral (i.e. after graduation from medical school) training in the primary care fields: family practice,

---

*Specialty status depends on a number of things: length of residency training, usually three to five years; additional study; experience; type of practice. Whether a physician shows up in the statistics as a specialist depends on the description of his practice that he himself supplies to the AMA, the organization that maintains the records. Board certified specialists are those awarded a certificate, or diploma, attesting to the fulfillment of the formal requirements of one of the twenty-four approved medical specialty boards. At the end of World War II, 24,752 certificates had been awarded. Since then, about ten times that number have been issued.

internal medicine, pediatrics, and obstetrics/gynecology.[7] Today, primary medical care reaches patients in a number of ways. Much, of course, is provided by specialists, especially by internists, pediatricians, and obstetrician/gynecologists. And a great deal is provided by specialists in family practice, including family physicians certified by the recently established (1969) American Board of Family Practice.

What triggered the abrupt rise in specialization? Certainly no other profession acted similarly. Lawyers, for example, spend no more time in formal academic training than they did thirty-five years ago. Nor do engineers or architects. The only parallel might be in dentistry, though the percentage of dental specialists is low compared to physician specialists.

The first great spur apparently came from the medical policies of the United States Army and Navy in World War II. At the moment a physician (under age thirty-seven) presented himself for military duty, it was immediately impressed upon him that there was a difference between someone with specialty credentials and someone without them. Those able to give evidence of specialty training—a year or two of residency work, for example—received a commission as captain. Those who were unable to do so took a step down, to first lieutenant. Not a shattering distinction, to be sure. But difference in duty assignments followed, and other distinctions were made that caused the military physician to be aware at all times that he was in a hierarchical structure where the upper rungs were, more often than not, reserved for those with specialty training.

"Let me try to outline the sort of experience that was then fairly typical," offers Richard L. Egan, M.D., the AMA's director of educational standards and evaluation, a member of the faculty at the Creighton University School of Medicine in Omaha from 1941 to 1971 and dean during his last eleven years.

> I had a friend at Creighton, whom I am going to call Riley. Let's say that Riley finished Creighton in 1938, did his internship, and went into practice in some rural community in North Dakota. America was coming out of the agricultural depression by then, and Riley had plenty to do. He was making a living. He got married, started a family.
>
> Then along came Pearl Harbor. Riley joins the Army medical corps. Here he first finds out the difference—in the military view—between himself and contemporaries who stayed in Omaha for an

extra year or two of residency training. Soon he is overseas with a tactical unit. As a battalion surgeon he has to see that the kitchen is clean, inspect the latrines, do the short-arm inspections, and in combat tend the wounded under fire and sleep in a wet foxhole. He probably is a captain by now. But his friends are majors and lieutenant colonels. And they're back in Paris, Honolulu, London, or Walter Reed doing interesting things in the advanced technology of military hospitals. Riley considers himself, at times, just a high-paid aid man.[8]

In the meantime, Congress passed the Serviceman's Readjustment Act of 1944, the famous GI Bill of Rights. Among other things provided for the soon-to-be-returning serviceman were educational benefits. And among the educational benefits for physicians in the service were post-graduate medical education benefits: in other words, residency training. The participants were assured subsistence allowances, and hospitals were promised modest financial support to conduct the programs. At the same time, hospitals were beginning to receive additional funds for the educational programs from the burgeoning prepaid hospitalization insurance plans, mainly Blue Cross.

As a consequence, when the Rileys of World War II arrived home, the road to specialty training stretched invitingly before them. Not all, but large numbers of them said good-bye to rural North Dakota. They traded it for the prospect of life in a larger city, better schools for the children, the chance to go to a concert every now and then, colleagues with whom they could trade on-call status over weekends, a better opportunity to keep up with medicine, the time just to sit down with a good book.

It is argued, by Egan among others, that even young physicians who did *not* go into the armed services during World War II experienced incentives to take specialty training. With a third of the profession in the military, a heavy workload fell upon those left to treat the civilian population. The general practitioner, serving a rural population alone, emerged from the war years thoroughly overworked, exhausted from being on call twenty-four hours a day, seven days a week. In the summer of 1945 many of them said to themselves, "Surely, there must be a better way." They too could see the rewards of entering specialized training.

At the time, no one foresaw the long-term consequences that grew out of the way military medicine was structured or out of the GI Bill. The Army and Navy medical corps were organized to serve a military emergency, and they did so admirably. The GI Bill was enacted to give extra compensation to those who had been in service, a thank-you gesture from a grateful nation. And it accomplished its purposes. Yet later the two decisions were to have a major impact on the character of our medical profession.[9] Who could have predicted in 1944 that the GI Bill would affect medicine? Maybe it didn't specialize American medicine overnight. But it did much to finance a trend just beginning to gather momentum.

Soon, additional and more powerful forces came into play. After passage of the Public Health Service Act of 1944, the federal government, for the first time really, went outside of the military and the Public Health Service to support biomedical research.[10] A massive—and massively growing—flood of federal dollars rapidly expanded the National Institutes of Health (NIH). And grants for biomedical research from this source sluiced into medical academe at a rate of acceleration that was truly astonishing. The start in 1945 was modest: $85,000 in total research grants for the year. But the figure leapt to ten times that just one year later, more than ten times that in 1950, and well over ten times that in 1960. The 1982 figure for federal research grants was nearly $2.5 billion.[11] Not all of this money went to medical schools or medical scientists doing research in medical schools. But most of it did.

The impact was profound. For it was these federal dollars that bankrolled the research that made the heart-lung machine possible, the research that had to be done before organ transplants became possible, and some of the research for the new, miraculous medicines. And, as scientific exploration spread, it created important side effects. The trend toward a specialized profession gained speed; the modern hospital, with new equipment, became the locus of more and more medical care.

In the chapter he contributed to *Advances in American Medicine: Essays at the Bicentennial*, John A. D. Cooper, M.D., Ph.D., President of the Association of American Medical Colleges, wrote, "The next three decades [following 1945] were to become the most tumultuous in the history of American medical education. During this period the schools underwent a transformation from simple educational institutions to huge, complex medical centers with a vast array of interrelated and interdependent programs largely supported by sources of funds outside the control of the universities or schools."[12]

The late Hugh H. Hussey, M.D., a former editor of *JAMA*, an ex-chairman of the board (1961-62) and dean of the Georgetown

University School of Medicine from 1956 to 1962, believed that the infusion of new federal money had its first significant impact on the size of full-time medical school faculties.[13] Medical schools have, of course, grown tremendously, both in size and in number. But between 1950 and 1975, while the number of students grew by a factor of something over two, the number of full-time faculty grew by a factor of more than ten.[14] Since the new faculty members were specialists, strongly oriented toward research, the students they turned out took on more of that coloration. The traditional balance between the art of medicine and the science of medicine shifted sharply toward the scientific. Since they were specialists, even super-specialists, the new teachers gave students a different model around which to shape their careers.

Hussey added an interesting point: that government policy made it virtually painless for medical school administrators to add these new teachers to the faculty. "Bright young men, working in any medical field, productive—as evidenced by publication—could come to a dean of a medical school of his choice and say, 'I'd like to become a member of your department of physiology with a tenure appointment. You needn't worry about a salary. I'll support myself out of the grant funds I can bring with me.'

"I had that happen to me," Hussey observed.

But it was not just research dollars—and faculty members—that the government was contributing. Construction money became available, then loan and scholarship assistance for students, funds to relieve financial distress, funds to construct hospitals owned by medical schools. From $20 million in 1950, federal obligations to medical schools grew to nearly two billion dollars in 1982.[15]

Of the many factors that pointed medicine toward specialization, probably none exerted more influence than the remarkable growth of scientific knowledge. As this grew and became more complex, it created new demands for expertise. There is a sort of natural law which says that the more a subject is analyzed, studied, and developed, the more it requires specialists. The phenomenon applies to sports, giving rise to the place-kicker and the designated hitter. And it applies to medicine.

The training milieu from which today's physician emerges is clearly changed from the milieu of 1945. It is more sophisticated, more intense, more focused on science and research. Medical care in the tertiary care facilities, in the large metropolitan teaching centers, has obviously changed. What may not be so obvious is that medical care has changed all down the line. Witness Blair Henningsgaard, M.D., a longtime AMA delegate, a former member of the Judicial Council, who, until his death in 1980, practiced where he started to practice in 1948, in Astoria, Oregon, a town of 10,000 serving a community of 55-60,000.

> When I came to Astoria the telephone would ring twenty-four hours a day. I made many, many house calls. People went to the emergency room only when there was a bona fide injury, something acute.
>
> That's changed now. The capabilities of the hospital to render service have improved a thousandfold. People know this, and when they become ill they head for the hospital, even here in a small town like Astoria.
>
> The upgrading of the equipment and the capabilities of the hospital and the paramedical staff...that's the big change. We didn't have intensive care units and coronary care units or respiratory therapy departments back in 1948, things like that. Our lab was run by a technician who did everything you could do there. A pathologist came down once a week.
>
> Now we are linked to a pathology group that gives us daily service on all our tests. Our respiratory department is as good as you'll find in the big cities. And we have ICUs and CCUs.

And what about the newer physicians now starting in practice?

> They are not encouraged to establish the kind of relationship that I established with patients thirty years ago. They tend to work in a group, see patients in rotation, by appointment. They do their job and expect to be unmolested after it is done. They are slow to develop the close personal friendships that I developed thirty years ago with my patients. By consequence, I think my patients demand more of me than [they would of] some of the younger doctors, who probably render better care. The approach to the patient has changed. A small town is not a small town any more.[16]

Part II

The Organization

MEETING TWICE A YEAR, the House of Delegates determines AMA policy. On the opening day of each meeting, the 200 or so reports and resolutions that constitute a typical agenda are divided for consideration among 8-10 reference committees, which conduct open hearings (right) where delegates and anyone else with something to contribute may speak. Later, at a plenary session, (below, right) the speaker presides as a reference committee chairman (in front of him) presents his committee's recommendations for action. The annual sessions of the house are now usually held in Chicago in June, the fall meetings at convention centers in different parts of the U.S. At the 1973 meeting in Disneyland (below), the delegates welcomed an unexpected visitor.

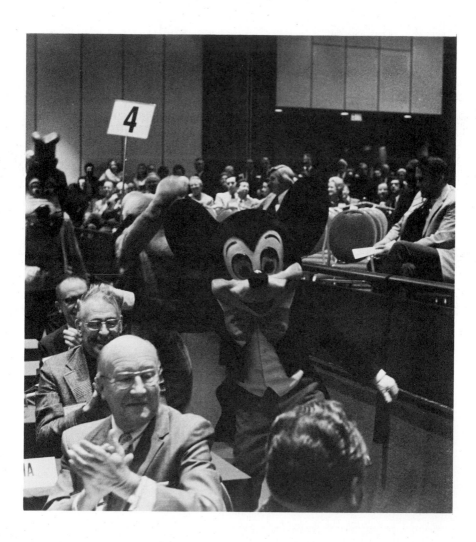

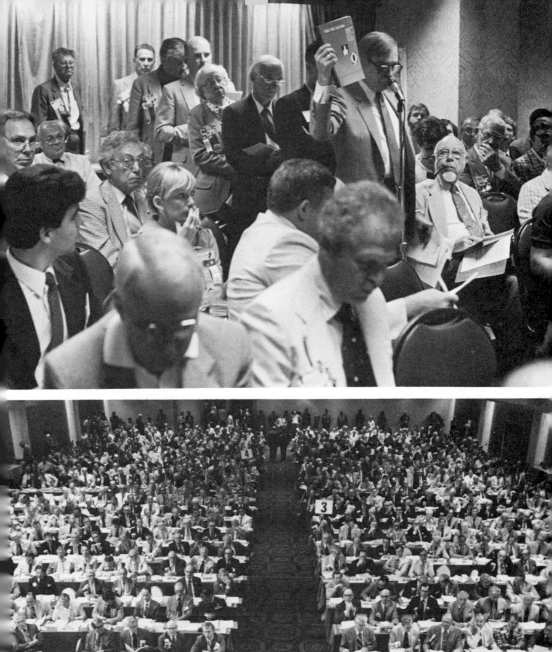
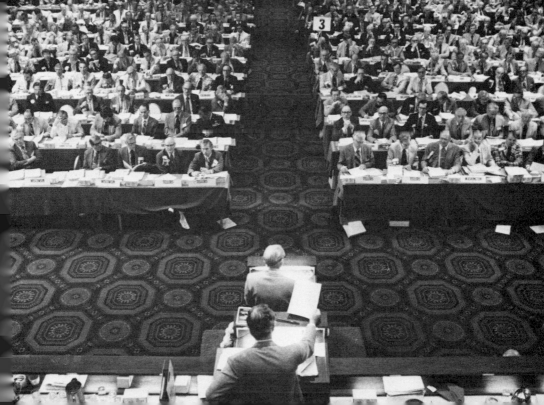

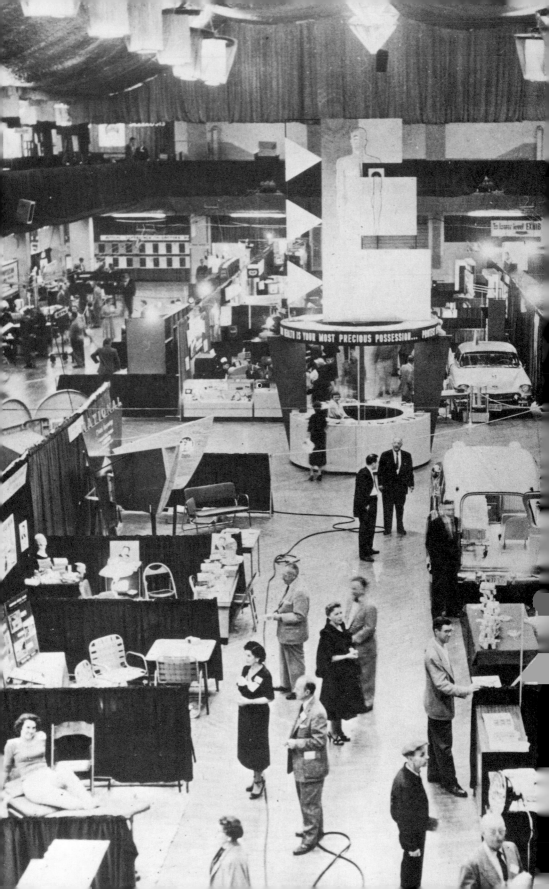

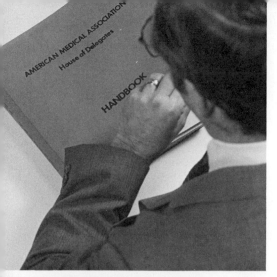

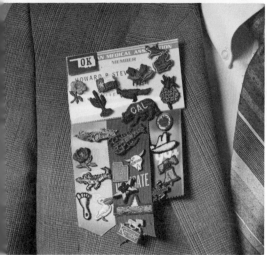

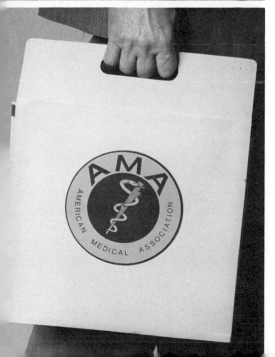

FAMILIAR SIGHTS at a meeting of the House of Delegates are the ring-bound Handbook (top), which contains the agenda items; the mementos of visits to the hospitality suites accumulating on the delegates' identification badges (center); and the gray, cardboard tote bag used by the delegates to carry the Handbook and other matters of convention business (bottom). Opposite page, an exhibition hall, part of the scientific assemblies held simultaneously with the sessions of the house through June 1978.

FOLLOWING PAGE: the AMA headquarters at 535 North Dearborn Street, Chicago. The front part of the building rests on land where the AMA established its first headquarters in 1902.

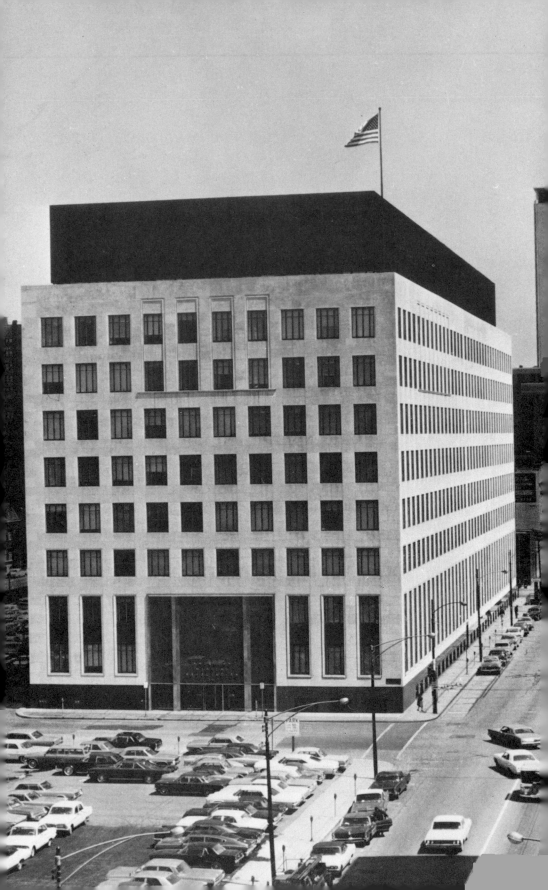

Chapter Five

The AMA:
What does it do?
Whom does it Represent?

Of the 1,339 health-related groups that are listed in the *Encyc-lopedia of Associations*, the American Medical Association is the largest, the broadest based, and the best financed. With a staff of 902 and annual operating expenses of $83,392,000, it is supported by 251,745 individual members (including about 45 percent of United States physicians), of whom 158,960 are regular members (annual dues of $285), 28,060 are physician resident members (dues of $35), 26,338 are medical student members (dues of $15), 36,500 are dues-exempt members (physicians over 70 or retired), and 1,887 are honorary or special affiliate members. The AMA policy-making body, the 305-member House of Delegates, includes representatives from the fifty state medical associations; the medical associations of the District of Columbia, Guam, Puerto Rico, and the Virgin Islands; sixty-one medical specialty societies; the residents; the students; the medical schools; the United States Public Health Service; the Veterans Administration; and the medical corps of the United States Air Force, Army, and Navy.*

It is, without question, the umbrella organization of American medicine. As a steadfastly liberal and activist physician wrote in a magazine article in 1972 when he finally decided to join, "So far as the future of medicine is concerned, the AMA is the only game in town."[1]

Legally classified as a professional association, the AMA is generally exempt from federal income taxes. However, the advertising revenues of its publications remain subject to such taxes because

*1982 figures throughout the whole paragraph; membership figures from the AMA Division of Membership.

the Internal Revenue Service considers them to derive from business unrelated to the AMA's primary purposes. These, according to Article II of the AMA constitution, are "to promote the science and art of medicine and the betterment of public health."

The simplest way to understand what the AMA does is to examine its own definitions of what it considers to be its major functions. These are described clearly in the organization's annual budget.[2]

Representation—representing the profession—is internally regarded as the key function; opinion surveys of the membership confirm this as the service physicians consider most important. The AMA represents the profession in many ways: before the press and the public; before the legislative and executive branches of government; before an assortment of academic, business, and medical groups—national and international. It develops policy positions on scientific questions, legislative proposals, and the socioeconomic issues that affect medical practice. It is continually active in determining and participating in the agenda of policy questions that have a bearing on the nation's health. In countless ways, the AMA is the doctor's advocate.

The second major function that the AMA identifies is providing scientific information. The association publishes ten journals and a multitude of other scientific and educational materials, including books such as the periodically revised *AMA Drug Evaluations*. The AMA sponsors scientific meetings and conferences on matters of professional and public concern. It has an extensive library, and, under a licensing agreement with the General Telephone and Electronic Corporation, provides the services of a national, computerized medical information network. Keeping its members alert and informed as to new advances, new techniques, and new scientific data, the AMA performs one of the traditional functions that characterize a profession: the dissemination of knowledge.

Another AMA function is providing socioeconomic information. For this purpose, the AMA publishes a weekly newspaper, *American Medical News* (*AMNews*), and other communications to keep the membership informed on non-scientific matters such as changes in medical practice, trends in medical economics, Washington developments, and organizational news.

The AMA also provides data on the profession. The association maintains a comprehensive electronic data bank of census-like information on all United States physicians. It includes their number, geographic distribution, specialty characteristics, and so forth, plus data on medical schools and hospitals.*

Maintaining educational standards is another of those functions that distinguishes a profession from a trade, calling, or occupation. The AMA performs this function by being involved in developing and maintaining standards of professional education and training—and, ultimately, performance. Together with other organizations, the AMA plays a major part in the accreditation of medical schools, residency training programs, and institutions that offer continuing medical education programs for physicians already in practice. The AMA participates in the Joint Commission on Accreditation of Hospitals; it is involved heavily in accrediting programs for the training of allied health professionals.

The remaining functions that the AMA lists in the budget concern the maintenance of the AMA's organizational strength (membership), the viability of the federation (relationships with the county, state, and specialty societies), and internal, corporate services (accounting, legal, personnel, etc.).

To carry out those functions, the AMA depends on a structure that seems somewhat diffuse in design. There are, for example, three identifiable seats of power. The House of Delegates, meeting twice a year, debates and determines broad policy matters; it sets the dues and elects the officers, including the president. The fifteen-member Board of Trustees, elected by the house, meets five or six times a year, usually in the AMA's Chicago headquarters. Far more so than the house, it becomes intimately concerned with the operations of the association and functions closely with the staff. The board has the fiscal responsibility and the authority to make policy decisions between the biannual sessions of the house. The AMA administrative staff also wields power through its chief executive officer, the executive vice president, who reports to the Board of Trustees. Its staff of about 1,000 people (in 1984) sometimes has a great deal to do with assembling information and generating background thinking for reports that underlie the policy formation.

Ultimately, of course, the real power of the AMA lies with its members. Many associations—the United States Chamber of Commerce, for example, or the American Hospital Association—derive their legitimacy and their income from corporate memberships. But others, like the American Bar Association, the American Dental

*See Appendix A

Association, and the AMA, have to rely on the support of many, many individual members of the profession.

A physician actually has to go a bit out of the way to become a full-fledged member of the AMA federation; joining is not a totally effortless process. Generally speaking, a prospective member is introduced by colleagues to the county medical society, proposed for membership by current members, subjected to a background check and an examination of academic credentials, and, if all is in order, elected. In many cases, the candidate's name is "posted"; if you pick up a county medical society bulletin, you will often see pictures and thumbnail biographies of candidates for membership.

In the process of being elected to many county societies a physician must attend one or two orientation sessions to learn the codes of behavior adopted by the county society (dealings with the press, for example), what is expected in terms of keeping abreast of medical advances, and a member's obligation to contribute part of his or her time to the community medical programs undertaken by the county society.

The restrictions on membership are few. A regular AMA member must have a degree of Doctor of Medicine or the equivalent, and be licensed by one of the states or an equivalent licensing jurisdiction. In 1982, the AMA lifted its long-standing requirement that a physician member also join the appropriate county and state societies, though only about 2 percent of regular members who belonged to the AMA in that year belonged directly, that is, without first joining the county and state societies. The AMA does not require that a member be a citizen. In fact, nearly a fifth of the foreign medical school graduates now in the United States are AMA members. Many of them have acquired citizenship. The AMA does not specify what form of medical practice a member engages in. He or she may be a solo fee-for-service practitioner, a member of a prepaid, closed panel group, a full-time member of a hospital staff, or a salaried federal government employee practicing medicine in, say, a Veterans Administration hospital. But the chances are that the next regular AMA member you encounter will be engaged in patient care (as opposed to full-time teaching, research, or administrative work) and will be office-based (as opposed to holding a salaried position with a hospital). The odds are roughly seven in twelve that he or she will have completed the extra training and passed the examinations required for board certification in a medical specialty.[3]

During the last thirty-five years, the concept of AMA member-ship has undergone a fundamental change. From something that was regarded casually, even off-handedly, until the late 1940s, it has become a matter that today is watched, studied, and sometimes worried over. From 1912 to 1949 there were two categories of mem-bership. A physician who was a member of the state association and county medical society was—without any requirement to pay dues—"logically" considered to be an AMA member. If in addition he decided to apply for membership and pay dues annually (initial-ly $5, then $6, $8, and $12), he received a subscription to *JAMA*, became a Fellow of the AMA, and, after two years, became eligible for elective office.* Since the dues for Fellowship members equaled the subscription price of *JAMA* to a non-member, there were, re-alistically speaking, no membership dues at all.

But in 1950, when for the first time in many years dues were required of members, the AMA gradually began to shift its finan-cial base from publishing revenues to a greater reliance on mem-bership dues. Income from Fellowship dues—after allocations to *JAMA* to reflect subscription cost—was a modest $73,185 for 1948. By contrast, in 1982 membership dues generated over $44 million in revenues, or 47 percent of the association's total income for the year.

A great deal has been written about the AMA's alleged power to coerce physicians into joining and then forcing them to abide by its policy decisions. By some accounts, the physician who fails to join the AMA federation and accept its strictures suffers devastating penalties, ranging from social ostracism to professional boycott. "No other voluntary association commands such power within its area of interest as does the AMA," an article in the *Yale Law Journal* stated in May 1954. "It holds a position of authority over the indi-vidual doctor...controls the conditions of practice...The doctor who challenges AMA authority to determine his method of practice is tried and judged by his fellow physicians who may have an eco-nomic interest in proscribing his allegedly offensive conduct."[4]

Although charges in the article have been picked up and repeated in articles and books about the AMA, they often are, where not actually untrue, badly overstated. Written by four students at the law school, the article based its conclusions largely on a somewhat spotty response to a questionnaire sent to state medical societies, from the evidence of court cases, many going back to the 1930s, and

---

*When his death was noted in the obituary listings in *JAMA*, a small mark—a Swiss cross enclosed in a circle—appeared after his name, indicating he had been an AMA Fellow. The obituary listings in *JAMA* now identify members thus: Ⓜ

a terrier-like search of library material. There are, in fact, 709 footnotes in the eighty-four page article. What is missing is any sort of journalistic description of the day-to-day workings of medicine.

No attempt to interview member or non-member physicians is evident, nor any effort to seek comment from people within medical organizations. The thrust of the article is further weakened by the authors' inclination to magnify single incidents and fragmentary evidence into broadly applied conclusions. Nor did the authors attempt to explain how a substantial percentage of physicians managed to prosper without membership or why antitrust actions had not been instituted.

A more realistic view of the reasons why physicians join the AMA may be derived from the results of an AMA survey of member physicians done in August 1980. The response rate to the questionnaire that was mailed to a random sample of members was 50.8 percent. The results (Table 1) provide a picture that varies sharply from the conclusions reached by the authors of the *Yale Law Journal* article.

By the actions of a county medical society—or a metropolitan society in the case of some large cities that spread over more than one county—organized medicine can exert an influence on physician behavior, but only up to a point. It is the state licensing board, not the county or state medical society, that has the authority to restrict a physician's license, impose fines, or revoke a license.* The worst a medical society can do is refuse admission to someone who is not a member or revoke the membership of someone who is. Medical society membership is not a condition of licensure. It is not a condition for hospital privileges, although in past years pressure of this sort was used to build membership in many county societies. It is not a condition of specialty board certification, although that was once proposed. "Joining the AMA," says one longtime member, "is like joining a church. You don't do it because it pays or because you have to. You join it because you believe in it."

Over the years, several writers and physicians have dwelt on a schism within the AMA between private practitioners and academic physicians; that is, those with research or teaching appointments

---

*Licensing boards are appointed by governors, sometimes with some of the nominees suggested by the state medical association. A majority of the boards today also have public members.

TABLE 1
Reasons Given by AMA Members for
Joining the Association.

Question: A number of reasons have been given by other physicians as to why they belong to the AMA. How important to you are each of the following reasons for belonging to the AMA?

Responses:

Reason for Joining	Very Important		Somewhat Important		Not Important		No Opinion/ Not Applicable		Total (100%)
	No.	%	No.	%	No.	%	No.	%	No.
The AMA effectively represents my interests on the national level	752	52.5	503	35.1	107	7.5	71	5.0	1,433
I belong to the AMA because it provides attractive membership benefits (e.g., insurance, publications)	146	10.2	480	33.4	727	50.7	82	5.7	1,435
I must belong to the AMA in order to belong to my local medical society	227	15.9	286	20.0	497	34.7	421	29.4	1,431
I belong to the AMA due to peer influence	46	3.3	266	18.9	874	61.9	225	15.9	1,411
It is important to me to belong to my professional association	538	37.2	585	40.5	259	17.9	63	4.4	1,445
I renew my AMA membership each year out of habit	135	9.6	277	19.8	590	42.1	398	28.4	1,400

Source: Study done for the AMA in 1980 by Market Opinion Research.

at medical centers (many of whom also provide patient care, generally of a highly specialized nature). During the first years of the century, medical academia and private practitioners worked in close association. They joined forces within the AMA to bring about the reform of the medical schools, for example. But "town" and "gown" (as they are sometimes categorized) began to go separate ways about the time of World War I, divided over the issue of "state medicine," i.e., legislative proposals calling for the financing of medical care for the working poor by the individual states. The AMA at first endorsed the concept, but after World War I withdrew its support. With that action, the gown segment of medicine tended to drift away from the AMA, and the town segment—the private practitioners—became dominant.

During the early 1960s, in the emotional heat that surrounded the legislation that became Medicare in 1965, the factionalism reached peak temperatures. In an analysis of the AMA published in the *New England Journal of Medicine* in 1964, John G. Freymann, M.D., describes an episode that suggests just how bitter the split had then become.

The year is 1962 and the scene is the 181st annual meeting of the Massachusetts Medical Society. The business before it is a proposal that membership in the AMA be made a condition of membership in the Massachusetts society.* The proposal has received a chilly reception. But at the invitation of the Massachusetts physicians, a representative of the AMA is present to make his case. Freymann wrote:

> The opening speaker for the proponents ran over his allotted ten minutes before advancing his arguments. The opening speaker for the opponents was the antithesis of the proponent. His presentation was articulate, precise and delivered in just four minutes. He stated that strong members of the AMA must be voluntary members and that they should be convinced, rather than forced, into membership.

*Beginning with Oklahoma in 1950, many state medical associations instituted unified membership, requiring their members to join the AMA as well. By 1970, Arizona, California, Colorado, Hawaii, Illinois, Kansas, Mississippi, Montana, Nebraska, New York, Nevada, Oklahoma, and Wisconsin had all become unified states. Because physicians tend to become county-state members more readily than AMA members, unified membership policies greatly benefited the AMA, and it encouraged states to adopt them. But during the 1970s all but two of the states, Oklahoma and Illinois, revoked their unified membership policies.

He released a parliamentary steamroller that closed off further debate and defeated the proposal by an overwhelming vote. The meeting was adjourned, and, well satisfied and triumphant, the cream of Boston medicine disappeared.

Freymann recounts the incident not to argue for or against the issue of unified membership but to show the polarity. "On the one side," he said, "are those whose chief endeavors are directed toward research and teaching, and on the other those whose primary occupation is private practice." He also wanted to make the point that both sides were taking negative positions on then-current legislative proposals.[5]

Although the political breakage of the 1960s has been repaired and the temperatures lowered, vestiges of an underlying difference still linger. Physicians in teaching and research do not always share the intensity of interest in socioeconomic issues displayed by private practitioners, who must build their practices, conduct them within a welter of governmental regulations, and protect them from a variety of encroachments. On the other hand, the practitioners do not always share the academicians' concern with research grants, hospital reimbursement policies, and their problems with regulatory agencies.

The gap between medical academia and private practice may well be exaggerated; by no means is it unbridgeable or final. In fact, the lines between are frequently and easily crossed. For example, as many as 95,000 volunteers—many of them private-practice, fee-for-service, office-based physicians—have medical school appointments and teach part-time.[6] By providing for a delegate to represent the medical school deans in 1976, opening the house to specialty society delegates in 1977, and authorizing a delegate for hospital medical staff physicians in 1983, the AMA has invited greater participation by the academic community.

Nevertheless, the AMA is often characterized as being overwhelmingly representative of the private practitioner. In a sense, that is correct, but largely because that category also dominates the profession. So that a fair judgment may be made as to how representative the AMA is in terms of physician activity, the comparative distribution figures for the 452,800 physicians who comprised the medical profession in 1979 and the 211,899 physicians who were AMA members* that year are listed in Table 2.

*Total does not include 17,672 AMA medical student members, who are not yet physicians.

TABLE 2

Professional Activities of AMA Members and the Medical Profession as a Whole by Percent.

Professional Activity	AMA Members	Profession as a Whole
Total physicians	100 %	100 %
Physicians in patient care	81.6	75.8
Office-based	67.2	52.8
Hospital-based	14.5	23.0
Physicians in other activity	6.1	9.1
Teaching	1.3	1.7
Administration	2.4	2.7
Research	1.8	4.1
Other activity	0.6	0.6
Inactive physicians, or address unknown, or non-classifiable	12.2	15.1

Source: AMA Center for Health Services Research and Development

A certain amount of controversy has also surrounded the AMA's choice of priorities. To what degree is its organizational energy focused on political and socioeconomic activities and to what degree is it concentrated on educational and scientific concerns? Non-member physicians in particular worry over the point, often saying they are willing to join a "scientific" medical organization but not one that is "political." That the AMA is and has been a mixture of both elements has been clear for a long time.

Even in the years when the academically oriented physicians tended to dominate the AMA, the legislative-political-socioeconomic function was clearly acknowledged as a key mission. In 1901, for example, when the AMA was organizing itself into its present form, the argument presented by the Committee on Organization for a restructured AMA was forthright on the point. "If the Association will give its sanction to these recommendations," the committee's report stated, "there will be good reason to hope that in five years the profession throughout the entire country will be welded into a compact organism, whose power to influence public sentiment will be almost unlimited, and whose requests for desirable legislation will everywhere be met with that respect which the politician always has for organized votes."[7]

At the annual meeting in 1910, the president, William H. Welch, M.D., one of the four physicians prominent in establishing Johns Hopkins as an institution for the rest of American medical education to emulate, chose as the subject of his address to the annual meeting, "Fields of Usefulness of the American Medical Association." When he got around to discussing the AMA's legislative role, he was quite emphatic. He said:

> The Association should assuredly keep aloof from politics in the customary significance of the term, and it should never resort to the arts of the politician. Its function and indeed its duty in relation to national legislation concerning health and medicine is to utter the voice of medical science as effectively as possible and to endeavor to have it heard by the lawmakers. It was entirely right and proper for this Association through its Committee on Legislation to aid in the defeat of the antivivisection bill before Congress ten years ago and to support the passage of the Food and Drugs Act, the pensions for the widows of our medical heroes, Reed, Lazear and Carroll, the introduction of trained nursing in the army, the various health bills, including the one under consideration now for a department of public health.[8]

Even then, and even from a man who might be called an academician's academician, the legitimacy of the AMA's political role was asserted with candor, emphasis, and wide agreement.

Intellectually, most physicians understand the need for political involvement. But temperamentally many of them are uneasy with politics. They would, for example, agree thoroughly with the first two sentences of the quotation above from President Welch's remarks on the AMA's fields of usefulness. Possibly because a physician's training is focused so intently on the sciences and so lightly on history and the humanities, politics as an occupation seems to rank well down on the physician's scale of values. Politics, many doctors feel, somehow carries a taint, and not all physicians are convinced that political activity is something that a proper medical society should get into. The feeling, of course, collides with the AMA's primary function—representing the profession—and it colors the attitudes of an appreciable number of physicians toward the AMA and membership in it.

Is the AMA of today "political" or "scientific"? An outside study of the AMA done in 1977 provides one independent perspective. In approaching the task Frederick D. Sturdivant, Ph.D., the M. Riklis

Professor of Business and Its Environment at the Ohio State University, together with two associates, decided to analyze three aspects of the issue. What would the budget—the allocation of resources—show? What would a comparison of the AMA's budget with those of other associations—manufacturing and educational associations, for example—indicate? What, finally, might be revealed by comparing the AMA's program of activities with the programs of six other associations?

Professor Sturdivant's findings leave little doubt as to what receives the major emphasis. An objective assessment of all three of the analyses, the report states, leads to the conclusion that "the American Medical Association is a professional association engaged overwhelmingly in scientific and educational activities." The AMA legislative activity, which Professor Sturdivant calls the "government interface," appears in his analysis as 3.7 percent of the total budget.[9]

Though it might be argued that parts of other activities—part of the public relations budget, for example—should be included as part of the government interface, the total still would not come to much more than 5 percent of the AMA's overall budget.

Yet that 5 percent attracts a disproportionate share of attention. The phenomenon is not peculiar to the AMA; it applies to some labor unions, to trade and business associations, and to other professional groups. Because political activity attracts attention and makes headlines, it can easily overshadow the visibility of other functions.

When polled on the emphasis given to "scientific" versus "political" programs, as they periodically have been, physicians give consistent evidence that they consider the AMA's direction to be responsive to what the majority wants. The AMA does reflect the profession's views, the polls say, and especially those of the membership.

Recent confirmation that the AMA works in tune with the membership—and in a general way with the profession itself—emerged from a survey done in 1972, when the AMA was backing its own national health insurance legislation. The survey measured support for the AMA proposal along with the extent of support for a far more sweeping plan introduced by Senator Edward M. Kennedy and a third proposal developed by the administration of President Richard M. Nixon. Sponsoring a bill of its own was a departure for the AMA; for many years it had usually taken a purely negative position, with no attempt to come up with alternative ideas.

How did the membership feel? Questionnaires went out to 172,882 members of the AMA. More than half of them filled in the answers, and a check indicated that those responding, except for giving some over-representation to internists, constituted a valid sample. Of the options described (which were *not* labeled Kennedy bill, Nixon Bill, or AMA Bill to avoid emotionally triggered responses) the concept of the AMA legislation received four times the support of the next most popular bill.

Another question in that survey sought opinions about program emphasis. Two-thirds said that the scientific activities of the AMA were receiving the proper emphasis. But only about 40 percent of the respondents thought socioeconomic issues and legislative issues were getting the proper degree of attention; about a third of the respondents said there was "not enough emphasis" on socioeconomic and legislative issues.[10]

In 1975, this time using a probability sample rather than the entire membership, the AMA surveyed both member and non-member physicians on the various approaches to national health insurance legislation. Again without labels, the Kennedy, the administration, and the AMA concepts were offered as choices.[11] The results, shown in Table 3, contradict once more those who charge that AMA policy is frequently divergent from the broad views of the profession. There have been and are physician organizations to the left of the AMA: Physicians Forum, the Medical Committee for Human Rights, Physicians for Social Responsibility. And there have been and are organizations to the right of the AMA: the Private Doctors of America (formerly the Council of Medical Staffs), the

TABLE 3
Physician Response to
National Health Insurance Legislation,
by Percent of Respondents

	AMA Members	Non-Members
Favor Kennedy approach	6.2%	12.1%
Favor Nixon approach	11.7%	13.6%
Favor AMA approach	60.6%	49.4%
Favor none of the above	11.1%	11.3%

Source: AMA Center for Health Services Research and Development

Congress of County Medical Societies, the Association of American Physicians and Surgeons. But over the years, none has really gathered strong support; the AMA occupies too wide a strip of central ground.

From time to time, especially during those periods when national health insurance legislation has come up for serious consideration in Congress, the AMA has been roughly handled by the media. Taking positions opposite to those embraced by organized labor and the liberal wing of the Democratic party, the AMA has periodically undergone sharp, partisan attacks from parts of the press.

The perception of the AMA by the general public, however, differs from the descriptions sometimes offered by the press and television. The more favorable public view is possibly colored by the public's impression of the quality of medical care it receives. An AMA study done in the mid-1950s, for example, found that among people who said they were familiar with the AMA 43 percent had an opinion that was "all good;" 26 percent had an opinion that was "more good than bad;" while 18 percent registered opinions that were either neutral or negative.[12] In 1976, and again at the end of 1979, the AMA engaged the Gallup Organization, Inc. to find out how the AMA rated relative to similar associations and institutions. Choosing the credibility of communications as an index, the Gallup pollsters asked members of a national probability sample to rank ten professional/trade associations and four societal institutions on a scale of 1 to 10, a response of 1 indicating "little confidence," a response of 10 indicating "great confidence." The results are reported in Table 4.[13]

Despite periodic immersions in political partisanship, the AMA has emerged with its public credibility largely intact; somewhat stronger, in fact, than that of its detractors.

TABLE 4
Ranking of Professional Trade Associations and Institutions by the Public, 1976 and 1979

Professional/Trade Association	1976	1979
American Medical Association	6.8	6.6
American Dental Association	6.8	6.9
American Bar Association	6.2	6.1
National Rifle Association	5.7	5.9
American Hospital Association	6.2	5.8
Pharmaceutical Manufacturers Association	5.9	5.8
American Trucking Association	5.9	5.8
National Association of Manufacturers	—	5.7
National Association of Realtors	5.0	5.1
American Petroleum Institute	4.2	3.7

Societal Institutions

	1976	1979
News media	6.1	6.0
Business corporations	5.0	5.1
Labor unions	4.9	4.9
Federal agencies	4.9	4.9

Source: The Gallup Organization, Inc.

Chapter Six

The Making of a Physician

No longer is it so easy to assert, as Ralph Waldo Emerson once did, that an institution is the lengthened shadow of one man. Until recently, the point could be readily illustrated: Jimmy Hoffa and the Teamsters; Louis B. Mayer and M-G-M; Richard J. Daley and the Cook County Democratic Organization. A plausible case could even be made that the American Medical Association of the 1930s and the 1940s was the lengthened shadow of Morris Fishbein, M.D., whose personality, energy, and persuasiveness appeared to dominate the organization. But times have changed. People now are more inclined to insist on their rights. Organizations stress participation and pay more attention to their bylaws. Even Congress has yielded, tempering the arbitrary system by which committee chairmanships were once decided.

With one-man rulers off the stage, what is it that now establishes the character of an organization? What is it, for example, that makes the Audubon Society one sort of organization, the American Civil Liberties Union another, and the Business Roundtable a third? Interest, of course, is a major determinant—sometimes economic interest, sometimes interest in a subject or a cause. But along with interest, a number of other elements must be considered: the style, tastes, education, and occupational experience of the people who constitute the organization. Neither the direction nor the personality of an organization stem from one person any more. More often, organizations reflect several factors, not the least of which is membership.

It is therefore helpful to consider some of the personality characteristics of physicians. They affect both the AMA's operational style and its policy-formation process. Above all else, the AMA is a *doctors'* organization.

Not that there is such a thing as a physician "type." The profession is, among other things, too large for that. It comprises so wide a sample of humanity that virtually all physical, psychological, and moral traits are represented. Within the profession and within the AMA membership you will find endomorphs and ectomorphs, introverts and extroverts, idealists and materialists, saints and sinners, and all graduations in between. There is a wide variation in the income of physicians as well (see Chart 1).

But that is not to say that this medical universe is a cross-section of the general population. It is, in fact, not even a cross-section of the college-educated segment of the United States population. It is, first of all, a narrowly selected population, the selection process tending to favor certain traits of personality over others. It is also a conditioned population, the education of a physician taking longer and demanding more than the training for any other commonly practiced profession or occupation.

As early as freshman or sophomore year in college, the first conscious step in the selection process usually confronts the physician-to-be. It is by no means formal; in fact, it is self-administered. And it comes as the answer to the question, "Should I major in pre-med?" Some students screen themselves out right away. Unless he or she is prepared to shoot for top marks, a student may as well forget a medical career. The competition for places in United States medical schools is so fierce that until 1983 there were usually two or three seriously considered applicants for each opening. To an extraordinary extent, it is academic standing—marks—that determines who is admitted. Of the first-year medical school students in 1978-79, for example, 50 percent had A averages in their pre-med studies; 45 percent had B averages.[1] "With the exception of the 2 percent or 3 percent of the population who are geniuses," says Ralph Crawshaw, M.D., a practicing psychiatrist in Portland, Oregon, "if you are going to get grades, you have to work like hell. That means the A and B students have to grind it out of the books. And that means they have to have a certain personality, which will sit them down at a desk with enough discipline and enough control over their instinctual desires to grind it out. There is a blistering competitive* experience in being pre-med."[2]

---

*Competition among medical students can at times be ugly. M. Therese Southgate, M.D., the deputy editor of *JAMA*, recalls going to her biology lab class one day and finding the remains of the cat she was dissecting had been stolen. Presumably, the student or students who took them figured that the resulting delay would cause her to do less well on the approaching exams and thereby enhance their chances of moving up in the scholastic standings. Dr. Southgate smiles about the incident today. "You forget how callow we all were."

CHART 1

Distribution of Physician Net Income, 1982
(After expenses but before taxes)

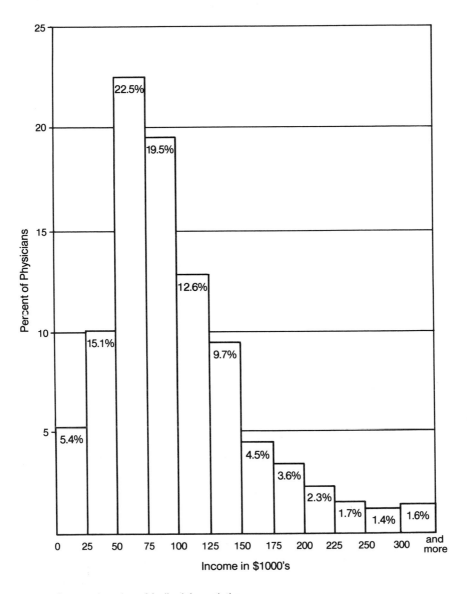

Source: American Medical Association

Thus, preparation for medical school in college serves as a first screen. It deals not only with mental capacity but also with depth of motivation. The student headed for medical school must be determined to work to the limits of his or her abilities and energies. A certain inner discipline is required to continue working at those limits.

That intensity of motivation often springs up beside an equally intense desire for independence. Few doctors fit the mold of the organization man. Hugh H. Hussey, M.D., who spent much of his medical career teaching at the Georgetown University School of Medicine, six years of it as dean, says, "Medicine is perceived as a career where you are your own boss. The physician has a distinct sense of independence, and it carries over into other things."[3] John W. Tarnasky, M.D., a practicing obstetrician-gynecologist, bears out Hussey's observation. "I grew up here in Portland," Tarnasky recalls. "My dad was a clerk for the railroad, with an annual income of something like $3,500. I was going to Portland University, living at home, paying maybe $52 a term in tuition. Dad, if he left me anything, left me with one thought. And that was, 'I don't care what you do. But do something where you work for yourself.' That's what decided me on medical school. And that's when I decided I'd hit the books."[4]

It is interesting to ask physicians what they might have been if they had not made it into the medical profession. First of all, the question causes surprise, as if the thought had never occurred to them, as if the idea of failure had never really crossed their minds. Then they respond with answers that again reflect the desire for an independent life. Tarnasky thinks he probably would have become a lawyer if he had been turned down for medical school. A fellow Oregonian, Thomas R. Reardon, M.D., says he probably would have become a rancher or a farmer.

The depth of commitment can often be measured by the age at which the determination to be a doctor first emerges. *Boys in White*, a study of medical students at the University of Kansas published in 1961, indicates that of sixty-two students, twenty had decided to be doctors while still in grammar school and another twenty-five had made the decision in junior high or high school. Only seventeen had waited as late as their college years to make their career choice.[5]

Often too, the commitment has strong personal and emotional overtones. The desire to emulate the physician who saved a seriously ill parent or brother or sister may be present. A personal experience often plays a role. Hussey attributes his own first stir-rings of interest in becoming a doctor to his admiration for the family physician who saw him through a somewhat sickly child-hood. "But," he smiles, "I was also fond of the veterinarian who took care of our dog. He sometimes used to take me along when he made his rounds."

As with many commitments made early in life, the decision to be a physician is usually accompanied by a streak of idealism. C.H. William Ruhe, M.D., an AMA senior vice president at the time of his retirement in 1982 but for many years before that the dean of admissions at the University of Pittsburgh School of Medicine, says:

It's not just that the applicants have a long-standing interest in medi-cine. It is an interest that is rooted in a strong inner commitment to serve other people. This may sound a little corny, but most of the applicants to medical school have a desire, which they do not express very well, to help others. This is not to say that they are all hopelessly altruistic and that everyone else is egotistic. In fact, this kind of altruism may, philosophically, be the purest form of egotism.

I am sure that most medical school applicants are aware that they will enjoy their share of the world's goods. But the motivation is not so much that, or even the desire for power or status in the commu-nity, as it is the gratification that comes from providing direct assis-tance to other people. It's the desire for this sort of gratification that brings most of them to the field.[6]

Once he is admitted to medical school, the student's sense of com-mitment, his inner discipline, and mental capacities are put to a severe trial. Crawshaw remembers:

The immensity of what I was about to do really hit me. I entered medical school in 1943, when I was still in the Army. My first day there, I was told, in effect, to report to the supply sergeant and draw my medical books. What I got were the books for the whole cur-riculum, everything, not just the books I'd need for the first few months. There was Gray's *Anatomy*, Best and Taylor's *Physiology*, Boyd's *Pathology*, books on biochemistry, pharmacology, physical di-agnosis. My God, those books would have filled a wheelbarrow. And all I could think of was, How am I going to put all of the information in all of those books into my head?

So much has been written about the ordeal of medical school that little elaboration is needed here. But two facts might be mentioned just to underscore the scale of the challenge. One has to do with vocabulary. First year students in medical school probably have to double or triple their vocabulary before graduation. They have to learn 5,000 anatomical terms alone. Then there is the workload. A college undergraduate, typically, may carry sixteen to seventeen semester hours. An exceptional program may run as high as twenty. For the medical school student, just the *norm* requires more than that. "I figured out one time," says Ruhe, "what the medical student load might be in equivalent terms. Based on the number of hours in the classroom and in the laboratory, it came to around twenty-five to twenty-six semester hours. Fatigue becomes a part of the medical student's life. There is always the feeling that no matter how long you study, you never can learn it all."

In response to that feeling, psychiatrist Crawshaw suggests that medical students develop a lasting "psychological warp" in their personalities that he regards as a form of compulsion. He says:

> In psychoanalytical terms, in order to have the necessary kind of discipline—the sitting down and dotting all the i's and crossing all the t's—you have to have a compulsive side to your personality. You can't get through medical school without it...The kind of thing I am talking about can be seen in the surgeon. He scrubs his hands for his ten or twelve minutes or whatever. He really enjoys making sure there are no germs there. That compulsion, that getting into the details of something, is one of the traits that a physician has. He becomes far more persnickety over details than an artist or an accountant. But if he matures properly, the physician isn't left with just getting the grades or getting his hands clean. He becomes the sort of person who wants to take things to completion. He does not like to leave anything up in the air. This compulsiveness underlies discipline, and the discipline leads to commitment. The physician is a deeply committed person.

What boot camp is to the Marine, medical school is to the physician, Ruhe observes. He says:

> It's the feeling of mutuality that springs from a shared test of character. It is a trial by fire, and it produces an unusually strong bond among those who have endured it. This is one of the reasons—that plus the vocabulary—that makes physicians feel most comfortable when talking with other physicians. The medical school experience does affect communications. When someone starts telling physicians what to do, they will listen if it is another physician. But if not, very frequently they won't.

After the first two years of medical school, the training site for students starts shifting to the hospital. Here again, the experience continues to be intense and demanding. And especially when it moves into residency training (which follows graduation from medical school), the experience takes on some unique psychological overtones. For now, again and again, when the physician is dealing with another human being, he is—literally and figuratively —dealing with someone who lies prone before him. "There is an abnormality in this relationship," Ruhe points out.

> People who are injured or sick or in need of surgery are not themselves. They are at the mercy of those people in the hospital who are taking care of them. And the developing physician finds that his most frequent contact with the general population is with someone in an explicitly dependent state, someone who is unwilling or incapable of making critical decisions about his own future. The experience has a conditioning effect, for it reinforces the physician's ego as a person who makes the decisions and gives the orders.

When a physician completes his training, society grants him extraordinary powers. Upon fulfillment of the requirements, the states license physicians—and physicians exclusively—to perform medical and surgical services for compensation.* Strict laws prohibit the practice of medicine without a license. A physician may prescribe controlled substances and other drugs. For someone seeking compensation for a disability, it is a physician who often evaluates the extent of it. Infrequently, and then usually in consultation with another physician, he or she may certify a person as mentally incompetent. A physician signed your birth certificate in all likelihood, and, depending upon the state, a physician may sign your death certificate.

As he or she enters the practice of medicine, what sort of person has the physician become? What, for example, has happened to the early idealism? Has the training process flattened it? Ruhe believes not:

---

*Generally speaking, to become a licensed doctor of medicine you must: (1) graduate from one of the 127 approved United States medical schools; (2) complete one post-doctoral year of graduate medical education, i.e., residency training; and (3) pass the state licensing examination. The word internship, which used to describe the first year of training after medical school graduation, is no longer used.

The studies which have been done do show change. The educational process is demanding, hardening, just by the nature of the workload. The repeated exposure to people in a subservient position, because of their illness, creates a superficial hardening. No one can take on the burden of every sick individual as a personal burden. You have to remove yourself by at least one step. Most of the psychological studies describe an increased level of cynicism. But I think it is more a building up of a set of defenses.

The late novelist (and physician) W. Somerset Maugham once described the emotional impact on the student. Writing about his own three years at St. Thomas' Hospital in London, Maugham said, "I must have witnessed pretty well every emotion of which man is capable...I saw how men died. I saw how they bore pain. I saw what hope looked like, fear and relief: I saw the dark lines that despair drew on a face: I saw courage and steadfastness."[7] Without question, the experience is bruising. "But," says Ruhe, "if you scratch the physician, I think you will find the dedication to service is still there. He's been hammered by the workload. He's been hardened by the pressure. We like to think of physicians as compassionate, and I think they are. But frequently the compassion does not show. The pressures of time and work sweep over it, and it gets pushed under, a little below the surface."

Something else happens to the physician along the way: he or she becomes a strong authority figure. This is expected by the patient and desired by the patient. And it is easy to see how the trait develops. The patient who presents himself or herself at a physician's office may or may not be truly sick. But he is worried, anxious. He suspects something is wrong, and he is frightened. It is to the physician that he has turned to find out what is wrong and solve the difficulty. Yet in an impressive number of cases, there is no clearcut, easy diagnosis to be made. A primary care physician probably sees as many cases of mental depression as any other one medical condition. Spend a day with a physician in general practice and you will come away with an appreciation for the insights expressed by Ann Landers in her introduction to her *Encyclopedia.* "I have learned how it is," she writes, "with the stumbling, frightened people in this world who have no one to talk to. The fact that my column has been a success underscores for me, at least, the central tragedy of our society. The loneliness, the insecurity, the fear that devils, cripples and paralyzes so many of us."[8] That is a large part of the vision of mankind that the physician sees every day.

Whether the patient's complaint is physically treatable or not, possibly the most important thing a physician can do consists of allaying the fears, easing the anxieties, and giving the patient psychological, emotional support. Of the few options the physician has—drugs, surgery, physical therapy—emotional support may be the most beneficial part of treatment. And in the process of giving that support, again and again, the physician cannot help developing a personality that exudes strength and confidence.

In the making of a physician there is also the making of a person with a "show me" mindset. The physician is trained to be skeptical, to be a doubter. Physicians want evidence, proof. Like people trained in other scientific disciplines, they are schooled in the process of inductive reasoning, with its emphasis on objective observation, the formation of hypotheses, the testing of those hypotheses through experimentation, and the acceptance of only those that can be proved scientifically. Three other characteristics may very well derive from this emphasis on the scientific method. One is the physician's celebrated liking for gadgetry, for things to tinker with and try out. The physician is an innovator. Another is the care with which physicians arrive at their conclusions, a deliberateness that may be accentuated by the life-or-death consequences of the decisions they must make. The third result is the physician's resistance to emotional argument on scientific matters. Physicians do not like to be swayed: they want to be shown. They become uneasy in situations that demand compromise.

Of all the personality traits that develop or emerge, the one that runs deepest seems to be the intensity, the sense of compulsion to study, to learn, to work, to excel. "Maybe not all physicians are compulsive," deadpans Crawshaw, "Maybe it's only 99.9 percent of them. You just can't get through medical school without a certain compulsivity in your thinking. You sometimes work until you are ready to drop, and then as soon as you get some strength you go back and do some more work, it's all so fascinating."

There are casualties along the way in terms of marriage and home life. A survey by the magazine, *Medical/Mrs.*, of 1,000 physicians' wives found that while they anticipated the problems, 53 percent of them said that the time and energy demands of the medical profession took a terrible toll in terms of family life.[9] In an

AMNews survey, a number of physicians said that they thought their family life had suffered.[10] Doctors become alcoholics, possibly more frequently than people generally. And, partly because of ready availability, it is easy for a physician to become addicted to drugs. Connected to the stress too is the physician suicide rate, believed to be seventy-seven per 100,000 versus fifteen per 100,000 for the population as a whole. In attempting to identify causes, at least one recent study of physician suicide emphasizes, in addition to the presence of emotional instability, such factors as a sense of professional failure and a sense of autonomy that prevents him from seeking help.[11] A physician's compulsion to excel can sometimes turn on him, with fearful results.*

On an entirely different level, the compulsiveness exhibits itself in the seeming inability of at least some physicians to stop being a doctor for more than a few minutes at a time. William R. Barclay, M.D., for example, confesses to a habitual difficulty in separating his social existence from his clinical instincts. "At a party, I'll count the number of drinks somebody takes. Or keep track of the number of cigarette butts he puts in the ash tray. If I see someone with large ears and prematurely gray hair, I can't stop myself from wondering whether the man might have pernicious anemia. I glance at fingernails, looking for ridges that might indicate pneumonia within the last year."[12] Physicians have a hard time letting go.

And what they want to let go least of all is their control over their professional decisions. Doctors begin with a deep, early commitment to provide their fellow man with the best of medical care. They spend long, arduous years learning how to do that, emerging from the process as individuals with more than normal quotients of intensity, independence, self-confidence, individuality, and ego. As they go to work on their own, finally, they resent anything that comes between them and what they perceive to be optimal care for their patients.

The experience may explain why such a preponderance of physicians has traditionally objected to what has been labeled as "socialized medicine." Strictly defined, the term refers to a totally federalized system, such as England's, in which care for everyone is financed by taxes. The patients receive care without charge, and the

---

*Together with county and state societies, the AMA is placing a renewed emphasis on programs to identify and rehabilitate impaired physicians.

doctors receive reimbursement from the government. Although no program as sweeping as the British national health service has been seriously considered in the United States, variations of it have. Bearing the label of national health insurance, these have been generally resisted by physicians—as a possible encroachment on their professional independence, as a threat to their authority to make medical decisions (and provide optimum care for patients), or as a politically motivated first step along the road to "socialized medicine."

As a spur to action, the desire of a professional to retain control over professional matters ranks high in the range of human motivation. Lawyers, architects, engineers, all professionals, resist encroachments from those who do not have equivalent expertise. A lawyer who specialized in union-management relations for many years equates physician responses in this respect to those of university faculty groups that he has observed. "Why do university teachers organize?" he asks. "The number one reason is their feeling that they are losing control over the way they teach students. They come to feel they have no voice in what happens, no say in the content of the courses they are teaching. They get the feeling they are being downgraded to employee status and losing their status as professional people. Physicians experience that same uneasiness."[13]

That line of reasoning may do much to explain the emotional intensity that has accompanied some of the AMA's battles over federal health legislation. Business, of course, has been the target of federal regulation for a far longer time, but it has not responded with the degree of anger and harshness that medicine displayed over the Wagner-Murray-Dingell bills in the 1940s and the King-Anderson bill that preceded Medicare and Medicaid in 1965. The difference is that the regulation of business usually deals with marketing practices or product standards; it does not interfere with the businessman's principal prerogative—to operate his business at a profit. That is, the regulations leave undiminished the businessman's authority to make profit-making decisions.

By contrast, physicians believe that in their case the government is going for the jugular by curbing their authority over medical decisions. Businessmen believe they are left with enough elbow room to maneuver; physicians think they are being fitted for a straitjacket. Arguable as that point may be, there is no disputing that in fervor of emotion and harshness of language—on both sides—the debates over health care issues during the Truman and Johnson Administrations reached peak levels.

Along with many societal institutions and the other professions, medicine today feels that it is under siege. Physicians feel badgered by the press. Most of them are wary of litigious patients, and suspicious of Washington. Most of them are uncomfortable, at best, with the new political buzz words—entitlement, social accountability, and consumerism. They are acutely aware of what Professor Emeritus Jacques Barzun of Columbia describes in *The Profession Under Siege* as "the animus [that] comes from the general unrest and impatience with authority in the Western world, coupled with the belief that anything long established is probably corrupt."[14] The physician may be learning how to respond better to that animus. But there is little in medical education, training, or experience—or in the traits of character thereby engendered—that makes it particularly easy.

Chapter Seven

The House of Delegates

It is Chicago. It is July, 1980. It is 2:00 p.m., Sunday. From a cloudless sky a hot sun burns down, sending the temperature to 101° F and softening the asphalt of the streets in the deserted Loop. At Wrigley Field a sweltering crowd cheers on the Cubs to what will be a 6-0 win over the San Diego Padres. The Park District reports that an estimated 400,000 people are at the city's beaches, seeking relief from the heat in the sparkling blue of Lake Michigan.

On upper Michigan Avenue, inside the new Marriott Hotel, there is gathering what is undoubtedly the only major business meeting of the day—the opening session of the annual meeting of the American Medical Association. On the seventh floor, the ballroom is suitably decorated for a group conscious of tradition. Across the south end of the room a dais extends from wall to wall, behind it, a gigantic, brightly lit American flag whose width reaches from floor to ceiling, its stars the size of hula hoops, its three-foot stripes dwarfing the figures moving about on stage. To the left and right, panels of red, white and blue set off the standards of the fifty states. Below the dais, in the well of the room, an amiable, well-dressed crowd of 1500 cheerfully mills about, waiting for the proceedings to begin.

It is mostly, but not entirely, a masculine crowd, and it is mostly, but not entirely, a middle-aged crowd. The hair tends to be silvery, a bit thin. But if you look closely you can see some long hair, a few bushy sideburns, a scattering of beards. The men are wearing suit-coats and neckties; the women are in dresses, not slacks. Occasionally, you see a face that is black, Oriental, Polynesian, or Hispanic. Virtually everyone wears glasses, and nobody is smoking. In fact, there are no ashtrays in the room.

The outward signs point to the presence of a familiar American institution: the convention. The names on the lapel tags are representative—Holden, Ortiz, MacLaggan, Chinn, Shapiro, Sweeny, Franzoni, Kochtitzky, Schreiber. The hometowns reflect the same diversity—Baltimore, Shreveport, Detroit, Patchogue, Toledo, Thief River Falls, Honolulu, New York, Memphis, Boston, Tulsa, Houston. To the badges everyone wears are attached ribbons of various colors—blue for elected officers of the AMA, brown for officers of state and county medical societies, light blue for specialty society officers, red for AMA staff members, maroon for state and county society executives, and green for the delegates who will be seated front and center in the ballroom and who will vote the decisions that, four days later, will constitute the actions of the convention.

Despite the trappings of Babbittry, it is not an average convention crowd. For one thing the income of the delegates is far higher, probably something close to the physician's average annual net income of $99,500 (1982 figure).[1] For another, the educational level is exceptional. In fact, 76 percent of the delegates are board certified in various medical specialties,[2] which implies several years of study in addition to medical school. Somewhere between a third and a half of the delegates practice in the primary care specialties: general practice, family practice, obstetrics-gynecology, pediatrics, and internal medicine. Between a quarter and a third of them are surgeons. Their average age is just over fifty-eight.

At 2:10 p.m. the Speaker of the House of Delegates, William Y. Rial, M.D., a family practitioner from Swarthmore, Pennsylvania, gavels the crowd to order. Glancing briefly at the seated, quiet audience, a minister reads from Psalm 139, reminding the physicians of a miracle they are all familiar with, "Truly you have formed my inmost being; you knit me in my mother's womb. I give you thanks that I am fearfully, wonderfully made..." Two stanzas of the Star Spangled Banner follow. After the AMA Auxiliary reports raising over $1.6 million for the AMA Education and Research Foundation (which helps support medical schools, student loans, and research), five awards are presented in recognition of scientific achievement, public service, and contributions to medicine. At 3:06 p.m., the ceremonial side of the meeting complete, the general session recesses.

Reconvened ten minutes later, the house hears from the Committee on Credentials that 274 of the 279 delegates are present, clearly constituting a quorum. With no further delay, the business of the meeting begins. The proceedings are public; a section of the floor is reserved for the press. The current AMA president, Hoyt D. Gardner,

M.D., of Louisville, Kentucky, makes a twenty-minute report, reminding physicians of the continuing need to participate in matters of public policy. "This is a time of great change," he warns, "that will largely be made either by us or against us." There are some brief remarks by the presiding officer, three other brief reports, and the adoption of the minutes of the previous meeting of the house, seven months before. Finally, the speaker takes up the 226 items of business on the agenda, consisting of the reports of the board and various AMA councils and committees and the resolutions submitted by various state associations and specialty societies and some individual delegates, and divides them for consideration among nine previously appointed reference committees. Those assignments made and other business concluded, the meeting is then recessed until Tuesday.

The intervening day, Monday, is given over to the meetings of the nine reference committees. These conduct public hearings at which proponents and opponents of various matters of business may argue their positions. Any physician member may speak, as may non-physicians and non-members so long as the chairman of the reference committee believes the speaker has something to contribute. At the end of the hearing each reference committee goes into executive session to draw up a report for the House of Delegates, stating its recommendations on the business items referred to it. Tuesday, Wednesday, and Thursday the House of Delegates is back in session to consider and act upon the reference committee reports. By combining related recommendations, clarifying language, and summarizing viewpoints, the reference committee reports reduce the agenda to manageable dimensions.

In advance of a meeting of the AMA, the delegates and those alternate delegates who attend devote considerable time to preparation. From the opening session on they can be seen carrying a gray cardboard tote bag that contains a two-inch-thick, ring-bound Delegate's Handbook. In it are copies of all the reports and resolutions that will be considered at the meeting. Altogether, the material weighs five pounds, eleven ounces. The reports are in typescript, single-spaced, with both sides of the individual sheets of paper used. Some of the material, the majority of it in fact, was distributed by mail three weeks earlier. The delegates have an opportunity not only to read the material ahead of time, but also to discuss the issues with their colleagues and the officers of their state or specialty societies. The remainder of material in the

Handbook, the late reports and resolutions, was distributed the morning of the opening session.

The typical delegate is a fairly busy person throughout the meeting. In addition to the day-long meetings of the house, there are early morning caucuses with other delegates from his state, if it happens to be a large one, or regional caucuses (New England, for example), if he represents a small one. At these, he reports on the hearings he attends and listens to other delegates report on the meetings he was unable to attend. Candidates for office appear at the caucus meetings, giving the delegates a closer look at those they will be voting for. An AMA meeting is not without its convivial side, but delegates are mindful that an appreciable amount of work and thought is expected of them.

Who are the delegates? The majority, 214 of them, are 211 men and three women elected by the state medical associations. Fifty-seven are physicians elected by specialty societies, one delegate per society. Five are delegates from the federal health services: one each from the Army, Navy, and Air Force Medical Corps, the Public Health Service, and the Veterans Administration. Finally, there is one delegate from each of three groups: medical students, resident physicians and the deans of American medical schools. The 214 delegates from the state associations (one for every 1,000 AMA members, or fraction thereof) are elected by the state houses of delegates, except in California and Oregon where the members of the state associations vote directly.

The typical delegate from a state association has come up through service in his county medical society and then his state medical association. In response to a questionnaire done by the magazine *Medical World News* in 1971, the delegates who responded said they had served a fairly lengthy apprenticeship: about five years active service in county society affairs, then about ten years in state association activities, and finally three years as an AMA alternate delegate.[3] That progression produces delegates thoroughly familiar with the workings of organized medicine but possibly older than many would consider desirable.

During the 1970s the average age of AMA delegates began to drop, from an average of 59.6 years in 1970 to 53.3 in 1978. But then the average headed upward again (58.2 in 1980), coinciding with the admission of the specialty society delegates. Figures for 1970 show a turnover rate in the house of about 15 percent of the delegates a year; at this 1980 annual meeting, 56 percent of the delegates had less than five years in office. Some state associations like to send their "comers" to the AMA, hopeful that they will go on from there to election to AMA councils, the AMA Board of Trustees, and the presidency of the AMA. Other states elect delegates whose influence within the state has begun to wane. Many states select whoever gives promise of being able to do the best job. Delegates serve a two-year term.

The position of AMA delegate requires a personal commitment of time. There are the two formal meetings of the house each year: the four-day interim meeting held in various United States cities in late November or early December, and the five-day annual meeting, usually in June in Chicago. To be effective, a delegate must study numerous papers and reports, and he must stay in close touch with what his state medical association or specialty society is doing and what its members are concerned about. At least one state, Kentucky, requires its AMA delegates to attend the county society meetings in their region of the state. In the 1971 *Medical World News* survey, most delegates estimated they spent twelve to twenty days a year on the business of being an AMA delegate. About a fifth of them said they devoted between twenty and thirty days a year to the job.[4]

Like other parliamentary bodies, the House of Delegates incorporates the classic strengths and weaknesses of the democratic process. It can find excuses to delay action. It can be persuaded into mistakes. It can use up time working itself out of them. There are casualties to parliamentary maneuvers. In voting, the delegates do favors for each other, and the favors are returned. There are coalitions of delegates, but they seem to form and dissolve on an ad hoc basis; the house is not dominated by powerful, enduring voting blocs. An estimated 10 percent of the delegates might be said to constitute a conservative wing, taking rigid, uncompromising stands on any matter that appears to impinge on medical "freedoms." At the other end of the scale is an equally strong but less visible liberal wing. In between is a majority of the delegates whose "liberalness" or "conservativeness" changes from issue to issue and from time to time.

While displaying the negatives of parliamentary government, the House of Delegates likewise exhibits its major virtue. The house is a means by which the medical profession can air an issue, debate its merits or demerits, and then articulate a consensus of sufficient power and legitimacy to gain strong attention. It is the policy-making body of the AMA.

From its founding in 1847 through the end of the nineteenth century, the AMA suffered for lack of a clear organizational structure. Only after a new constitution and new bylaws redefined the House of Delegates in 1901 was the AMA able to grow into a strong, effective organization.

Before then, business was conducted with an informality that increasingly aroused objections. The AMA was a representative organization—as it is today—but the linkage between many of the delegates and the constituencies they supposedly represented was too flimsy. In addition to the state medical associations and county medical societies, all sorts of regional, auxiliary, and affiliated medical societies claimed delegates. And there were delegates both from individual medical schools and from staffs of individual hospitals and clinics. Toward the end of the century, as the profession grew in size, it became more and more difficult to verify a delegate's credentials and be sure of the number of AMA members in the organization he claimed to represent. Each AMA annual meeting drew a disproportionate number of delegates from the particular region of the country where the meeting was being held. Often, when it came time to settle an issue, there were either too many delegates (all wishing to speak) to make a decision possible or too few to make a decision that was representative.[5]

An 1887 criticism is illuminating. "Perhaps no other part of the practical working of the association," noted *JAMA*, "has occasioned so much adverse criticism as the hasty and imperfect method of selecting, after the commencement of each annual meeting, the Committee on Nominations by such a little group of delegates from each state and territory as could be gathered in some corner of the room in the brief recess of fifteen minutes, and on whom devolved the paramount duty of nominating all the general officers of the association, of seven members of the Judicial Council, three members of the Board of Trustees, and the selection of the next place of the annual meeting."[6]

To replace such offhand actions, the AMA adopted a revised constitution and new bylaws at its 1901 annual meeting. The key element in this reform was the creation of a House of Delegates consisting (basically) of delegates from the state or territorial medical societies, at the time one delegate for every 500 members (or fraction thereof) in each society. Provision was made also for delegates from each of the thirteen scientific sections* then extant. What was created was a formally structured legislative and executive body empowered to elect the officers of the AMA, oversee its business affairs, and develop its policies.

The committee that developed the plans for the restructured AMA pointed out at the time that the AMA would now be "a confederation of the state societies of the country, which in turn must be a confederation of the local societies of the state." The AMA had transformed itself from an amorphous, town-meeting sort of organization into a different entity. It now became an organization in which the state and territorial medical societies were federated.

Improvements quickly became apparent. Membership, for example, spurted sharply ahead, from 11,121 in 1901 (slightly under 10 percent of the profession at that time) to almost six times that a decade later (about 50 percent of the profession). No longer burdened by an unwieldy policy-making apparatus, the AMA could deal better with controversial matters. "Under the old order," *JAMA* observed in 1902, "all subjects which were likely to develop an interminable debate were laid on the table...Vexed questions, such as that pertaining to the Code of Ethics, etc., which were liable to develop acrimonious discussion, were not allowed to come before the large meeting..."[7]

The AMA's effectiveness as an organization dates from the 1902 annual meeting at Saratoga Springs. Here, for the first time, a House of Delegates chosen by well-defined rules was seated, giving a new legitimacy to the decisions of organized medicine. Since then there have been changes in the composition of the house, making it more representative. But its basic form has not changed, and the process by which it conducts its business is fundamentally the same.

During the first decades after World War II, very few changes were made in the House of Delegates. One of them took place in 1946 when, to handle the growing number of reports and resolutions and to deal with increasingly complex issues, the house went from one to two sessions a year, one an annual meeting in June or July, the other a supplemental session in November or December. This was called the "clinical meeting" from 1946 through 1976, the "interim meeting" after that. Another change had to do with medical students. Following the founding of the Student American Medical

*described later in this chapter

Association in 1950,* the house provided for two ex-officio student delegates who were given the privilege of the floor. They could be recognized and speak, but had no vote and no authority to introduce resolutions. The representational base of the house stayed the same.

With the social upheaval of the late 1960s, however, came a general demand for wider participation in institutions. The pressures began to build—both without and within organized medicine—for the inclusion of students and residents in the policy-making process of the AMA. The two ex-officio delegates from the Student American Medical Association grew more active at this time, speaking up with greater frequency at the reference committee hearings, for instance, and getting their resolutions introduced through sympathetic state delegations. Marvin Rowlands, who was then the editor of *AMNews* and kept close but semi-official liaison with the students, recalls, "These guys were smart. They wanted in and they knew where to go to find allies. They knew the right people in the house to talk to, how to swing key people over to their side. And they were persistent." Terrence S. Carden, M.D., a former editor of the Student American Medical Association journal, *The New Physician*, dates the medical student drive for added recognition from 1968. "A group of students elected to office in SAMA about that time became interested in what you could call the left-wing health care issues—medical care delivery in Appalachia, for instance, the over-emphasis on tertiary care specialty training, medicine's failure to meet the needs of the public. They came forward and challenged a lot of conventional thought about health care delivery and, more important, about medical education."[8]

At the fall meeting of the AMA in 1969, President Gerald D. Dorman, M.D., the memory of a protestors' invasion of the AMA meeting that spring still in mind, told the opening session, "Although we don't like the criticism of us by some of the younger members and would-be members of our profession—and perhaps we don't approve of the leftward lean of some of their politics—these young professionals are nonetheless as much, or more, patient-

*Started by the AMA in 1950, the Student American Medical Association became independent in 1954 and moved its headquarters out of the AMA building. It became self-sufficient financially through dues and the revenues of its own journal, *The New Physician*. It did, however, accept grants from the AMA, mostly for specific programs. In 1975, to emphasize its independent status further, it changed its name to the American Medical Student Association.

oriented than some of us." The AMA must, he said, find ways to attract students and residents into becoming members.[9] As an example of what could be done, he cited the action of the Colorado Medical Society in giving students representation in its house of delegates on the same basis that physicians were represented, one delegate per twenty-five members. Reacting to a resolution introduced by the California Medical Association three days later, the house adopted this resolution:

> Whereas, Fragmentation of the medical profession will weaken the Association and will ultimately lead to a decrease in the effectiveness of its leaders; therefore be it
> RESOLVED, That the American Medical Association continue its study of trends of membership in the Association; and be it further
> RESOLVED, That these studies include the involvement of students, interns and residents in the ranks of organized medicine; and be it further
> RESOLVED, That the Board of Trustees direct a task force to develop a realistic program to correct any cause which may result in a loss of potential physician members and carry forward an active recruitment effort.[10]

Without specifically saying so, what the resolution did was suggest to the Board of Trustees that it develop a procedure by which students and interns/residents could become AMA members.

Two obstacles stood in the way. First was the problem of county-state membership. Until 1981 regular physician members usually had to be county-state members before becoming eligible for AMA membership. Should student and resident members be exempted from the requirement? At the time few county and state societies provided for student or intern/resident memberships, and the AMA had no power to force their doors to open quickly. Obstacle two consisted of the presence of already existing organizations, the Student American Medical Association in the case of the students, the Committee on Interns and Residents and the Physicians National Housestaff Association in the case of interns/residents. As things were then organized, there was strong likelihood that a future student delegate might, in effect, be a delegate from the student association, and a future intern/resident delegate might, in effect, be a delegate from either of the two housestaff associations.

"We did not want to look solely to those organizations for participation," says Theodore R. Chilcoat, Jr., then the chief AMA staffer concerned with relationships with the students and residents. "The Board of Trustees, all of us, were more interested in getting student and intern/resident involvement through the whole federation structure, from the county level on up. We wanted people participating in the AMA rather than people participating in the AMA through outside organizations."[11]

Despite the tense adversary positions taken in many of the meetings that ensued, agreement did evolve. At the June meeting in 1971 special provision was made for resident membership and for a delegate with full voting privileges. Similar action for students followed at the 1972 annual meeting. Where county and state societies provided for student and intern/resident membership, they could join through the federation. Where provision for local membership did not exist, they could join the AMA directly. Dues for students were set at $15 per year. Resident dues were originally set at $20 per year, later raised to $35 and then $45. In addition to delegates, both groups soon gained positions, in many cases voting positions, on important AMA councils and committees. As a result, student and resident membership in the AMA skyrocketed, with more than 24,000 students and more than 21,000 residents joining the AMA as dues-paying members in 1982.

What is more important is the degree of participation. Both the students and residents have elected persons to AMA offices who have won the respect of the older physicians. They have become a powerful new voice in the policy-making process of the AMA. In AMA policies regarding health manpower and medical education, they have been especially influential.

Carden looks back on the experience as a healthy one. "There was always a struggle," he recalls, "between those who thought the AMA was too hidebound to change and those who thought that the AMA was truly representative and thus could be changed. It is interesting that some of the people who were most doubtful that anything could be accomplished have been working with the AMA."

So successful has the integration of students and residents been that at the June 1983 meeting the house adopted a board recommendation to add a voting resident member and a non-voting student member to the board.

Five years after swinging its doors open to students and residents, the AMA made another momentous change in its structure. After authorizing a delegate to represent the medical schools in 1976, the

AMA significantly expanded its constituent base in 1977 by seating some fifty new and additional delegates representing the major medical specialty societies. This was formal and direct recognition that American medicine had become organized along medical specialty lines as well as along the lines of the geographically defined medical societies.

Radical as the change was, it was not as abrupt as one might assume, for the AMA had acknowledged the growing specialization of the profession in many ways and had gradually increased the opportunity for input from the specialty societies through several actions. Rather than a sudden turn in policy, the provision of delegates from the specialty societies in the house was the culminating step of an evolutionary process.[12]

At the time the AMA was founded, one of its first goals was the upgrading of the quality of American medicine through the upgrading of the physician's knowledge. From the start, the AMA functioned as a vehicle by which new scientific information could be reported, discussed, challenged, validated. Within a few years of its formation, the AMA became the clearinghouse for new medical knowledge. But as early as 1859 it was evident that not all physicians were interested in all aspects of medicine. As a consequence, the AMA divided its membership into "scientific sections." Originally, there were six: anatomy and physiology, chemistry and *materia medica*; practical medicine and obstetrics; surgery; meteorology, medical topography and epidemic diseases; and medical jurisprudence and hygiene. Physician members of the AMA became members of a section at the time of the annual meeting when they would register and declare which of the sections they would join, the choice presumably reflecting their primary areas of interest and practice.* At the meeting, they would attend the educational sessions arranged by that section, and the business session of the section. At the business session they cast their votes for the section officers (whose main job was to develop the scientific program for next year's meeting) and delegate. When the House of Delegates was reorganized in 1901, provision was made for delegates from the state medical associations *and* two from each of the scientific sections.** Since there were thirteen of these, instead of the original

---

*This was accomplished in more recent times through the *American Medical Directory*. On a questionnaire, each physician was asked to list his or her primary specialty. The answer determined the section he or she belonged to.

**One delegate per section after 1903.

six, the first meeting of the new house included twenty-six section delegates.

From the standpoint of organization, the scientific sections left a great deal to be desired. They were autonomous. They were defined in only the most general of terms. How do you deal with an entity which is, in actuality, a "section" of your membership? In 1914 the House of Delegates created a Council on Scientific Assembly to oversee and coordinate the work of the separate sections. By and large they performed their principal function reasonably well during the early decades of this century and even into the 1960s. Physicians attending the AMA annual and clinical meetings—a high of 24,268 registered for the educational-scientific sessions at the 1965 annual meeting—would hear papers on the latest medical developments and listen to reports of new techniques, new modes of treatment. The sections—twenty-eight of them at the end—were well established elements within the AMA. Through their scientific sessions, they were providing an important forum where research-oriented physicians could report their findings to practice-oriented physicians. Partly through the activities of the section organization, the AMA had grown into a major force in the continuing education of physicians. But two problems had begun to appear.

The first arose from the acceleration in the rate at which American medicine was becoming specialized. Simultaneously—and consequently—the medical specialty societies were growing in numbers, in size of membership, in finances, and in professional loyalty. They were developing more scientific meetings of their own, and they were starting to take the play away from the educational sessions developed by the AMA scientific sections. William R. Barclay, M.D., editor of *JAMA* from 1975 to 1982, points to the growing breadth of medical technology as the underlying cause for the shift. To handle the sheer volume of new knowledge, physicians were finding it increasingly necessary to divide it into segments, that is, specialties, and to develop their own expertise around one of them. "If a physician wanted to make a report on his work in hematology," Barclay says, "and if he decided to give it before a general audience of physicians, he might find only a handful of physicians who would know what he was talking about. On the other hand, if he gave his paper before a hematological society, he would have a smaller total audience, but one with far, far more people who would know just exactly what he was saying."[13] For a long time medicine had not been specialized to that extent, but now it was.

The second problem stemmed from the odd organizational status of the scientific sections. On policy matters they were not responsible to the AMA Board of Trustees; they were not a part of the House of Delegates. Questions arose about the validity of their leadership. That was decided at the AMA annual meeting simply by the section members who happened to attend the business meeting of the section. And the number of section members at the business meetings could be small, well under a hundred physicians in many cases, as few as a dozen in one documented instance.[14]

Not unnaturally, the matter of proportional representation arose. Delegates from the states were now authorized on the basis of one delegate for each 1,000 AMA members or fraction thereof in the state association. Why should a section delegate, possibly elected by only a handful of section members, have an equal voice and vote? At one time, in 1942, it was proposed (though not adopted) that section delegates be reduced to ex-officio, non-voting status. Dependent on an ill-defined organizational base, the sections were finding that what underpinnings they did have were being eroded by the swelling of power of the specialty societies.

This did not, however, prevent the sections from proceeding in their old, independent way. And this behavior continued to irk the more formally defined elements in the AMA hierarchy, the House of Delegates and the Board of Trustees, whose members bridled at occasional acts of *lese majeste* committed by the section officers. Jurisdictional rows broke out over who should nominate the AMA representatives to the specialty boards, the bodies that set the standards for certification in a specialty. Disputes arose over the issuance of offical opinions, the sections insisting on their autonomy, the house and board asserting their authority over policy-making and policy pronouncements. Tempers frayed over the handling of non-scientific business. The house and board thought the sections should stick to science; the sections did not consider themselves limited to just the narrow, scientific concerns of their specialty areas. In 1956 the house felt constrained to state, with some asperity, that the scientific sections were to "provide a forum for discussion of the scientific aspects of medical practice. All other aspects— sociological, political and economic—are within the purview of the House of Delegates." That should have settled the matter, and it did. But only for a while.

In 1961 the House of Delegates began to address the problems raised by the sections with a new sense of urgency. A virtual continuum of studies and reviews erupted. The Appel report was followed by the Wheeler report, which was succeeded by the Gundersen report to be followed by the Quinn report and then, after only the briefest pause, by several major studies by the Council on Long Range Planning and Development. At first, attention focused on the jurisdictional disputes between the sections and the board and the sections' loss of scientific stature to the specialty societies. But in time the issue changed, and the reports began to zero in on a broader issue: how the AMA could adapt structurally to the increasingly specialized character of the medical profession.

From 1961 to 1969, the house wrangled over several ways to change the scientific sections. Finally, a plan developed under a committee headed by William F. Quinn, M.D., a delegate from California, attracted enough support to win adoption. What it suggested was the creation of a new leadership for each section, a new council of six to ten physicians to take charge. These leaders would not be elected at the annual business sessions of the sections, nor would they be appointed by the Board of Trustees as had once been suggested. Instead, they were to be named by the appropriate specialty societies—except for one council member, who would be elected by the section members at the business session. As for the section delegate to the House of Delegates, he or she would be chosen by the six to ten members of the section council. The councils would also nominate representatives to the specialty certifying boards and transmit their choices to the Board of Trustees.

The effect of the Quinn report and the creation of the new section councils was to transfer the traditional powers of the AMA scientific sections to the medical specialty societies. "There is an acknowledged need to support these national specialty societies," the Quinn report stated, "and to stimulate their interest and allegiance to medicine as a strong, unified profession under the 'umbrella' of the AMA." The House of Delegates evidently agreed, and it adopted the report at the 1969 meeting.

This new arrangement removed many of the old sources of confusion and irritation. The new section councils gave the specialty societies a greatly increased measure of participation in the AMA, and it gave them easier access to the House of Delegates. But they were still one step removed from direct representation. The specialty societies did not appoint their delegates; they appointed the people who did the appointing.

In some instances, the new section councils worked well; in others, the mechanism proved to be cumbersome. Especially in the sections where a multiplicity of specialty organizations existed—internal medicine, for example, where there are at least two major societies, the American College of Physicians and the American Society of Internal Medicine—the old questions arose again. Whom does the delegate represent? To what constituency is he responsible? Is he just talking for himself? The section councils were not really giving the specialty societies what they most wanted: representation in the House of Delegates *as organizations*.

With encouragement from many quarters, including the AMA's newly appointed executive vice president, James H. Sammons, M.D., the Council on Long Range Planning and Development tackled the problem again in 1975. At the interim meeting in Honolulu late that year, the council submitted a bold, new concept of the AMA organization. The plan stressed organizational rather than individual membership, envisioning an "organization of organizations" concept. This provided that various medical organizations would be the basic AMA members, with the individuals belonging to these societies becoming individual AMA members. The state medical associations would be members, as would the specialty societies and the Association of American Medical Colleges. The house gave the concept a chilly reception and sent it back to the Council on Long Range Planning and Development for further consideration. But one positive result stemmed from the proposal. Just a year later, at the 1976 fall meeting, a section for medical school deans was established, much in the manner in which the students and residents were structured into the AMA, with provisions for a voting delegate in the house.

By the beginning of 1977, the specialty society issue had become far more urgent, especially in the minds of the AMA leadership. If the AMA was going to be the "umbrella" organization of American medicine, a place would quickly have to be found underneath it for the specialty societies. In March 1977 the Board of Trustees and the Council on Long Range Planning and Development convened a meeting at a hotel near O'Hare airport in Chicago, with the presidents and the executive directors of the major specialty societies, approximately fifty of them. What came out of that meeting was reported to the House of Delegates at the annual meeting in June. "The overall message," read the report of the Council on Long Range

Planning and Development, "was that organized medicine as a whole must begin to operate with a greater sense of unity. The pluralism that grew out of the trend toward specialization has tended to result in factionalism, and organized medicine owes it to its collective physician constituency to pull together to help ease the pressures facing the profession. It is critical, therefore, that the AMA and the specialty societies establish a more formal mechanism for interaction."[15]

When the report of the Council on Long Range Planning and Development reached the floor of the House of Delegates, Trustee Jere W. Annis, M.D., put the proposition more bluntly. "Do you want the specialty societies to organize themselves inside the AMA or outside the AMA?" he asked.[16] When the vote was taken, the house approved direct specialty society representation as a concept. Later, at the December meeting, the delegates made the decision final. Trustee Joseph F. Boyle, M.D., argued the positive side of the case. "No other organization," he said to the house, "is as capable of providing strength and leadership as the AMA. The specialty societies do want to become active participants. You have a real chance—that may be fading—to accomplish the long-term objective of a strong federation of American medicine in this house."[17] Within an hour, the house adopted a plan that did away with the section delegates and gave each of approximately fifty specialty societies a delegate.*

It was a change of major dimensions. Looked at one way, the AMA dramatically extended its power base from the traditional geographic foundation of county and state medical societies to include the base of the scientifically oriented organizations. Looked at another way, the AMA gave direct representation to a segment of medicine that hitherto had no direct, formally recognized status in the nation's principal medical establishment. By expanding its House of Delegates to include first the students and residents and then the representatives of the specialty societies and medical schools, the AMA transformed itself into a far broader federation and strengthened its position at the center of American medicine.

*Dissatisfied with representation by only one delegate, the 48,000 member American College of Surgeons did not send a delegate to the meeting of the house in December 1979 and continued that policy for at least the next four years.

Chapter Eight

Moving Through the Chairs

Among the peculiarly American phenomena that caught the interest of that shrewd nineteenth century observer, Alexis de Tocqueville, was the way Americans would invariably turn to voluntarily organized efforts as a mechanism to solve whatever problems they felt needed solving.

"Americans of all ages, all conditions and all dispositions," he wrote in his perceptive study, *Democracy in America*, "constantly form associations. They not only have commercial manufacturing companies, in which all take part, but associations of a thousand other kinds—religious, moral, serious, futile, general or restricted, enormous or diminutive. The Americans make associations to give entertainments, to found seminaries, to build inns, to construct churches, to diffuse books, to send missionaries to the antipodes..."[1]

Unlike Sinclair Lewis a century later, who focused on the parochialism of such organizations, de Tocqueville thought them essential to the functioning of a truly democratic society. Particularly in a new nation lacking the traditions of a monarchy, an aristocracy, or a strong central government, de Tocqueville maintained that associations played a leadership role that would have otherwise gone unfilled. "Whenever at the head of some new undertaking," he wrote, "you see the government in France or a man of rank in England, in the United States you will be sure to see an association." Elaborating on his point, de Tocqueville described how quickly they could acquire power. "As soon as several of the inhabitants of the United States have taken up an opinion or a feeling which they wish to promote in the world, they look for mutual assistance; and as soon as they have found each other out, they combine. From that moment they are no longer isolated men, but a power seen from afar, whose actions serve as an example, and whose language is listened to."[2]

De Tocqueville's analysis is applicable to American medical societies. Many, including several state medical associations, were already in existence at the time of de Tocqueville's visit in 1831. The AMA was founded just sixteen years later. In the way they were formed, in their enduring zeal to elevate the standards of medical education and care, in their drive for laws to protect the public health, and in their perception of themselves as having a rightful say in determining national health policies, American medical societies exemplify what the observant de Tocqueville noted.

Intent on broader perspectives, de Tocqueville says little about what was—and is—the main thing needed to keep an association going: interested people. If an organization has a long-term objective, then, *ipso facto*, it must develop a long-term viability, a continuity. And to achieve that, several requirements must be met. First, there has to be a continuation of the original goal, or need, for the association. Second, the desire to accomplish the original purpose must remain sufficiently intense to assure continuing membership and financial support. Third, there should be some sort of reward for the backers, signs of progress toward the stated objectives, or some material benefits and services, or all three. Fourth, the bonds of involvement must be kept strong, through publications, conventions, committee activities, visits by the national leaders. And finally, there must be an adequate number of able people willing to participate in the affairs of the association in a more than perfunctory way. There must be people—a large and dependable core of people—willing to volunteer that most valuable gift of all: large amounts of their own time.

This is difficult under any circumstances. In medicine, it would be logical to expect special problems. Because they work a longer week than most people (57.1 hours vs. 35.3),[3] physicians have less time to volunteer than the average person. Physicians are presumed to be deeply involved with their professional work and thus less inclined than others to pursue avocations. Furthermore, a sizeable minority of physicians ostensibly scorns politics of any sort, including those of their own professional societies. There is a part of the physician psyche that says politics is scut work; that is, work that does not require medical training to perform and, therefore, somehow, work that is to be left to others.

But despite such assumptions physicians participate in their professional society activities as intensely, or more intensely, than other professionals participate in theirs. One reason is the nature of medical practice itself. Because so many doctors practice singly or in small groups, they lack the buffers—those of a corporation, for example, or of a union—that usually intervene between an individual and the major forces that can affect his livelihood. For the strength that comes from numbers, physicians turn to their professional associations, and at the same time often demonstrate a willingness to give their medical organizations a generous amount of time. There is an isolation to the practice of medicine; the medical societies help compensate for it.

Consider also that medicine, though not the most recondite branch of science, is still quite special. A physician's training and experience condition him to rely heavily on peer judgments in evaluating new medicines, technology, and methods of treatment. Often these judgments grow out of the deliberations of a committee appointed by a medical society, the results reaching a practitioner through a medical society meeting or a medical society journal. Thus, the science of medicine draws a physician into involvement with his professional societies.

Finally, there is the stimulus arising out of the changed relationship between government and medicine. Before 1940, government played a minor role, comparatively speaking, in the formation of medical policies. But where once it was a shadow on the wall, government today has grown into an inescapable presence. Physicians have reacted variously, a few with approval, a few with fear, the large majority with concern. And as they have watched more and more medical decisions being made in the political arena, more and more of them have decided that they themselves must become more active in the political process. Accordingly, they have turned to their medical societies as the best way to do so.

The work of a voluntary association is not for everyone. It requires patience to endure a certain amount of drudgery; it requires poise to take a certain amount of flak. Specific skills are needed: the ability to argue a point convincingly; a good organizational sense; a talent for parliamentary tactics; knowing how to run a meeting; and, above all, an understanding of the political process. And it takes time, especially at night and on weekends. Young physicians, struggling to get a practice started and involved in raising a family, find it especially difficult to participate.

But like people in other walks of life, physicians develop the ability to get things done within the context of the voluntary association. And many of them, especially those who become adept at it, develop an appetite for the work. Those so inclined, particularly the more competitive among them, often win a succession of elective offices, finding themselves rising steadily into positions of wider and wider responsibility. To describe that phenomenon, medicine has borrowed a term from the Masons: "moving through the chairs." In some quarters it has been common to downgrade such physicians as "politicians." After all, runs one argument, why should those without exceptional scientific or academic achievements be qualified for positions of medical leadership? But organizationally-oriented people are necessary. Without them, without their interest and energy, an association withers, loses effectiveness, and dies.

Many physicians delve into the business of organized medicine with enduring gusto and a variety of motives. A perfectly typical example is hard to find. But to suggest the level of energy and the base of motivation that is sometimes evident, it is instructive to retrace the path of a recent AMA president through the chairs.

Robert B. Hunter, M.D., the 1981 president, began both his civilian professional medical career and his organizational medical career in 1946 in the small town of Sedro Woolley, Washington (population: 3,705), some sixty miles north of Seattle. Hunter grew up there, his father a physician, his mother a school teacher. In 1939 he graduated at age nineteen from the University of Washington and then traveled east to his father's medical alma mater, the University of Pennsylvania. In 1945, at age twenty-five, he found himself a battalion surgeon in the United States Army on a shell-torn island in the Carolines. He recalls:

When we came home, that is to say, myself and my contemporaries who had gone directly from medical training into World War II military service, we found that the county medical societies had been kept in business by physicians who had stayed home from the war and had worked themselves into advanced stages of fatigue. As we began to practice, we found ourselves very welcome to participate in hospital staff affairs and county medical society affairs.

My own father, who practiced in Sedro Woolley throughout the war, was glad to have me back both for personal and professional reasons. It was a touching moment for both of us when he took me to my first meeting of the Skagit County Medical Society and introduced me. I would guess that there were about 55,000 people in the county then, with maybe forty-five physicians.

Those of us back from military service were promptly elected to various county society offices. I was the president of Skagit County Medical Society in 1951. Then after we had gone through the chairs at the county level, the natural momentum involved swept us on to the activities of the Washington State Medical Association, where we repeated the process. We served on various committees. We became county delegates to the state association house of delegates. Some of us went on the state board of trustees. In my case, I was elected president of the state association in 1962. When that term was over, in 1964, I was elected a delegate to the AMA.[4]

In analyzing his motives for such active participation in organized medicine, Hunter frankly acknowledges the personal satisfactions. He also stresses a sense of obligation to the profession as a source of motivation in his case. He says:

Power and prestige are involved, of course. Some of the perks, especially the travel, have their appeal. But probably the greatest pleasure I have gotten out of it is the friendships formed. Some of the finest and some of the smartest people I have known in my life I have encountered on the same track I've been on—the leadership track in organized medicine. When you're from a small town, as I am, you don't always find such opportunities at home.

Organized medicine has really been my avocation. I have concentrated on it just as other physicians I know have concentrated on golf or fishing or stamp collecting.

But a lot more than ego is involved. Like my father, I have wanted above all to be a good physician. But I have also wanted to do some things on behalf of the profession and some things that I would consider to be on behalf of the people as a whole. I've always felt a genuine desire to perform a community service to contribute somehow to society. I also feel obligations to the profession. Just as teachers value their academic freedom, doctors value the integrity of their profession. Many physicians, myself included, plunge into medical society activities as a way to preserve that.

In 1970, during his third two-year term as a delegate to the AMA, Hunter started his move through the chairs at the national level of medicine by running for the AMA Board of Trustees. He points out:

This is not the sort of decision you make all by yourself. It involves the other delegates from your own state, because they have to play an active role in your campaign.

It also takes commitment. In my instance, the first experience was traumatic, because I got beat. I decided to run again the next year. By virtue of a lot of button-holing, talking to people, having other people work on my behalf, I was elected. Then I had to turn right around and run again the next year because I'd only been elected to the unexpired part of a term. Then I had to run again three years after that.

By the time he decided to run for president-elect of the AMA in 1979, Hunter had earned such respect that he ran unopposed, a rare, though not unprecedented, set of circumstances.

As such things go, the AMA does its campaigning for internal political office with restraint. Nominating speeches are permitted only for those seeking a general officer's position (usually only seven vacancies a year), and those speeches in the House of Delegates are now limited to two minutes. No seconding speeches are permitted. State delegations backing candidates run hospitality suites, open at lunch time and after adjournment of the house in the late afternoon. The most visible sign that some campaigning is going on: tiny, fabric emblems distributed by those running the hospitality suites and, as time goes on, gathering in clusters on the delegates' lapel badges: a crab for Maryland, a mule for Missouri, a bee for Utah, a cactus for Arizona, an ear of corn for Iowa, a baked potato topped with a melting pat of butter for Idaho, and so forth. Wearing the small emblems may indicate political inclinations. But more often they identify only the hospitality suite where the delegate stopped off during the preceding evening.

At times, a state association pushing hard for a candidate will stage an elaborate reception or luncheon for the candidate. Over the years these have generated mixed results. In one case, a leading candidate for president lost out, presumably because the delegates thought his campaign efforts were too lavish. At the 1980 annual meeting, the speaker, William Y. Rial, M.D., asked for a review of the election process, reflecting concern that campaigning took too much of the delegates' time and cost too much money.

In response, a report from the Council on Long Range Planning and Development recommended that expenditures be limited ($18,000 was a figure cited in the report as being unconscionably high), that electioneering at the interim meetings be sharply curtailed, and that the elections (held during the annual meetings) be moved up two days to get them out of the way earlier. The report met with general approval, though the elections were advanced by only one day.

The experience of running for AMA office strikes candidates differently. Hugh H. Hussey, M.D., elected to the board first in 1956, recalled his candidacy as being rather innocent.

> Some of the friends I had made in the house urged me to run. They thought I had been a good spokesman, that over the years I had made a good impression at the reference committee hearings, that I had a chance. I felt a little lost in the effort of running. But there had been some omens. Earlier in the week, the New England states had invited me up to their hospitality suite for a buffet lunch. At the time I did not recognize what these invitations meant. But of course it turned out that they meant a lot.[5]

Donald E. Wood, M.D., an unsuccessful candidate for president-elect in 1964, a successful candidate for trustee in 1971 and then an unsuccessful one in 1974, equates his experience to the tough, horse-trading world of real politics. "As I made my rounds of the hospitality suites and the caucuses," he remembers, "I recognized that at least the major states—California, New York, Illinois, Texas—all had their own axes to grind, their own candidates to get elected. It was just as it is at the national Republican or Democratic convention. You back my candidate. I'll support yours."[6]

Hunter downplays the role of coalition politics in the AMA House of Delegates. In his opinion, the coalitions that exist, exist to evaluate candidates rather than to back them. "The caucuses," he says, "the Rocky Mountain states, the New England states, the North-Central states, make the elective process more efficient. They round up small delegations so that you can talk with them all at once. This means that if you are running for office, you don't have to get up at 5:30 in the morning to talk to just one state."

If moving through the chairs of organized medicine is likened to the ascent of a pyramid, the apex consists of the seventeen places ranked around the horseshoe-shaped table in the boardroom on the third floor of the AMA headquarters in Chicago. There is a chair for each of the twelve trustees, elected by the House of Delegates to staggered, three-year terms.* There is a chair for the AMA

---

*From 1923 to 1962 the term was for five years, with a limit of two consecutive terms.

president-elect, the president, and the immediate past president. (Once elected by the House of Delegates, the same individual serves one year in each office). Those fifteen general officers of the AMA constitute the Board of Trustees, although two additional general officers, the speaker and the vice speaker, sit regularly with the board. They enter into the discussions, they participate fully, but they do not vote.

Among the general officers—to take 1980-81 as an example—there is a strong and predictable weighting in favor of the active physician engaged in patient care and office-based practice. It is also clear that they reached their positions after considerable elective experience at the state and county medical association level. There was only one man who had *not* been president of either a state or county society. Five of the general officers had been both. All but two had served in the House of Delegates.

Beyond that, it is difficult to make generalizations, except to observe that it was a diverse group. No two were from the same state: seven lived in the Midwest, three in the West, three each in the South and East. One, who was part Polynesian, lived in Hawaii. Ten of them graduated from medical schools in the Midwest, seven from Big Ten university medical schools. Five received their medical education in the East, two from Ivy League universities. Two went to medical school in the South. Most of the officers were in their fifties; the oldest was sixty-five, the youngest forty-eight. All but one was board-certified in a specialty; all but three had clinical teaching appointments; one was a member of the Institute of Medicine of the National Academy of Sciences, a well regarded honor. Nine of them were surgeons; four were family practitioners; four were internists. Two of them could be classified as small-town general physicians, though both were board-certified family practitioners. A third practiced surgery in a small town. The rest of the general officers practiced in or near big cities—Philadelphia, New York, Atlanta, Chicago, Dallas, St. Louis, Los Angeles, Phoenix—or medium-sized cities—Norfolk, Louisville, Salt Lake City, Hammond, Honolulu, Dayton. Most were in solo practice or in small partnerships. But at least two were in group practice, and one was salaried. One had a degree in engineering as well as medicine. One was a state senator (Republican). One was an unsuccessful, former candidate for the United States House of Representatives (Democratic, Midwestern state).

The wide power that the board exercises is something that evolved gradually. For the first thirty-five years of the AMA there was, in fact, no board at all, nothing that might even be called a forerunner. In 1880, however, as the desirability of an AMA medical journal grew, that began to change. Up to this time, the scientific papers presented at the annual meetings were brought together and published annually as the *Transactions*. To speed this process and expand the AMA's role as a disseminator of medical information, AMA leaders urged the founding of a periodical.[7] A Committee on Publications was charged with exploring the feasibility and, after a short study, proposed a weekly journal to be called *The Journal of the American Medical Association*. The delegates adopted the proposal in 1882.

Part of that recommendation established a nine-person Board of Trustees, the members to serve staggered, three-year terms.[8] So closely was the Board of Trustees then identified with the finances and business affairs of the new journal that it was usually referred to, even in offical documents, as "the Board of Trustees for Journalizing the *Transactions*" or "the Board of Trustees for Publishing *The Journal of the American Medical Association*." When the delegates adopted a new AMA reorganization plan in 1887, the Board of Trustees' broader fiscal responsibilities were emphasized,[9] though references to the board as "the Board of Trustees of the Journal" can be found as late as 1891.

With the chartering of the AMA under the statutes of Illinois in 1897,* the Board of Trustees had its powers even more clearly defined. The Illinois Not-for-Profit Corporation Act specifies that "the affairs of a corporation shall be managed by a board of directors," that body being defined as "the group of persons vested with the management of the affairs of the corporation irrespective of the name by which such group is designated." The restructuring of the AMA in 1901 confirmed those managerial responsibilities of the board. As the AMA grew and as new needs arose, the house widened the scope of authority delegated to the board: the power to

---

*A vote of the membership conducted by mailed ballot established Chicago as the AMA's headquarters in 1896. By that time, the city was already something of an operational base because it was the location for *JAMA*. That, in turn, had been determined by the fact that *JAMA*'s first editor, Nathan S. Davis, M.D., was a resident of Chicago. Thus, many members may have concluded that Chicago, with its central location, was already the AMA's hometown.

form an executive committee for the purpose of keeping in closer touch with all work at the headquarters office, its liaison function with other organizations, its role in the articulation of policy and in supervising public relations.

For almost thirty years after 1882 the nine-member composition of the board remained unchanged. Then in 1909 the house adopted a suggestion that the president and president-elect be invited to attend the board meetings. In 1923 those two officers, plus the speaker, became ex-officio members of the board, though still without the right to vote. Finally in 1951, the president and president-elect were made fully privileged members of the board. The speaker continued in his ex-officio, non-voting status, the vice speaker joining him more and more frequently at the board meetings. In 1956 the vice speaker and vice president were given ex-officio, non-voting status. In 1963 the number of trustees was raised from nine to twelve, and the immediate past president joined the president-elect and president as a voting board member. Four years after being given voting privileges, the vice presidency was abolished in 1976, creating the present seventeen-member composition: twelve trustees (voting); the president, president-elect and immediate past president (voting); the speaker and vice speaker (ex-officio, non-voting). Over the years a number of resolutions have been introduced to provide that the trustees represent defined geographical areas, but they have all been rejected.

Immediately after the House of Delegates adjourns to end the AMA's annual meeting in June, the Board of Trustees—including those just elected—assembles for an organization meeting. To serve throughout the year ahead, the members elect a chairman (who customarily is elected to two one-year terms), a vice chairman, and a secretary-treasurer. Those three officers plus the president, president-elect, and two trustees elected at the time become the executive committee of the board. The board meets five times a year, sometimes six, each session usually extending over three days. The executive vice president and other senior staff executives attend and are frequently invited to take part in the discussions. Other staff members attend as well, usually to supply information.

About every two years, the board schedules a special meeting not to conduct routine business but to think over some of the broader issues—societal trends, the problems of cost, continuing physician education. Quite frequently, outside experts are brought in to give presentations.

At its meetings, the board makes its decisions by taking a vote, the business being conducted according to the rules in the *Standard Code of Parliamentary Procedure* by Sturgis. Although matters of almost every sort come before the board, probably the most frequently considered areas of concern have to do with corporate planning, finances, legislative positions, medical education, and responses to federal regulatory action.

To attend an AMA board meeting is to be impressed with the amount of work required of a trustee. For starters, there are twenty-three to twenty-six days a year taken up by the two meetings of the house and the regularly scheduled meetings of the board. Then there is the work of several intra-board committees such as finance, nominations, candidate selection, and awards. Trustees also receive a generous amount of homework; the agenda books, distributed ahead of each board meeting, sometimes run to three, inch-thick, volumes. On top of that, there are special assignments: serving on a task force to handle an issue like peer review organizations, for example; or representing the AMA on a Department of Health and Human Services advisory committee; continuing a liaison with other medical organizations; filling in a speaking engagement; representing the board at a state, specialty, or county medical society meeting. An informal study done in the 1970s indicated that a trustee could expect to spend fifty-six days a year on AMA business. A trustee can easily log 100,000 miles of travel on AMA business in just one year.

The duties of the chairman inevitably make him a figure of power. He presides over the board meetings; he sets the agenda; he is the person who makes sure the work gets done. Another source of the chairman's power is knowledge. As someone who deals regularly with the leaders of the house, the heads of the councils and the executives of the staff, the chairman—of all the elected officials— quickly becomes the most knowledgeable about the AMA's policy positions. This makes him a logical witness before a congressional committee; it makes him a well-prepared spokesman to the press; it insures a steady flow of invitations to address both lay and medical audiences. Most of all, his intimate relationship with the organization helps him to establish his leadership in the board, whose powers go beyond those that are officially defined.

As they developed over time, the duties, responsibilities, and privileges of the Board of Trustees have been incorporated in successive versions of the constitution and bylaws. They are spelled out in clear, simple language, and they have been summarized in the preceding section. But to gain a more realistic picture of the role that the Board of Trustees plays and a more realistic appraisal of the power it wields, some interpretation is helpful, especially with respect to the board's relationship to the staff and the other power elements within the association.

One of these elements consists of the councils of the AMA. Historically, many of the widely recognized accomplishments of the AMA stemmed from the studies and reports of various AMA councils and committees. This is especially true in the fields of drugs, medical service, foods and nutrition, and medical education. Because of the way the AMA was structured until 1975, the councils (and sometimes committees) were often able to build themselves into autonomous fiefs, operating without a great deal of regard for the rest of the organization. That is not the case today. The lines of authority have been drawn more tautly, leading through the board to the house. The councils remain an important part of the AMA; they receive wide responsibility and make significant contributions. But their relationship has changed so that there is a more sharply focused direction to their efforts. The requirement that they report "through" the board to the house serves to channel their efforts and give their work an overall cohesiveness that was frequently absent in the past. Going through the board does not give the board a veto. But it does mean that the trustees can ask a council to explore a different aspect of a problem, reconsider a judgment, or clarify facts. The board cannot stop a report of a council from going to the house, though it can—if it disagrees—send the house its own recommendation on the question. Most often, though, the board takes a supportive, positive position.

In 1983 there were seven councils of the AMA, which were, in effect, standing committees. Generally speaking, they are composed of eleven members. In many cases, members are nominated by the board and elected by the house. Generally, the members are elected to three-year terms, with a limit of three terms. Most of the councils include a voting, resident member; most have, additionally, a student member whose right to vote is determined by the council itself; voting rights are almost always granted. Two of the councils—those on scientific affairs and medical service—conform exactly to that description. There are variations in the others.

The Council on Medical Education has eleven members, including a resident with the right to vote and, in addition, a student who may be enfranchised by the council. The variation here is the specification in the bylaws that at least one council member *not* be a salaried member of a medical school faculty. In actuality, there is usually more than the one required non-faculty member, though the council generally has a majority of medical educators.

The Council on Constitution and Bylaws has seven regular members, including a resident. There is, in addition, a student member, whose voting privileges are decided by the council. The council also includes four more members, all ex-officio and none entitled to vote: the AMA president, a trustee selected by the board, the speaker and vice speaker of the house.

The Council on Long Range Planning and Development consists of ten members. The speaker appoints five of them: two from the House of Delegates; two from either the AMA membership at large or the membership of the house; and one resident member. The board appoints four: two from the board and two from the membership of the house or the AMA membership at large. The students appoint a member with full voting privileges, the choice being subject to the concurrence of the board.

The Council on Legislation is composed of the usual eleven members, including a resident. The board appoints a member of the AMA Auxiliary and an ex-officio member nominated by the students, whose voting status is determined by the council. A representative of the American Dental Association may serve on the council, with the understanding that an AMA representative serve on that association's Council on Legislation. The terms of office are one year. The Council on Legislation does not report to the House of Delegates. It acts instead as a review, advisory, and referral committee to the board.

The Judicial Council is more of a court than a council, acting independently of the house and board on matters of ethics, discipline, and constitutional interpretation. It is made up of five members, nominated by the president and elected by the house to five-year terms, with a limit of two terms.

Except in the case of the Judicial Council, the board solicits state and specialty societies for the names of candidates they would recommend for various openings on the councils. The board considers these names for the vacant positions it is empowered to fill and for the nominations (two candidates) for each position filled through election by the delegates. Other nominations can be made from the floor of the house. But the normal channel is through the

Board of Trustees, a procedure that enables the board to exert a strong though indirect influence over the councils.

In appraising the board's strength, one must also take into account its relationship to the AMA staff, a relationship that is close, continual, and generally cordial. Given the authority to make policy decisions between sessions of the House of Delegates, the board is in frequent consultation with the executive vice president and the senior staff. On the authority of the executive vice president, a standing rule of the board is specific. "The Executive Vice President, in carrying out the duties of his office," it reads, "shall consult with the Chairman of the Board, or in his absence, the Vice Chairman of the Board in making important decisions. In general, the Executive Committee shall be the group to be contacted by telephone when urgent matters arise."

According to the AMA constitution, it is the House of Delegates that is charged with deciding AMA policy. It is the Board of Trustees that supervises its implementation. And it is the staff that carries out the directions of the board. But policy formation within the AMA is seldom that orderly a process. It does not proceed in the linear fashion, originating at Point A, moving through Point B, and emerging, tidily packaged, at Point C. Policy formation is, rather, an interactive process, a back-and-forth, give-and-take process, in which all four of the AMA's power elements—the house, board, councils, and staff—usually play a part. As subsequent chapters will show, the relationships among those four power elements are by no means static. They have changed from time to time, sometimes shifting gradually, sometimes clashing acrimoniously, with occasional breakage.

The point to be stressed here is the central position of the board. With two-way channels radiating outward to the other power elements of the organization, the Board of Trustees is uniquely positioned at the center of the AMA's decision-making machinery.

If the chairmanship of the board has traditionally been regarded as the AMA's most powerful office, the presidency is usually seen as its most prestigious.* The president begins his year under the spotlight

*The president and chairman receive equal annual honoraria from the AMA to compensate for practice income lost because of time spent on AMA business. The president-elect receives a smaller honorarium. The other general officers receive honoraria plus per diem allowance for days spent on AMA business. All are reimbursed for travel and other expenses.

of an inauguration ceremony at the annual meeting that is attended by his family, his friends from home, the delegates, and other visitors to the convention. After he is sworn in by the chairman, he gives an inaugural address, and after that there is a convivial reception. Throughout his year in office he acts as medicine's principal spokesman, traveling around the country, speaking to the various medical societies as well as to the public audiences of various sorts. Until the next annual meeting of the AMA, he is regarded nationally and internationally as the leader of American medicine.

During the first part of this century, the AMA tended to favor physicians prominent in education, research, or clinical practice for the presidency. Among such figures were persons like Frank Billings, M.D., who was largely responsible for building the University of Chicago into one of the great medical teaching centers of the country. William H. Welch, M.D., one of the four physicians who brought Johns Hopkins to prominence, was a president, along with both the Mayo brothers and Frank H. Lahey, M.D., founder of the clinic bearing his name in Boston. William C. Gorgas, M.D., famous for his work with yellow fever and the Chief Sanitary Officer of the Panama Canal, was a president, as was Ray Lyman Wilbur, M.D., chancellor of Stanford University and President Hoover's Secretary of the Interior. Several of those physicians (though not all of them) were active in the AMA, serving on AMA councils, in the House of Delegates, or on the Board of Trustees.

After World War II, with the increasing politicization of medicine, a change in the type of person who was elected president became apparent. What came to the fore first were often politically-oriented conservatives whose crusading zeal frequently backed the AMA into corners where it had no room to turn. Then in the 1960s, as the pressures for what became Medicare and Medicaid mounted and as the AMA found its legislative efforts more and more frequently frustrated, those coming into leadership positions within the AMA stressed the need for presidents who could speak more effectively to non-medical audiences, presidents more adept with the press, better equipped to make a good impression on television, more pragmatic and flexible in dealing with the political issues. This is not to say that you can mark off specific periods when this or that type of person was elected to the presidency. That cannot be done. But over the long run a change has taken place.

Since 1945, it is noticeable also that the presidency has gone with great regularity to physicians who have risen through the elective offices of medicine to the position of trustee, chairman, or speaker. Of the thirty-nine individuals who served as president in 1944-80, twenty-four were former trustees, eleven of them former chairmen; eight had been either speaker or vice speaker. Since 1960 it has become an informal custom for the house to elevate the speaker to the presidency every three, four, or five years. Of the remainder, six have become president after filling other AMA offices, such as the vice presidency or various positions on the councils. The one exception is Edward R. Annis, M.D., president in 1963, who was elected from the membership at large, having held no prior elective office at all—county, state, or national. What Annis had was a well-merited reputation as an attractive, articulate public speaker and debater, something the AMA urgently sought in the years immediately preceding passage of Medicare and Medicaid.

As specified in the bylaws, the president's duties are few: an inaugural address; a speech to the opening session of the annual meeting of the house; participation in the business of the House of Delegates, but without vote; the nomination of candidates for the Judicial Council; and the nomination of committees to meet an emergency or other short-term need. Much of the job is ceremonial.

In 1982, the Board of Trustees changed its standing rules to expand the powers of the president within that body, placing him more nearly in a position of parity with the chairman. Starting in June 1983, the president nominated the candidates for chairman at the board organization meeting after the annual meeting. In instances where the president's initial nominee failed to win election, he provided successive nominees until one was. This replaced the system whereby the chairman was elected by the board members by written ballot without any nominations. The president, in consultation with the chairman, started approving board member travel on behalf of the association and the selection of witnesses to appear before congressional hearings, something the chairman alone had previously done. The chairman continued to appoint the intra-board committees and their chairmen, but in consultation with the president.

In addition to being a major figure in the deliberations of the board, the president carries considerable weight in the house. He is in demand as a speaker to medical society audiences, and, since he is often what the local physician member sees of the AMA, he can do much to bring a sense of cohesion and unified purpose to the diverse medical federation. He is widely welcome as a speaker to business and civic groups. He has access to background sessions, editors' lunches, and the press generally. He has what Theodore Roosevelt called a "bully pulpit."

The impact of an AMA president on the profession, on organized medicine, or on the public varies with his warmth of manner, the force of his personality, the validity of his ideas, and his ability to articulate them. There have been successful AMA presidents and there have been failures.

In the mid-1970s, when the AMA was struggling out of a financial crisis and re-examining nearly all of its assumptions, the incoming president, Max H. Parrott, M.D., took the occasion of his inaugural address to suggest that the office of president might be redundant. He recommended abolition of the offices of president, president-elect, and immediate past president and a new role for the chairman. He would be elected not by the board, as was (and still is) the practice, but by the house after nomination by the board. "Hence," Parrott argued, "the chief leaders and chief spokesmen of the AMA would be the chairman of the board of trustees, acting for the elected officers and the house, and the executive vice president, acting for the staff. Both those offices invariably represent a continuum of what we need if our voice is to be clear and distinct..."[10]

The proposal was not adopted, and Parrott, in retrospect, thinks that his suggestion was misunderstood. "Having been on the board for nine years," he says, "I thought they could do away with the president-elect, president, and immediate past president at a saving of about half a million dollars a year. My idea was to make the chairman and the president the same person. I was not suggesting, as some people think I was, that we make the executive vice president the president of the AMA."[11]

It was not long, however, before the suggestion was made to provide for a full-time, salaried president. A resolution introduced at the 1976 interim meeting by A. Halnan White, M.D., a delegate from California, in effect called for the elevation of the executive vice presidency into the office of AMA president. At the reference committee hearing, according to the reference committee's report, the discussion was "wide ranging." The idea that the AMA needed "one clear voice" gained "tremendous support." The enthusiasm may also have reflected the extreme pleasure with which the house was reacting to the decisive way the new executive vice president, James H. Sammons, M.D., had picked up the reins of the then financially troubled organization following his appointment in 1974. The house voted to refer the matter through the board to the Council on Long Range Planning and Development.

Reporting to the house at the 1977 annual meeting, the council gave the proposal its endorsement. It recommended that "the current position of the chief executive officer (the executive vice president) carry the title of president and that this position continue to have the responsibilities of the chief executive officer as well as those of the chief, but not only, spokesman of the AMA. The president should be selected by the Board of Trustees, serve at its pleasure, and be responsible to it." The offices of president-elect, president, and immediate past president would be replaced by three new trustee positions on the board. The house did not take to the idea of losing its power to elect the president each year and referred the report to the board. Six months later, after consultation, the board and the council could see no way of carrying out the sense of the original resolution while allowing the house to retain control over the election of the president.

The board report, adopted by the house at the 1977 interim meeting, argued that recent administrative changes "toward a more modern corporate management structure have strengthened and clarified the role of the executive vice president and that this position currently provides the continuity of leadership and spokesmanship...." The board also expressed its agreement with the house that "a president who is elected by the house provides a close and valuable link between the membership and the association's most visible officer. The elected president has performed both a ceremonial role and a spokesmanship role that has served the AMA well in the past."[12]

Neither Parrott's proposal nor White's resolution changed anything. But the episodes are nevertheless significant, for they reveal how the power elements within the AMA interact. By insisting on its right to choose the president, the house showed its reluctance to surrender power to the board. In recognizing the need for "one clear voice," all concerned—the house, the board, and the Council on Long Range Planning and Development—acknowledged an organizational weakness: the absence of a single, well-known, tenured leader—a permanent president. No one in organized medicine, for example, enjoys the sort of stature the late George Meany enjoyed within organized labor. But the words in the board's report about "a more modern corporate management structure" are not empty,

for important changes were later made in the organizational structure. While the association was willing to identify the handicap of a
presidency without continuity, the AMA nonetheless reasserted its
long-standing preference for a parliamentary, rather than an executive, control over its affairs.

Part III

The Events

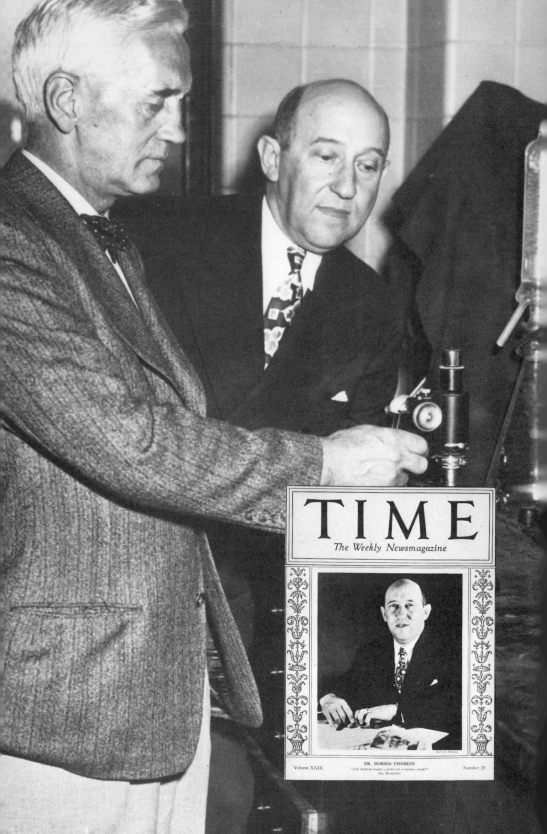

TIME

The Weekly Newsmagazine

DR. MORRIS FISHBEIN
"Shall Medicine remain a profession or become a trade?"
(See MEDICINE)

Volume XXIX   Number 25

UBIQUITOUS, MALIGNED, INFLUENTIAL were words *Time* used to describe Morris Fishbein, M.D., (opposite page, right and inset) As the editor of *JAMA* from 1924 to 1949, he came to dominate the meetings of the Board of Trustees and took over the role of spokesman for both medical and socio-economic policy questions. At left, he gives Sir Alexander Fleming, M.D., the discoverer of penicillin, a tour of the AMA chemical laboratory in 1946. Below are two physicians who figured importantly in Fishbein's downfall. Elmer L. Henderson of Kentucky (left) won election as president-elect in June 1949, promising to curb the activities of the editor. John W. Cline (right) led his fellow Californians in opposition to Fishbein, introduced resolutions in the house to limit his authority and followed Henderson into the AMA presidency.

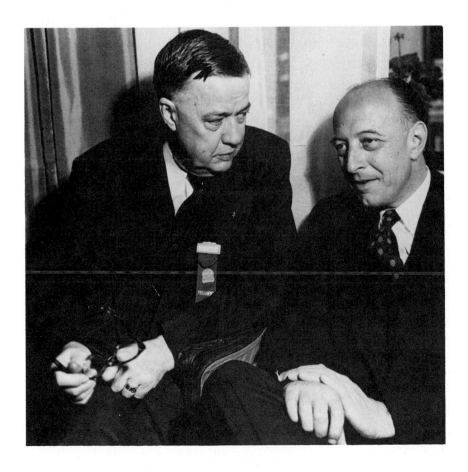

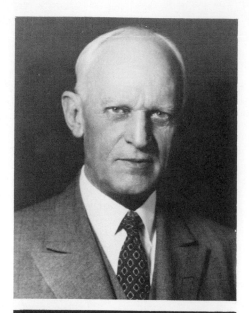

EARLY CHIEF EXECUTIVES,
Olin West, M.D., (top) and
George F. Lull, M.D., (bottom)
each held a dual title. They
were annually elected secretary
of the AMA by the house and
appointed, on a more permanent basis, general manager
by the board. West became
secretary in 1922, the secretary-
general manager in 1924, serving until his retirement in 1946.
The house then voted him president elect, but ill health forced
him to resign before he could
take office as president. Lull, a
former deputy surgeon general
of the U.S. Army succeeded
West as secretary-general manager and held office until 1958,
when he was retired.

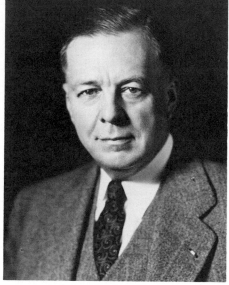

Chapter Nine

The End of an Institution

If you boarded a sightseeing bus in Chicago in the 1940s, as thousands of visitors did in those years, your tour would encompass such famous landmarks as the Union Stockyards, the Museum of Science and Industry, the Board of Trade building, Marshall Field's, the Gold Coast, and the Water Tower, a Gothic survivor of the fire of 1871. The bus would also swing by the AMA headquarters building on North Dearborn Street, at which point the guide would say, "And this, ladies and gentlemen, is the American Medical Association, founded by Morris Fishbein."[1] Both the association and the man were well recognized at the time, fused somehow into a single, nationally known identity.

Morris Fishbein, M.D., was not of course the founder of the AMA. For that matter, he was never the president nor the chairman. He was not even an elected delegate or a trustee. But from the mid-1920s until his dismissal in 1949 he dominated the organization. If you played word association games during those years and someone said, "American medicine," you replied, "Fishbein." He held only one office: editor of *JAMA*, a position to which he was appointed by the Board of Trustees in 1924. (He joined the editorial staff of *JAMA* immediately following his graduation from Chicago's Rush Medical School in 1913.) Over the years Fishbein not only established himself as the gifted editor of the most widely read medical journal in the United States; he also learned how to extend his editorial position, how to project his opinions nationwide. He became, as the saying went in those years, a "personality." *Time* referred to him as "the nation's most ubiquitous, the most widely maligned, and perhaps most influential medico."[2]

To someone familiar with the present AMA, with its trim administrative lines and its well-defined power elements, it is hard to understand how one man could so deeply stamp his personality on such a diversified organization. But, for over two decades, Fishbein *was* the AMA. As you might expect, he had charm, drive, and wit. He was a speed reader, a speed talker, and a speed writer— usually dictating his material. He was a courageous scrapper when it came to exposing medical fraud and fakery. Though subject to hundreds of attacks from every quarter, no one successfully challenged his ability as an editor or questioned his loyalty to medicine and the AMA. But he did have an ego. And he operated from a power base, *JAMA*, that then overshadowed its parent.

The AMA of 1945 differed from the AMA of today in significant ways. At the end of World War II, for example, a physician joining his county/state organization "logically" became a member of the AMA. He did not have to apply for AMA membership, and he did not have to pay dues. For its financing, the AMA was almost totally dependent on the subscription and advertising revenues of *JAMA*. It was thus, to a great degree, financially dependent on Fishbein. Of the association's net revenues of $1,687,452 for 1945, all but $242,736 were generated by activities under the control of Fishbein. More than 70 percent of the AMA's payroll dollars went to the people (most of them in the AMA printing operations) who worked under him.[3]

The non-Fishbein part of the AMA was responsible to a 71-year-old physician named Olin West. West actually had two jobs. He occupied the position of secretary, to which he had been elected annually since 1923 by the House of Delegates; and he carried the title of general manager, a position to which he had been appointed by the Board of Trustees in 1924.[4] He had policy responsibilities for which he was accountable to the house, and he had financial-administrative responsibilities for which he was accountable to the board. His authority was diffused, however, and he had none over Fishbein, who reported independently to the Board of Trustees. The employees under West performed the staff duties connected with the eight existing councils of the AMA and carried out the work of the various departments and bureaus: health education, quackery investigation, legal medicine and legislation, the chemical laboratory, exhibits, and public relations. Early in 1946, West announced his intention to resign, and in June he was elected president-elect. Poor health forced his resignation before he could take office. He was succeeded as secretary-general manager by a retired Major General (Medical Corps), George F. Lull, M.D., who had been Deputy Surgeon General of the United States Army. Lull was fifty-nine at the time.

In contrast to West and Lull, the flamboyant Fishbein sparkled at stage center. He relished his celebrity role and maintained that the limelight in which he bathed was inevitable. He wrote in his autobiography:

> Both the Board of Trustees and myself recognized by the very nature of my work and by the position that I held I must perforce be in the public eye. Nevertheless even a blind man could see that because of this the president of the association, the president-elect, the chairman of the board, and the secretary-general manager would simply not be news to the extent that I was as editor of *The Journal* and *Hygeia* (an AMA consumer magazine), writer of a daily column in newspapers, writer of many articles for periodicals, speaker via radio and in person to anywhere from 50 to 100 public audiences each year including doctors, public health officers and students from elementary schools through college, participant in debates, and witness appearing before various public hearings of local, state, and national bodies.
>
> This was my job and I enjoyed it.
>
> When the press asked for an interview I gave one; when they asked a question, I gave them an answer. When a feature writer came to prepare an article about the American Medical Association and its work, he was at liberty to interview anyone he wished, but he usually started and ended with me simply because many of the others in the headquarters office referred him to me with questions which they perhaps did not wish to answer.[5]

Although Fishbein's public role was more the outgrowth of his own ego than the product of his position, a word should be said about the status of *JAMA* at that time. Much more so than today, when medical reading interests tend to be specialized, as the profession itself is, *JAMA* had much of medical journalism to itself. With a circulation of 109,828 in 1945, *JAMA* was as big as the next six medical periodicals combined. Its prestige and readership were proportionately high. A study of its members by the Michigan State Medical Society indicated that 89 percent of them read *JAMA*; less than 30 percent read other medical literature.[6] Reinforcing its editorial and circulation strengths, *JAMA* enjoyed a strong advantage over its competitors as an advertising medium because of something known as the "Seal of Acceptance."

Despite passage of the Pure Food and Drugs Act in 1906, drug regulations in 1945 were, by today's standards, loose. The 1906 statute required only that a medical product be pure and unadulterated, assuring the purchaser that if he bought aspirin, say, he got aspirin, not a bottle of tablets that were 10 percent aspirin and 90 percent something else. Labeling restrictions were also put into effect, designed to eliminate false claims. Additional legislation in 1938 required that a pharmaceutical product be safe if used as directed. But there was no requirement, as there is now, that a product be effective.

Nor did the Food and Drug Administration have the power, as it does now, to approve or disapprove—word for word—what is said in the advertising copy for a prescription drug product. What policing was done then was done by the AMA through its Council on Pharmacy and Chemistry, which often relied on the findings of its chemical laboratory, its Council on Physical Therapy, which reviewed medical devices, and its Council on Foods and Nutrition. Well before the AMA councils began awarding Seals of Acceptance in 1930, *JAMA* had a strict advertising code.[7] Physicians had confidence in the products they saw advertised in AMA journals and tended to prefer prescribing them rather than non-advertised drugs. The fact was lost on neither Fishbein nor the advertisers.

"The Seal of Acceptance program was the brainchild of Morris Fishbein," says the AMA's retired general counsel, Bernard Hirsh. "He believed, and it worked out this way, that if the AMA put its seal on medical or medically related products, that would be a great advantage to the seller, to the purchaser-user, and to the AMA because there would be an inclination to advertise in AMA publications. It was a formalizing of the advertising review process, and from a financial viewpoint it was successful for many years."[8]

Fishbein's editorship also gave him access to the boardroom. The AMA bylaws then specifically stated that the editor had the privilege of attending meetings of the Board of Trustees, and from 1924 on, for a quarter of a century, Morris Fishbein did so. He became an imposing figure, the almost permanent nature of his presence there adding weight to the vigorously argued opinions he had to offer.

Ernest B. Howard, M.D., the AMA's executive vice president from 1968 to 1974 and its second ranking staff executive from 1948 to 1968, had a good opportunity to observe. He recalls,

> I attended every meeting of the board during the year and a half Morris and I both worked for the AMA, and there was hardly an important decision made in which he did not participate actively

and make strong recommendations. He had a strong personality. I think everyone, no matter what his persuasion, would agree that he was a man of enormous experience. When he made recommendations, they were generally accepted. It was a most extraordinary event when the board, unanimously or otherwise, rejected a recommendation made by the editor of *JAMA*.

And yet there was clearly developing a resentment by the very trustees who voted to accept what he recommended. There was resentment that a member of the staff was having such extraordinary control over the whole organization.[9]

Francis James Levi Blasingame, M.D.—Bing to almost everyone in medicine—knew Fishbein as a delegate during the 1940s, as a trustee in the early 1950s, and as the AMA executive vice president from 1958 to 1968. He confirms Howard's impression. "Morris Fishbein was a strong personality, an entertaining man, a quick wit, a highly unusual speaker. He was a powerful man, by intellect and by energy. He had many, many friends."[10]

In time Fishbein's ego got him into trouble. Physicians came to resent what they perceived to be his use of *JAMA* for his own aggrandizement. In his regular humor column in *JAMA*, "Tonics and Sedatives," Fishbein often inserted a feature, "Dr. Pepys' Diary," which chronicled his personal doings and came compleat with ye antique spellings, bathroom humor, and celebrity items. It raised an easy target.

Physicians cheered—but later winced—at his editorial haymakers, overstatements that came back to haunt him and the AMA. When, for example, the prestigious, well-motivated, independent Committee on Costs of Medical Care reported the results of its five-year study in 1932, Fishbein, in an editorial, pounced savagely on its advocacy of group practice. One of his sentences began, "The rendering of all medical care by groups or guilds or medical soviets..." His summation was equally inflammatory. "The alinement (*sic*) is clear—on one side the forces representing the great foundations, public health officialdom, social theory—even socialism and communism—inciting to revolution; on the other side, the organized medical profession...urging an orderly evolution..."[11]

Fishbein was by no means alone in his opposition. Several members of the committee, including eight physicians, signed a minority report. But that editorial, at least in Wilbur Cohen's mind, did much to set the harsh tone for the public debate over medical issues that has lasted for years;[12] it created what became a highly charged atmosphere that, in the opinion of many physicians, enormously complicated the job of presenting medicine's position.

But what launched the effort to topple Fishbein were two events that took place in California. In late 1938, in order to head off a plan for compulsory health insurance advanced by the Democratic governor, Culbert L. Olson, the California Medical Association put together a voluntary insurance plan (now California Blue Shield). When the California Medical Association met in mid-December to formally adopt the proposal, Roscoe G. Leland, M.D., director of the AMA Bureau of Medical Economics, appeared uninvited to lobby the California delegates in their rooms, advancing Fishbein's arguments against any system of prepaid insurance. To vote otherwise, Leland argued, was heresy. The California Medical Association delegates ignored Leland, adopted the proposal 100-4, and adjourned in a mood of smoldering resentment over Fishbein's insensitivity to their political needs.

The wounds were deepened in 1943, this time over the issue of osteopathy. Unlike many osteopathic schools that were operating in the United States, the one in Los Angeles had for many years tended to rely on the tenets of conventional medicine rather than strict osteopathic doctrine. As a result, medical physicians in the state had a higher regard for osteopathic physicians than existed elsewhere, and in 1942 the California Medical Association formed a committee to discuss the possibilities of a merger of medicine and osteopathy.

Howard Hassard, a San Francisco lawyer, an influential advisor to the California Medical Association for many years beginning in the late 1930s and counsel to California Blue Shield, recalls a visit from Fishbein in the fall of 1943. Hassard says,

The CMA hosted a reception for him at which the officers and members of the council (i.e., board of trustees) were present. I was there, and I remember Dr. Fishbein seating himself on an old-fashioned radiator, dangling his legs and lecturing his hosts on their folly vis-a-vis osteopathy. He was arrogant, condescending, and showed not the slightest knowledge of, nor interest in, the factual situation in California. He simply said the osteopaths were inferior and he had not let the AMA or anyone in medicine have anything to do with them. At that time Edwin L. Bruck, a San Francisco internist, was chairman of the council of the CMA and he was so incensed at Fishbein's attitude that he later authored a resolution demanding his removal. Two other AMA delegates, Dwight H. Murray, M.D., and E. Vincent Askey, M.D., were present and shared Bruck's sense of outrage.

Dr. Bruck was not an AMA delegate, but his good friend, John W. Cline, M.D., was, and Cline was willing to see to it that Bruck's resolution, adopted by the California Medical Association, reached the AMA House of Delegates.[13] The next June, at the 1944 meeting in Chicago, the Californians fired a double-barreled blast. Charge one was aimed at Olin West, M.D., the secretary-general manager. This took the form of a California resolution proposing that he be commended for long, faithful, and valuable service, that he be assured of affection, and that the board "be memorialized to appoint him as Secretary Emeritus for life on the expiration of his present term of office." The other was leveled at Fishbein. This resolution is worth reproduction in full, for it expressed both the resentment against the editor and the lack of confidence in the AMA leadership that pervaded the organization during the 1940s.

> Whereas, The medical profession in America finds itself facing the most critical period of its existence; and
> Whereas, Because of lack of understanding of basic issues and problems by certain officers of the American Medical Association, public opinion is turning against organized medicine; and
> Whereas, These changes of public opinion allow various and certain pressure groups to advance their own selfish causes; and
> Whereas, The political adherents of socialized medicine have seized on the rising tide of public criticism against organized medicine in an effort to accomplish their own desires; and
> Whereas, The unnecessary, continuous, defensive attitude of some of the officers of the AMA makes it impossible for them to take the leadership in bringing about proper general understanding of the real public needs with respect to medical care and progress; therefore be it
> RESOLVED, That the House of Delegates requests the Board of Trustees to replace the present editor of *The Journal.*[14]

That put the cat among the pigeons. The reference committee to which the resolutions were referred asked for "unity" and called upon physicians to "give their loyalty and support" to those selected by the house for the board and those selected by the board in turn for various positions. The reference committee recommended that the resolutions not be adopted.

The first, the one relating to West, was not adopted. As for the second, there was, as the minutes of the meeting noted, "discussion." Much of this took place in an executive session of the house; that is, a meeting closed to the press and public. California delegate Dwight L. Wilbur, M.D., son of Ray Lyman Wilbur, M.D., a former AMA president (1923) who headed the Committee on the Costs of Medical Care that Fishbein attacked in 1932, led off. "There is nothing personal in this resolution," he began, "but the editor has assumed in the eyes of the public a position of spokesman with or without the consent of the board...The rank and file membership does not believe that he truly represents them or their views...Many of you have heard from the lips of your own congressman, as we have, that it is high time for medicine to change its spokesman before Congress and governmental agencies."

Speeches pro and speeches con followed, none very long, but many drawing rounds of applause. Then, upon invitation, Fishbein spoke. Briefly, he reviewed his history with the AMA.

> I have done my utmost to produce a series of scientific publications which would represent the association properly to the medical profession of the world...There have been greatly added to my duties by the Board of Trustees certain other tasks having to do with scientific publications for the public, the handling of a certain amount of the activities of the association directing contacts with the press and public. I have carried on as efficiently as possible, and during that period of time, I have been compelled frequently to fight—in the open—quackery, to fight—in the open—those who would bring down the standards of medical education, to fight those who would compromise with ignorance to carry the message of scientific medicine wherever I could and as well as I could.

Some parliamentary maneuvers came next. It was proposed that the unusual procedure of vote by written (secret) ballot be followed. A Fishbein supporter, Edward H. Cary, M.D., of Texas, called instead for a rising vote, "that we stand up and be counted." Cary wanted to force the anti-Fishbein delegates to identify themselves. Cary's motion carried the day, and in the rising vote that followed Fishbein won 144-9.[15]

But within six months, toward the beginning of 1945, what might have passed into the record as a personal vendetta between Fishbein and the California Medical Association turned into warfare over a matter of principle.

Governor Olson's 1938 proposal for compulsory health insurance had gone nowhere, but his successor, Republican Earl Warren, elected in 1942, was now pushing for it. In fact, he had asked the California Medical Association to inform him of the type of tax-financed medical plan, if any, that the association would approve. The California Medical Association rejected all compulsory plans, proposing instead that the state give aid and assistance to existing, voluntary, non-profit plans, such as the California Physicians Service (which became California Blue Shield). The California Medical Association was taking the path of political realism, mounting opposition to undesired legislation but offering an acceptable alternative at the same time. It was following a hallowed tenet of political wisdom: You don't beat something with nothing.

But Fishbein was having none of it. In a *JAMA* editorial on February 17, 1945, he argued his own view of voluntary health insurance, even though the House of Delegates had unequivocally endorsed Blue Cross hospital insurance in 1938 and the equivalent of Blue Shield insurance for physician charges in 1942.[16] He wrote, "The problem of establishing medical care for all under prepayment plans, whether voluntary or compulsory, is complex and susceptible to various detrimental influences. Much carefully controlled experimentation with voluntary plans such as now prevails in many parts of the country is needed before anything resembling a real answer to the problem of medical care for all the people will be forthcoming."[17]

Offended again by what they perceived as Fishbein's obliviousness to their problems and more convinced than ever that his was the way to political suicide, the Californians went at him again. The resolution they introduced at the 1945 annual meeting requires a brief second look, for it did not mention Fishbein by name. Because the AMA was in "need of the most efficient organization possible," it stated, and because "employees who participate in activities outside of the association cannot render their best service," it proposed that employees "be required to devote their full time to the activities of the association and not engage in outside activities from which they derive financial income."[18]

As at the 1944 meeting, the reference committee recommended that the resolution not be adopted. Again, the minutes note, there was "discussion." John W. Cline, M.D.,* a California delegate, confessed right away that "this resolution is aimed at the activities of the editor." Among the many things on Cline's mind was the matter of the AMA's public relations. "We hope a positive program, bearing sufficient evidence of the desire and ability of the AMA to meet the medical needs of the people of the United States and destroy the demand for compulsory health insurance, will come out of this session. But that is not enough. Such a program and our ideas concerning medical care must be presented to Congress and the people in a manner that will convince them of our sincerity and the truth of our position."[19]

To Fishbein's defense again came Cary of Texas. "Why," he demanded, "should we strike down a man who has served this organization, who has possibly contributed so much information to the public, whose great editorial in last week's issue was one of the greatest pieces of literature on the subject (the Wagner-Murray-Dingell proposal for national health insurance) that anyone could read?"[20] More to the point, another Californian, Lowell S. Goin, M.D., brought up the external realities, his state's recent battle over compulsory health insurance with Governor Warren very much on his mind. "I don't know how much experience some of the speakers have had with the forces of the CIO," he said. "One would think sometimes...that we delegates from California were a kind of cross between medical communists and ivory tower theorists. As a matter of fact, we are those persons who like the Hittites, [fought] in the forefront of the battle, and we don't lack the experience you gentlemen lack but which you are going to have very shortly."[21]

When the debate subsided, tellers passed out ballots. The voting was to be by secret ballot this time. Fishbein won again, but the margin narrowed, 106-60. The anti-Fishbein feeling was beginning to spread.

Though beaten, the Californians were not finished. Wilbur and Goin immediately came back with resolutions that would, in effect, take his public relations functions away from Fishbein—end his more or less self-appointed role as the AMA spokesman—and hand them over to the Council on Medical Service and Public Relations. The House of Delegates did not accept this proposal either. But

*It is interesting to note the number of anti-Fishbein California delegates who later became presidents of the AMA. They include Cline in 1951, Dwight H. Murray, M.D., in 1956, E. Vincent Askey, M.D., in 1961 and Dwight L. Wilbur, M.D., in 1968.

upon learning that the Board of Trustees had already engaged an outside public relations consultant to make a sweeping analysis of the AMA's performance in this area—something the Californians had sought—most of the California delegates, though not all, were satisfied that progress had been made.[22]

It probably should be said here that in the lexicon of the Californians, the term "public relations" included a number of activities. The usual things—press releases, answers to media queries, the news generated by the activities of the AMA's scientific councils— were part of it. But the term spilled over into policy matters, into questions of legislative tactics and political strategy.

The truce, as Fishbein called it, lasted only a year. As the delegates assembled in San Francisco for the 1946 annual meeting, California was ready with another resolution to trim the activities of the editor. It was a rehash of criticisms made earlier, but this time it was introduced "by title only," meaning that the various whereas's and resolved's were not revealed.[23]

This resolution was to serve as a bargaining card, one to be played only if other desired actions were not taken.[24] In 1945 California had pushed the AMA into getting an outside appraisal of its public relations. Now in 1946 it wanted to be sure that the recommendations of the outside consultant, Raymond T. Rich and Associates, were acted upon. On the surface, the major recommendations, which were adopted, appeared to put more distance between Fishbein and the public relations-political-legislative processes of the AMA. Since the intent of the resolution was to do just that, limiting Fishbein to editorship of *JAMA*, Cline withdrew the resolution, thus ending the executive session of the house. Before the meeting, *Time* magazine reported, "The Californians put on their rubber gloves prepared at last for a Fishbeinectomy."[25] Now, it seemed to most of them, the chances had improved that the political strategy they had successfully used in California to defeat Governor Warren's health bill would supplant Fishbein's act, with its clumsy humor, its shoot-from-the-hip statistics, its give-me-liberty-or-give-me-death rhetoric.

Yet the issue was not settled. The AMA was unable to build a public relations operation powerful enough and effective enough to force Fishbein into the wings. There was little evidence that the Washington operation had grown stronger. No clear leadership emerged, which was the real problem. And Dr. Fishbein was still Dr. AMA.

When the shooting war finally broke out over President Truman's health bill in 1949, Fishbein's exit became inevitable. To handle political public relations, the Board of Trustees quickly sent for the high-powered, San Francisco-based public relations firm of Whitaker and Baxter, the successful duo that had won battle after battle in various California political wars and had shown the California Medical Association how to defeat Governor Warren's health insurance bill in 1945. Once and for all, the AMA had made its choice of political strategy—the California strategy, not Fishbein's. His role as a public relations figure for the AMA was over.

If there was any doubt left, it ended on February 22, 1949, when Fishbein stepped into a trap he baited himself. Arguing the issue of national health insurance on the Town Meeting of the Air, a popular radio forum in those days, Fishbein said, "I was in England in September. I spent eight days...I visited the offices of general practitioners...I saw doctors try to handle forty patients in two hours, so that this assembly-line medicine consisted in most instances of the patient voicing his complaint, a question by the doctor, and a made-to-order prescription." England had launched its National Health Service the previous year, and Fishbein liked to point to it as the sort of impersonal, government-run medical system that threatened the United States. His point drew applause.

Then Nelson H. Cruikshank of the American Federation of Labor, a leading supporter of the Truman health bill, got the microphone. He said: "In *JAMA*, there is a complete diary of Dr. Fishbein's covering not his eight days but his six days in England, not in September, but in August...He went to the theater, he had all kinds of dinners, he sat next to Lord Moran (Churchill's doctor), he went to the Olympic games, he passed out CARE packages, and spent one morning in Sandringham Road visiting a practitioner..."[26]

It was a devastating rejoinder. It was vintage Fishbein. And it was precisely the sort of public relations fiasco that spurred the mounting demands that Fishbein stick to his editing.

For a man with an ego of ordinary dimensions, the editorship of the largest medical journal in the United States would seem to be a position of satisfactory scale. But not for Morris Fishbein. In his autobiography, he described just what happened at the end of his thirty-seven years with the AMA. Early in 1949, he wrote, Elmer L. Henderson, M.D., then the chairman of the Board of Trustees and a friend, came to him and asked his support in his effort to run for the presidency of the AMA that June. Fishbein replied: "You know, Elmer, I don't get involved in the election of the president."

Then Henderson said, "Morris, the western delegation assures me that I will have their support if I agree to their proposal that you should be limited to editing *JAMA* and forced to give up all your other activities."

Rather than bow to that, rather than accept the pleas of friends that he confine himself to what he did best—edit *JAMA*—Fishbein replied: "Elmer, what you do is between you and your conscience."[27]

At the annual meeting of the AMA in Atlantic City that June, Henderson submitted to the house a report from the board announcing formal limits on the editor's activities and his forthcoming retirement (effective in December). There was no discussion and no executive session, for the bylaws gave the board, not the house, the authority to appoint the editor of *JAMA*. The report that Henderson read to the house did, however, go to a reference committee. In reporting back, it said, "Your reference committee feels that this organization, together with the whole civilized world, owes Dr. Fishbein a debt of gratitude. His contributions to the advancement of medical science as editor of *JAMA* have earned him international acclaim. *JAMA* is an enduring monument to his genius and devotion."

The only thing resembling a vote came on a blind resolution in which the house stated it had "full confidence in the Board of Trustees to carry on the duties imposed on it by the constitution and bylaws." When the speaker asked if there were any discussion, an uncomfortable silence fell over the house, and he declared the resolution adopted unanimously.

The next day the *New York Times* gave the story a two-column headline at the top of page one. Henderson went on to win the election as president three days later. Fishbein made his exit with class—no bitterness, no recrimination.[28] He led an energetic, productive life as a writer, editor, and lecturer until his death in 1976, at the age of eighty-eight. While the manner of Morris Fishbein's termination was criticized as brutal, his departure was not mourned —even though it took the AMA many years to determine what sort of leadership should succeed his.

Chapter Ten

Political Challenge and Response

Even when viewed from a perspective no more distant than the next decade, the AMA of the 1930s sometimes seemed remote from the realities of that time. While certainly aware of the social and political turmoil stirred by the Great Depression, its members nevertheless remained uncertain as to what changes in policy or structure might be appropriate to the new circumstances. The AMA's programs still centered on its traditional activities—the accreditation of educational institutions, the promotion of public health, the publication of scientific journals, the health education of the public, the exposure of quackery. It still relied on its array of committees and councils to develop its thinking, and, though some new councils were added, even they were confined in scope to intraprofessional concerns. Except in spasmodic outbursts, the organization chose not to deal with issues outside its established orbit of medical and medical-educational interests. There was no thought of a Washington office, and in 1937 the House of Delegates even rejected a suggestion that the AMA start a public relations department.

But if the AMA seemed transfixed by events, the omens of change were easy to read. One was the report in 1932 of the Committee on the Costs of Medical Care, with its recommendations for group practice and voluntary health insurance plans, ideas that for a while at least drew the AMA's opposition.* In 1935 the idea of putting substantial medical benefits into the original Social Security

---

*Although the committee was independent of the AMA (it had foundation sponsorship), its chairman was Ray Lyman Wilbur, M.D., a former president of the AMA (1923) and chairman of the AMA's Council on Medical Education and Hospitals (1929-1945). Wilbur was also president and later chancellor of Stanford University and President Hoover's Secretary of the Interior.

Act first appeared—and was quickly abandoned. Then in 1938, in response to a federally initiated National Health Conference, the AMA House of Delegates called a special meeting at which, among other things, it gave its unequivocal endorsement to voluntary, prepaid hospital service insurance; that is, Blue Cross.[1] Senator Robert F. Wagner of New York introduced his health bill in 1939, and, as the war clouds darkened over Europe in 1942, Sir William Beveridge released his plan for a postwar, socialized England.

Domestically, both the thrust of New Deal politics and the lofty declarations of United States political leaders seemed to be laying the groundwork for radical changes in the way American health care was to be delivered and financed. The AMA, disturbed by the trend since 1935, viewed events with mounting alarm. In 1943 when Senator Wagner, now joined by two Democratic colleagues, Senator James E. Murray of Montana and Representative John D. Dingell, Sr., of Michigan, introduced a bill that would provide medical and hospital benefits through Social Security, many physicians thought they heard the first shot in an ideological war over national health care policy.

The Wagner-Murray-Dingell bill of 1943 was a seminal piece of legislation. It called for a compulsory system of medical and hospitalization insurance for all persons (and their dependents) covered by the Social Security Act. The system was to be financed by social security taxes and administered by the Surgeon General of the United States under the direction of the Federal Security Agency. Among other things, it would "approve" a fee schedule by which doctors would be compensated for services rendered. Senator Wagner did not press the legislation aggressively; it was being offered for "legislative study and consideration," he said. Nevertheless, the bill quickly won labor support, and in the months following the introduction of the bill one national labor union after another voted its endorsement.[2]

Organized medicine wasted little time in voicing its objections. Fishbein thought the proposal would turn the Surgeon General into a "gauleiter" (Nazi party district leader).[3] The AMA feared the legislation would overturn the traditional, predominantly private system of medical care, gradually destroy private initiatives and freedoms, reduce physicians to the status of government employees, and eventually dictate medical decisions.

When the 1943 meeting of the House of Delegates opened that June 7—only four days after the introduction of the Wagner-Murray-

Dingell bill—a total of seventeen resolutions were presented for consideration, seven of which proposed actions related to the new legislation. Three of these resolutions proposed an "executive," a "legislative," or an "information" office in Washington. Four sought the establishment of a committee or a council on "medical care" or "medical service."[4]

Quite clearly, the delegates recognized a new challenge. For nearly a century, the AMA had concentrated on the quality of care, the quality of physician education and training, the competence of hospitals, the quality of medicines, the quality of the environment. Now it had to deal with a different set of issues, having to do with the availability, distribution, and financing of physician and hospital services; in other words, access to medical care.

Furthermore, the milieu had changed. Up to this point, the AMA had won its battles without doing a great deal more than developing factual reports and putting its case before a respectful public. The reforms it had accomplished in medical education, public health, drugs, and combating quackery usually gained immediate and wide public support. But now it was different. The medical profession had stepped into a tough political fight. The public was by no means instinctively on its side, nor were the opinion-makers deferential. The politicization of American medicine had begun in earnest.

The delegates who wanted to take arms against the new federal legislation found the raising of support slower than they expected. Not everyone in the House of Delegates was convinced of the need for a Washington operation or a council devoted to socioeconomic and political matters. In addition, some delegates feared that AMA political partisanship would only invite reprisal in the form of a federal review of the AMA's status as a tax-exempt organization. In fact, the AMA had just lost a long antitrust battle with the United States Department of Justice, and some leaders hesitated to tangle with the federal government again.

In 1938, the United States Assistant Attorney General, Thurman W. Arnold, obtained criminal indictments against the AMA, the District of Columbia Medical Society, the District of Columbia Academy of Surgery, the Harris County (Texas) Medical Society, and twenty-one individuals, including Morris Fishbein, M.D., editor of *JAMA*, and Olin West, M.D., the AMA secretary-general manager. The charge was that organized medicine had denied hospital privileges to physicians associated with the Group Health Association of Washington, a prepaid health insurance plan, by denying them membership in local medical societies. In an initial lower court decision, the judge's opinion said that medical practice is not a trade within the meaning of the Sherman Antitrust Act, and the AMA won the case. However, the association lost an appeal. Then it stood trial again and lost, and finally lost an appeal of that decision in the Supreme Court in 1943. The final result: fines of $1,500 for the District of Columbia Medical Society and $2,500 for the AMA. The individuals and the other medical societies were found not guilty.[5]

The question as to what sort of organization the AMA should be dominated the debate in the house in 1943. The case for staying away from political involvements was eloquently presented by the secretary-general manager, Olin West. In an executive session of the house he said,

I fear that the adoption of these reports is again going to raise what to me is a very serious question, and that is the classification of the American Medical Association as a scientific body or as a trade organization. I can tell you in executive [i.e., closed] session that there are certain departments of the federal government that still have their eye on every activity of this association.

I get a letter, for instance, wanting to know why a certain advertisement was rejected, and when I explain to the United States Department of Justice why it was rejected, I get another letter informing me that the Department of Justice has advised the organization which sent the advertisement to resubmit it, but the Department of Justice declines to state whether there is any law that requires the American Medical Association to accept an advertisement. We finally accepted it because we didn't want another lawsuit that cost the association $150,000...

What I am trying to impress upon you is that there are still some animosities that may get us into serious trouble, and I am very much afraid that with the adoption of all these resolutions you are going to see that the AMA is reclassified not as a scientific organization but as a trade organization, and I maintain that the AMA has no excuse for existence except as a scientific and educational organization.[6]

It was an argument that would be heard again and again in future debates. Sometimes it was voiced sincerely. Sometimes it was used tactically, as a smokescreen to stall the initiatives of delegates convinced that the AMA had to counter political threats and undertake non-scientific programs.

But West's idealistic plea, motivated by his fear of government retaliation, was a last stand. When the issue came to a vote later in the session, the AMA authorized a Washington office and committed itself irrevocably to a new body, the Council on Medical Service and Public Relations, which had clear, non-scientific objectives.

In the way the council was established, there was little question as to the extent of its power. As a standing committee of the house, it did not have to send its reports and recommendations through the board, where they might be edited, toned down, or altered. The council was allowed to select its own staff secretary; it was authorized to use the personnel and functions of all AMA staff departments. If it felt the need for additional personnel or a larger budget, it could take its case to the house, which in turn could exert its influence on the board to see that the requests received the proper consideration.

In later years, AMA Senior Deputy Executive Vice President Joe D. Miller, whose first position with the organization in 1957 was that of research assistant to the council, recalled, "It was my impression, which has been confirmed many times since, that the Council on Medical Service was one of the strongest policy-making and political groups in the association. At that time some even said that the council had more power than the Board of Trustees and had actually been created by the House of Delegates to balance the authority of the board."[7]

Along what lines was the new council to proceed? As is the case with legislation passed in an elected body, it is sometimes difficult to understand the real intent from the official language alone. The six-point charge to the new council, as stated in the board report adopted by the house at the 1943 meeting, is laced with those vague verbs that often characterize committee reports: "to make available"..."to investigate"..."to study and suggest"..."to develop and assist." For that reason it is helpful to examine the record preceding and following the action of the house.

What, for example, did the board intend by the last three words of the council's full name, "and Public Relations"? Minutes of the Board of Trustees indicate that it wished to reflect some of the thoughts expressed in a resolution submitted by Delegate E.H. Skinner, M.D. This was one of seven resolutions that were finally merged into the board's report calling for the establishment of the council.

Early in his resolution, Skinner mentioned the AMA's duty and right "...to make available scientific facts, data and medical opinion with respect to the provision of medical services." He was, in other words, talking about a greater participation by the AMA in the public dialogue on the issues relating to medical services. Later in his resolution he spoke about the need to "assist and coordinate committes on medical care and public policy originating within state and county societies."[8] He was, in effect, saying that the time had come for the AMA to step into the public arena and join in the debate over the national health insurance.[9]

An even clearer picture of the council's direction can be seen in two key reports that the council submitted to the house a year later, at the 1944 meeting. In discusssing its general policies, the council stated unequivocally that it "recognizes the desirability of widespread distribution" of medical care. It said the "removal of economic barriers [to medical care] should be an end in itself." It reaffirmed the principles of voluntary, prepaid, medical and hospital insurance. It announced its intention to analyze future legislation dealing with matters of medical service, to share that analysis with the state medical associations, and to work with legislative committees on the subject of medical service.

In terms of accomplishment, the reports mention the council's analysis of the first Wagner-Murray-Dingell bill, the publication of its statement thereon in *JAMA*, and its wide distribution to the association. It is important to note that it was the new council, not the board, that developed the AMA's policy position on the Wagner-Murray-Dingell bill, and on compulsory sickness insurance generally. The council said it had begun fortnightly publication of a bulletin for medical leaders and announced that it soon would release a question and answer pamphlet on the Wagner-Murray-Dingell bill designed for public readership.

And finally, the council announced the opening of an AMA office in Washington "for the collection of information and data concerning medical care and its distribution, its availability, its costs and its control in various parts of the United States."[10]

Although the house positioned the council across the path of the new political issues, the exact jurisdictional lines were still fluid. Even at the 1944 meeting, when the two reports from the new council were adopted and a resolution commending the council's work was passed, the house nevertheless asked the board for a further definition of the council's status.

At least three major friction points marred the working relationship between the council and board. First, there were all the predictable administrative problems. The board took strong exception to the negotiations that the council conducted with regard to salary, employment, and other actions normally controlled by the secretary-general manager. An understanding had to be reached that the council's recently hired Washington representative, Joseph S. Lawrence, M.D., was responsible *both* to the council and to the board through headquarters in Chicago.[11]

Another trouble spot surfaced when the council asked that the AMA Bureau of Medical Economics be transferred to its control. In making the request, the council had recommended that the bureau undertake a vigorous program to expand voluntary, prepaid medical insurance plans—most of them sponsored by state or county medical societies. The bureau was also to create an informational clearinghouse on prepaid medical plans and appoint a qualified executive to take charge of it.[12]

That may sound like an unexciting piece of administrative business, but it was more than that. This was, in fact, what was soon to become the national Blue Shield organization, and both the board and the council recognized its importance. The board argued successfully that the bureau should remain under its jurisdiction because the bureau serviced the needs of many elements within the AMA. But later, after a number of meetings, the board agreed that the council's functions should include the direction of a division of prepaid medical care plans.[13]

Much of the council-board difficulty came down to simple rivalry. Which group had charge of the AMA's response to the broad socioeconomic issues raised by the Wagner-Murray-Dingell bill? Which had the authority; who was to be the spokesman? When the house went into executive session in 1945, Delegate Lowell S. Goin, M.D., one of the Californians who was convinced that Fishbein's (and, by association, the board's) leadership promised only disaster, spurred the council on. "Keep on expanding the activities of this council," he cried. "Make it more and more our spokesman. Make it the voice of American medicine."

That was too much for the vice chairman of the Board of Trustees, Roscoe L. Sensenich, M.D. Taking the floor, he said, "I think it would be most unwise, and as a trustee I should not care to assume responsibility for acts or expressions of the council independent of the direction or supervision of the Board of Trustees. To say that they...were to be the only spokesman or the only ones to define policies would be...difficult...impossible."[14]

Undaunted, the council came right back at the annual meeting in the following year with a report recommending that the house designate the executive committee of the council and the executive committee of the board to jointly handle urgent legislative matters between the meetings of the house. "Interim authority," which had always been a board function, was now supposedly going to be shared fifty-fifty. Both sides bristled. In the discussions, the council's backers criticized the lethargy of the board by arguing the need for "prompter action than has occurred in the past." But the board won out when Sensenich, now chairman, reminded the delegates that the board's interim authority derived from the Illinois not-for-profit corporation statute.[15]

This, however, was not the only fight going on within the AMA. Led by the same Californians who were gunning for Fishbein, strong elements in the house were critical of both the council and the board. In an executive session of the house in 1944, Dwight H. Murray, M.D., a California delegate (who became a trustee the next year), said that several of the Western states sensed a lack of adequate representation in Washington. "We felt that the legislative affairs in Washington were being let go by the board at the time (late 1943, early 1944). We therefore proceeded to organize ourselves—six Western states—and establish ourselves in Washington and put a man in charge of our office who will be there permanently or until we see that the job is being done adequately by somebody else. We have offered heretofore to cooperate with [the AMA] office in Washington and we expect to do so. But until such time as [the AMA] office in Washington is a distinct reality and until it functions as we believe it should we expect to stay there."[16]

If there was doubt as to what the Californians considered "adequate" in Washington, Delegate Lowell S. Goin, M.D., clarified things in 1945. Again at an executive session, he told the house: "To say that this organization [the AMA] has no function except as a scientific assembly is, in my opinion, nonsense. I think 160,000 doctors all over the United States look to this body to defend them from the encroachment of economic planners and to keep it free from the chains and fetters of a national socialist state."[17]

But the council and the board took a more restrained view of the Washington operation. There were many joint meetings to "clarify" or "define" the duties of the council. The following excerpt is from a report developed by the executive committee of the Board of Trustees and read at the board meeting in June 1945: "...the duties of the Washington office are wholly related to the gathering of information to constituent and component associations, and the maintenance of study of medical service plans throughout the nation. It should also be clearly understood that it is not the function of the Washington office to influence legislation."[18]

To the Californians, this sort of thinking was idiotic. Referring to the words about gathering information and disseminating it back to the state and county societies, Delegate Goin was, as usual, blunt in his criticism. He told the house, "When this council was formed, there was considerable talk...about the dissemination of information—a pleasant and harmless phrase—with an eye cocked on the Department of Internal Revenue. I thought everyone in this house understood that the dissemination of information was to be in the opposite direction...namely, that the intent was to inform legislators and government agencies of the opinions of medicine, of its beliefs, its wishes and desires, and not to inform the members of the AMA of things they can very readily read in the newspapers."[19]

A year later, at another executive session of the house, California Delegate John W. Cline, M.D., echoed Goin's objections to the AMA's hesitant actions. "I think it is time that we wake up to the fact that until and unless we move into Washington, with a real coordination of effort there, we are going to continue to be at a disadvantage..."[20] But the house voted down a California resolution to establish a Washington lobby; it preferred to stay with the Council on Medical Service terminology for its Washington office, the bureau of information.

Beneath the turmoil, underlying the repeated jurisdictional fights, the power struggles, and the misunderstandings of direction lay a simple fact: the AMA lacked leadership. Neither the new Council on Medical Service nor the Board of Trustees was able to assert it. The house was divided. Largely by default, Fishbein continued his spokesman's role. An editorial in the May 1943 *Medical Annals of the District of Columbia* deplored the failure of the AMA's elective process to establish firm direction. "What the profession needs at this time above anything else is leadership—able, constructive leadership. It needs the confidence that is inspired by *elected* leaders who can speak for them effectively, without arousing unnecessary antagonism."

Before the Council on Medical Service was organized and grew strong enough to be effective, organized medicine's opposition to compulsory national health insurance came from two sources. One was Fishbein with his booming attacks on "socialized medicine" in *JAMA*, speeches, radio broadcasts, and press conferences. The other was an organization called the National Physicians' Committee for the Extension of Medical Service. Started in 1938, it was brought to the AMA's attention in 1939 by Fishbein through an editorial, which had board approval and blandly said, "Their work is in the nature of public relations activities."[21]

Actually, few introductions were necessary, for the leaders of the National Physicians' Committee included two former AMA presidents and several former trustees. Its guiding spirit was a current delegate and former president (1932), Edward H. Cary, M.D., the Dallas opthalmologist who, when needed, rose to Fishbein's defense in the house. Born in Alabama, Cary exuded the outward mannerisms of the antebellum South. But inside lay the instincts of a two-fisted frontiersman: a fierce determination (he was one of those largely responsible for getting the Southwestern Medical School launched in Dallas during World War II), a highly individualistic outlook on society, and a zest for political hardball. In contrast to many physicians and the AMA delegates who thought that a professional medical society should not "stoop" to political campaigning and techniques, Cary was a born gunfighter.

Raising 90 percent of its funds from the pharmaceutical industry and the rest from 22,000 individual physicians, the National Physicians' Committee picked up a cudgel that for a long time the AMA refused to wield. Endorsed by the House of Delegates in 1942 and again in 1945, the committee spent $905,359 in the six years from 1940 through 1945 on pamphlets, speeches, radio talks, and print advertisements denouncing the Wagner-Murray-Dingell proposals.[22] A leaflet titled, "Do You Want Your Own Doctor or a Job Holder?" featured a reproduction of a sentimental, nineteenth century British painting by Sir Luke Fildes called "The Doctor," which achieved a considerable notoriety in the 1940s.* One of the committee's ads pictured a frail, worried woman confronted by an overbearing doc-

---

Originally commissioned by Queen Victoria and once distributed by the makers of Petrolagar, a laxative frequently prescribed in the 1930s, the painting was chosen by the United States Post Office in 1947 to decorate the stamp commemorating the AMA's 100th year. It was picked up again for use in the AMA's 1949-50 campaign by Whitaker and Baxter.

tor who is telling her, "Make it snappy, sister." The text of the ad warned that political control would depersonalize medical care. The National Physicians' Committee favored blunt, even crude, material, reflecting the anger that surged through some segments of medicine. But the harsh tone offended many others; the press and parts of the public.

During the middle 1940s, the AMA was content to let the National Physicians' Committee wage the propaganda battle. The committee could raise its own money and spend it without the possibility, then so feared, that the AMA might jeopardize its status as a tax-exempt corporation if it engaged in political campaigning.

But in time the committee wore its welcome thin. What little credibility was left vanished after a mailing to AMA physicians in December 1948. This consisted of a Washington letter written by an ultraconservative of no particular distinction named Dan Gilbert whose "prophetic news-of-the-month" usually went to a list of Protestant clergymen. Quick to spot communist plots, remarkably careless of facts, and given to savage language, Gilbert called the health insurance bill a "made-in-Moscow importation" that violated the ideals of religious liberty and advanced the ambitions of "power-mad politicians." Although the letter itself was not anti-Semitic, the salutation, "Dear Christian American," struck most physicians that way.

Although the AMA disavowed the letter, stating that no AMA official had seen it or read it before distribution,[23] it alienated thousands of physicians. The strain it created between the AMA and the Medical Society of the State of New York lasted well over twenty years. In 1951 the National Physicians' Committee disbanded, voting its remaining assets of $11,222 to the American Medical Education Foundation, an AMA offshoot dedicated to the support of medical schools.

Despite its impact on the AMA, the 1943 Wagner-Murray-Dingell bill did not go anywhere. President Roosevelt, occupied with the conduct of the war, did not endorse it, and it expired in committee. But with the death of President Roosevelt and the succession of President Truman in the spring of 1945, followed by the end of World War II later in the summer, the Congress and the new administration could focus attention once again on domestic legislation that had received a low priority during wartime.

In a message to Congress on November 19, 1945, just two weeks before the annual meeting of the AMA that year,* President Truman swung the full weight of his office behind a national health insurance program. He opened his case with a ringing declaration of human rights. Every American citizen, he said, had "the right to adequate medical care and the opportunity to achieve and enjoy good health." Furthermore, Americans had "the right to adequate protection from the economic fears of sickness." Health is a national concern, he argued; financial barriers should be removed.

He proposed a "system of required prepayment" by everyone to finance "a health fund to be built up nationally." A citizen's payment to this fund would be made through higher Social Security contributions, the earnings base going from $3000 to $3600. There might also be increased taxes, depending on whether Congress contemplated the use of general revenues as well.[24] Simultaneously with the presidential message, Senators Wagner and Murray and Representative Dingell re-introduced their compulsory national health insurance bill. This time they had a powerful new ally at the other end of Pennsylvania Avenue.

As the new year began, President Truman reaffirmed his determination to secure passage of national health insurance. That January, when White House advisor Judge Samuel Roseman removed some strong words supporting health legislation from the draft of his State of the Union message, Truman penciled them back in. He meant business. He instructed the director "to mobilize all the resources within the Federal Security Agency for vigorous and united action towards achieving public understanding of the need for a National Health Program." At one meeting, a White House advisor told an interagency staff meeting, "The whole matter is rather close to the President's heart and he wants to put steam behind it."[25]

Reacting to the second Wagner-Murray-Dingell bill and responding specifically to language used by Senator Wagner in introducing it, Fishbein—with Board of Trustees approval—published another of his widely quoted editorials. He wrote, "No one will ever convince the physicians of the United States that the Wagner-Murray-Dingell bill is not socialized medicine...By this measure doctors in America

---

*It was late because wartime restrictions on travel and the general unavailability of convention facilities made the usual scheduling in June impossible.

would become clock-watchers and slaves of a system."[26] Strong words. But they reflected other actions on government health insurance that had physicians deeply concerned. In England, the National Health Act of 1946, which finally did socialize British medicine, was taking shape. In California, only a vigorous, professionally-managed campaign underwritten by the state medical association headed off Governor Warren's compulsory health bill, defeated in the lower house of the California Assembly by just one vote. Similar legislation for compulsory, state-financed health insurance, usually backed by the politically powerful Congress of Industrial Organizations, was introduced (and defeated) in several other states: Connecticut, Massachusetts, Michigan, New Mexico, New York, Washington, and Wisconsin.[27]

To feel the high emotional heat that already surrounded the compulsory health insurance issue in 1946, one has to look no further than the hearings on the second Wagner-Murray-Dingell bill conducted by Senator James E. Murray (D.-Montana), Chairman of the Education and Labor Committee of the Senate, beginning April 2, 1946. After inserting President Truman's recent State of the Union address in the record and entering copies of correspondence containing suggestions from William Green, president of the American Federation of Labor, Senator Murray embarked on a preamble aimed at keeping discussion in the hearings on a lofty plane.

He began, "I would like at this time to call attention to an editorial in the *Washington Post* this morning which discusses this situation in the country, where people sometimes instead of discussing these [health care] problems intelligently and dealing with the facts, sometimes go outside the facts and attempt to charge that some of these progressive measures that are being advocated in the Senate are communistic or socialistic. I would recommend that everyone read that editorial in the *Post* this morning. I am confident that..."

At this point, Senator Robert A. Taft (R.-Ohio) broke in angrily. He wasted no words.

"I think it is very socialistic," said Taft. "I disagree entirely with the editorial. I think you might have that to start with; if you are going to make a partisan statement, I am going to make one...I consider it [i.e. the Wagner-Murray-Dingell bill] socialism. It is to my mind the most socialistic measure that this Congress has ever had before it, seriously..."

The wrangle continued.

Murray: You had so much gall and so much nerve that you would not let me complete my statement.

Taft: You started it. You started your statement with an attack on the opponents of the bill, and I have a perfect right to reply.

Murray: You have been impertinent and insulting.

Taft: Mr. Chairman, I am not going to attend any more meetings of your committee. We are through, and I think that everyone will know that the report of this committee will be a partisan report which can command no support or respect.[28]

So began the hearings. Taft's walk-out doomed the legislation. He not only held great power over the Republicans in Congress; he also enjoyed the respect and support of many conservative Southern Democrats.

Years later, Odin W. Anderson, Ph.D., a University of Chicago sociologist, wrote, "Unless one was an adult during the 1940s, it is difficult to believe that the polemical battles between the proponents of voluntary health insurance and government health insurance were as intense as actually was the case. Self-righteousness characterized all the groups, not least the AMA hierarchy and the proponents of government health insurance."[29]

Often lost in the angry rhetoric was what President Truman proposed and what the AMA offered in reply. The President's November 19, 1945, message to Congress, the first in United States history to be devoted exclusively to the subject of health, advanced five basic proposals.

With the first—federal aid for the building of hospitals and health centers all over the country—the AMA had no quarrel. In fact, the Board of Trustees had previously approved the principles of this legislation (called the Hill-Burton bill); the house at its December 1945 meeting confirmed that action.

The second, dealing with the extension of maternal and child health services, was involved in a jurisdictional battle in Washington. Should the program, which was once related to early child labor laws, remain under the administration of the Department of Labor? Or should it be transferred to the Federal Security Agency? The AMA said it favored aid to extend such maternal and child health programs, but in this instance it opposed what was suggested because the program envisioned new medical functions that should not be under the jurisdiction of the federal government.

The third dealt with development of a National Science Foundation; this represented a vast, new federal commitment to biomedical research. It was a program that would grow rapidly and have a tremendous impact on American medicine. The AMA reaffirmed its earlier action approving such a foundation now that it was to operate under the direction of a scientific board rather than a single, presidentially appointed director.

The fourth proposal, which called for compulsory national health insurance, was strenuously opposed. The house adopted the sharp words in Fishbein's editorial, the one that called the Wagner-Murray-Dingell bill "socialized medicine" and said it would turn physicians into "clock-watchers" and "slaves of a system." Voluntary prepayment medical plans, said the House of Delegates, would accomplish the major objectives with far less expense and give the public the highest quality of medical care, without regimentation.

On the fifth proposal, compensation for loss of earnings due to sickness, the house, after first supporting the idea, reconsidered and decided to take no action.[30]

The hearings of the Senate Education and Labor Committee on the Wagner-Murray-Dingell bill extended from April into early June. April 16, 1946, was the AMA's day in court; its lead witness was the chairman of the Board of Trustees, Roscoe L. Sensenich, M.D. He submitted the official action of the House of Delegates for the record and then accepted questions from the committee members. Senator Claude D. Pepper (D.-Florida) went after him like a cross-examiner, interrupting, trying to trap him in contradictions. Sensenich barely managed to hold his ground.

Lowell S. Goin, M.D., a California delegate to the AMA but testifying as the president of the California Physicians' Service (Blue Shield), made a more effective witness. He was quicker on his feet, sharper with his answers, and emphatic enough in his statements to avoid the interruptions that hurt Sensenich. His arguments against Wagner-Murray-Dingell were forceful. The need for it, he said, was established more by emotional statements than by logic or documented fact. There was no evidence to demonstrate that it would bring on the health benefits promised. The cost was unpredictable. Factors other than medical care, he pointed out, affected public health in significant ways. Voluntary hospital and medical insurance plans, with which the nation had some experience, were more in the American tradition.

In response to an earlier report by Senator Pepper on the high rate of World War II draft rejections, Goin asked how any medical care system could be expected to correct the defects of the "manifestly disqualified;" that is, men who were missing an arm or a leg or were blind, deaf, or mute. What can medical care do about mental defectives, he asked. He pointed to medicine's inability to prevent congenital conditions such as those leading to hernias and defective vision. He effectively challenged Senator Pepper's argument (one that had also been used by President Truman) that it was a failing of the nation's medical care system that accounted for the high rejection rates.[31]

As medicine's witnesses voiced their doubts and fears regarding compulsory health insurance, Senators Murray and Pepper expressed theirs regarding voluntary insurance plans, saying that these would prove too expensive to attain any sort of wide application.

Chairman Murray also cited a request from William Green, president of the American Federation of Labor, that the financial sources for the public relations campaign against Wagner-Murray-Dingell be investigated. And, indeed, later in the month, Edward H. Cary, M.D., was asked to testify about the National Physicians' Committee's work and funding. While he was candid about the organization's finances, Cary offended the committee and antagonized the Washington press.

As the summer of 1946 wore on, however, the steam began to go out of the drive for national health insurance legislation. A surprising number of other organizations expressed to the senators the same view of national health insurance as the AMA: the American Hospital Association, the American Bar Association; the American Dental Association, the Protestant and Catholic Hospital Associations, the Chamber of Commerce, the National Grange, and others. President Truman, beset with other difficulties, fell silent on the issue. The public remained unaroused; the editorial pages were unsupportive.

That fall Republican candidates for Congress, running under the slogan, "Had Enough?" preyed on the public's weariness with the shortage of consumer goods and the continued wartime controls on wages and prices. When the election returns came in that November, the Republicans had recaptured Congress for the first time since 1932. The AMA thought the cause of national health insurance was as dead as a dodo.

While its external dificulties simmered down, the AMA's internal discords continued to boil. The Californians were still committed to the removal of Fishbein. The Board of Trustees still sparred with the Council on Medical Service and Public Relations. The house was distrustful of the board. The whole problem of leadership was still unresolved.

Shortly before the July 1946 meeting, the report of the outside public relations firm, Raymond T. Rich & Associates, was submitted. This was the report that the board had promised in late 1945, leading the Californians to drop the two resolutions that if adopted would have given the AMA's spokesman role to the Council on Medical Service and Public Relations. The Rich report went first to the executive committee of the board, then to the whole board, and then, in part, to the house.

As such things go, this diagnostic study of the AMA's public policies was remarkably candid. The report recommended first that the AMA re-emphasize its medical-scientific activities. These, said the report, had become lost to view, causing the association to become "widely regarded as primarily concerned at this time with the economic interest of the doctor." Rich thought that Fishbein should be given overall responsibility for upgrading the AMA's scientific public relations and that he should revitalize *Hygeia*, the AMA consumer health magazine. In a dig at Fishbein's output of magazine pieces published elsewhere, Rich recommended that the editor "reserve exclusively for *Hygeia* an appropriate number of his most vivid and popular articles."

Turning to economic matters, Rich urged that the Bureau of Medical Economics be rebuilt. Its activities had dwindled, and there had been no staff director since 1944. To be effective, Rich said, the bureau should be headed not by a physician (Roscoe G. Leland, who directed it from 1931 to 1944, was an M.D.) but by an economist with outstanding credentials. Furthermore, he thought this executive should also develop material for economic sections in *JAMA* and *Hygeia* that would provide, additionally, for the publication of diverse ideas. The report continued, "If minority viewpoints could be given opportunity for expression within the channels of the association, the raison d'etre of many of the separate minority groups would vanish."

As for the public relations operation, Rich saw it as a staff function more than a council function. A new position, executive assistant, responsible directly to the secretary-general manager, was

recommended with emphasis on broadening "the system of interpretation of the association to the public on matters other than
scientific medicine." At the same time, Rich stressed that the AMA
"must deal first and foremost with the needs of the public; second,
with the welfare of the physician."

In appraising the scope of responsibility for the Council on Medical Service and Public Relations, Rich tried to reduce the overlap
between the duties of the council and those of the board. Emphasizing that "the extension of adequate medical service is unquestionably the most urgent task for organized medicine today,"
he advocated an intensive program of professional relations with
state and county societies. To fix the responsibility clearly, he urged
changing the name of the council to the Council for the Extension of
Medical Care and charging it with two main responsibilities: (1)
enlisting medical society support for voluntary medical prepayment
plans; and (2) assisting in the public relations and promotional
aspects of their development.[32]

In transmitting Rich's ideas to the house, the board smoothed
over the rough spots. It questioned the wisdom of Fishbein saving
all his best articles for *Hygeia*. The board said it was already negotiating with a top-notch economist to "reactivate" the Bureau of
Medical Economics. It stated that AMA publications were always
open to diverse opinions. The new name for the council was not
accepted, but the old title was shortened in favor of the name that
exists today, the Council on Medical Service.[33]

What the board submitted to the house at the July 1946 meeting avoided the real bombshell in the Rich report: a recommendation that the AMA break with the National Physicians' Committee.
"With the exception of a few individuals, most of whom were interested parties," the report read, "no one whom we have consulted
has anything favorable to say about the National Physicians' Committee. The charges regarding gross inaccuracies and other inappropriate contents in the committee's publications are too widespread to be ignored."

It was an embarrassing business; it could be delayed but not
buried. Chairman Sensenich went to the house with "something to
suggest which so far as I know has not been previously done." He
wanted a special committee of delegates appointed to meet after
the current meeting adjourned to go over the remaining sixty pages
of the Rich report and "help us in considering the recommendations

made." After some maneuvering in the house, Sensenich got his committee, but California Delegate John W. Green, M.D., raised the question that Sensenich hoped would not come up. Green asked, "How may the membership of this House of Delegates be informed on the information contained in the Rich report so that they may ask intelligent questions with reference to it?" The speaker then said, "I will ask the Chairman of the Board of Trustees to answer that question." Sensenich said he would be happy to do so, though he obviously was not. He said, "I don't think it would be wise for every member of the House of Delegates at any given time to be furnished with a report containing confidential material. If you haven't the confidence in your board and your committee…"

The transcript of the meeting at this point reads, "Exclamations and whistles from the delegates."[34] The delegates felt that the trustees were leading them down the garden path, or treating them like children, or both.

At the meeting in December, the delegates did receive complete copies of the Rich report, along with an analysis by the committee of delegates requested by Chairman Sensenich. The recommendations on the National Physicians' Committee were, however, not acted upon until the June 1947 meeting. At that time the committee announced conclusions precisely opposite to those of Rich. Rather than "no one having anything favorable to say about the NPC," the committee, relying on studies of public attitudes and physician attitudes done by the Opinion Research Corporation, Princeton, New Jersey, interpreted the data to "show a majority favorable to the National Physicians' Committee." The report found that some statements and activities "might not have been dignified or appropriate had they emanated from a scientific body such as the AMA." But they were not out of line from an organization combating "vicious or unfavorable legislation."[35] The report did not, however, enjoy the credibility that it might have, for the group appointed at the request of Sensenich to develop it included Edward H. Cary, M.D., the man who had as much to do with founding and running the National Physicians' Committee as anyone else.

Simultaneously, and not suprisingly, Rich and the AMA parted company. The public relations staff executive recruited by Rich and appointed as the AMA's first executive assistant for public relations resigned too, Rich complaining that the financing for the programs he had originally suggested had been withdrawn.

But the Rich report and the AMA did agree on the need to expand, and expand rapidly, voluntary prepaid medical insurance plans— Blue Shield. The AMA required no prodding. In 1945 the house had, in fact, instructed the board and the council to establish a nation-wide organization for the local plans, and in February 1946 they did so. Standards were adopted, including a guarantee that participants would have a free choice of physician, and an AMA Seal of Acceptance was authorized for plans meeting the standards. An independent new corporation was created under the laws of Illinois, Associated Medical Care Plans, Inc.* It was to act as the accrediting agency for the growing number of physician-sponsored plans, to coordinate their operations, and to establish reciprocity among them so that an employer with nationwide operations and a joint employer-employee health benefits package could use Blue Shield to cover employees in different states. The new organization received $50,000 from the AMA initially, with $25,000 additional voted in the fall to be used as a loan fund to assist state organizations to get plans underway. A division of prepaid medical care plans was also established as an AMA staff unit under the council to promote the concept among physicians and help state medical associations develop the programs.[36]

At the time, an accusation was made by the magazine *Medical Economics* that the board's heart was not really in the drive for voluntary medical insurance, that it was not going to follow through, that it was only paying lip service to the concept. During the executive session of the house in July 1946, the council chairman, Edward J. McCormick, M.D., brought up the charge and answered it. "With all the power that is in me," he said, "I want to say that the council has received fine cooperation from the board...We have had our arguments, of course, but we are friends...They have supported us and we are supporting them...The editorial which had recently appeared is entirely false and without foundation... "[37]

Subsequent events proved McCormick's sincerity. Six months later, at the December meeting, the Council on Medical Service was able to report that so far in 1946, seventeen additional plans had been started in fifteen states. This brought the totals to eighty Blue Shield

*The name was changed to Blue Shield Medical Care Plans, Inc., in 1950 and to the National Association of Blue Shield Plans in 1960. It is now merged with Blue Cross. Though a separate corporation, Associated Medical Care Plans, Inc., was located in the AMA building during its early years.

plans in thirty-three states, with an enrollment nearing five million people.[38] In 1940, there had been only eleven plans.[39]

The war years had given voluntary health insurance an extraordinary boost, especially Blue Cross hospital coverage, which benefited from an earlier start than physician-fee coverage under Blue Shield. The vital contribution came from the National War Labor Board, which had jurisdiction over wartime wage and price controls. Since wages were frozen, union negotiators had little to talk about at contract time except fringe benefits, such as employee health insurance plans. When health insurance benefits were exempted from the strictures on pay increases, the unions could demand employer-financed health insurance plans. These were rapidly established, first through the auto and steel industries, then elsewhere. According to Health Insurance Institute figures, the number of people with private health insurance rose from twelve million in 1940 to more than thirty-two million in 1945.

Later, when the courts ruled that employer payments for employee health insurance premiums could be deducted from tax liabilities as a business expense, private health insurance received what amounted to a federal subsidy. Those decisions established the basic pattern by which health care for most of the working population of the United States would ultimately be financed.

Voluntary health insurance in the immediate post-World War II years was clearly an idea whose time had come. More and more unions pressed for health insurance programs each year, and management did not fight back too strenuously because the cost was deductible as a business expense. Labor liked the health insurance coverage because it was a way to obtain what amounted to a tax-free increase in employee income. Employers found such plans useful in recruiting labor or in holding on to labor in periods of shortage. They also found medical insurance programs good talking points when recruiting people for management jobs.

As a way to finance a growing demand for more hospital and medical services, the concept of voluntary insurance was a characteristically American response. It was locally organized, private, flexible, and respectful of the individual. And it received strong support from diverse sources: from organized medicine, which valued its private character and recognized its political ramifications; from government, which granted tax incentives; and, above all, from the marketplace, where voluntary health insurance won rapid acceptance not only from labor and management but also from patients and physicians.

THE DOCTOR, commissioned by Queen Victoria and painted in the late 19th century by Sir Luke Fildes, became the focal point for two political campaigns to sidetrack the Wagner-Murray-Dingell legislation in the 1940s. It was used first by the National Physicians Committee (a group technically independent of the AMA), then by the AMA. In 1947, it graced a U.S. postage stamp commemorating the AMA's 100th anniversary.

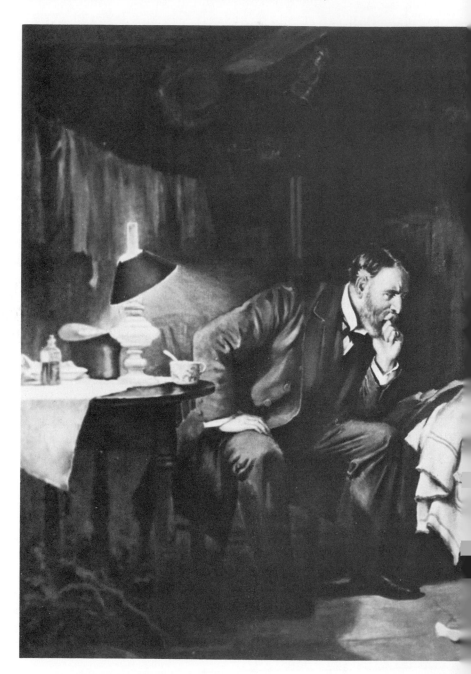

The picture reproduced here is actually a commissioned painting by Joseph Tomanek *after* the Fildes painting, with some minor differences in the details. The orginal Fildes work is in the Tate Gallery, London.

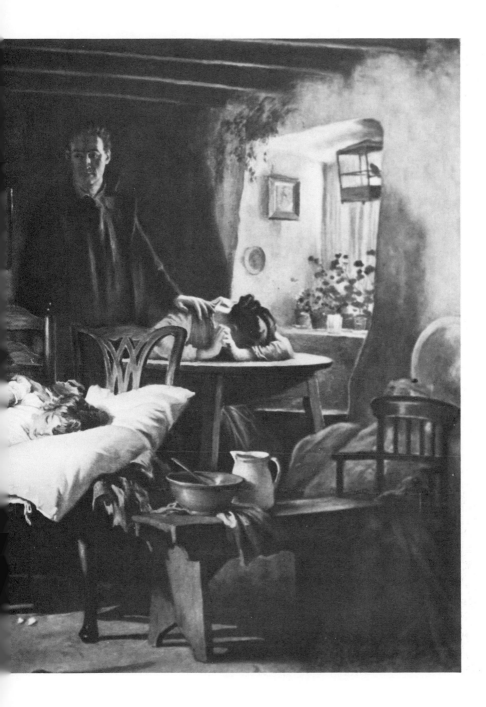

STRATEGIST for the AMA campaign against the Truman health bill in 1949 and 1950 was Clem Whitaker (opposite), shown addressing the House of Delegates. He and his striking, red-headed wife, Leone Baxter, headed the San Francisco-based firm of political consultants, Whitaker and Baxter. They developed hard-hitting materials (this page) for the AMA to distribute and mounted such a successful campaign of endorsements of the AMA position by other organizations (opposite, inset) that chances for passage of the bill, never strong, quickly vanished.

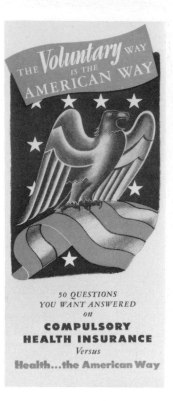

THE *Voluntary* WAY IS THE AMERICAN WAY

50 QUESTIONS YOU WANT ANSWERED on COMPULSORY HEALTH INSURANCE *Versus* Health...the American Way

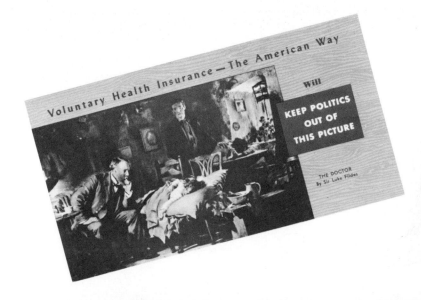

Voluntary Health Insurance — The American Way will KEEP POLITICS OUT OF THIS PICTURE

THE DOCTOR By Sir Luke Fildes

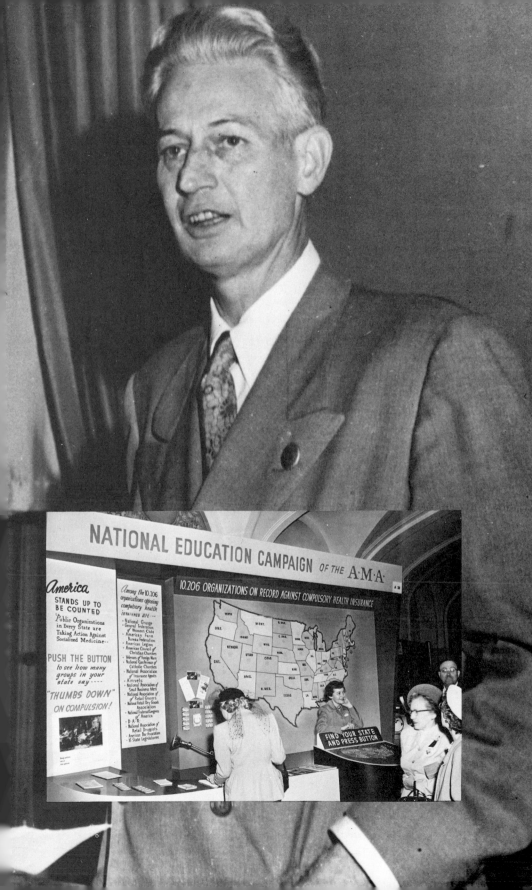

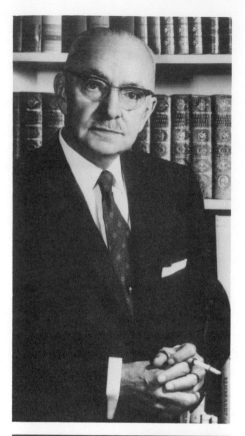

MEDICINE'S SPOKESMEN against the Truman health bills faced a determined U.S. Senate Committee on Education and Labor. It was headed by James E. Murray (D.-Montana), and its leading advocate for health legislation was Claude D. Pepper (D.-Florida). Lowell S. Goin, (top picture), president of the California Physicians Service and a member of the AMA House of Delegates, made a convincing witness against the legislation. Roscoe L. Sensenich, chairman and then president, (below) gave the AMA testimony. Divided over competing health proposals, the committee never did report out a bill.

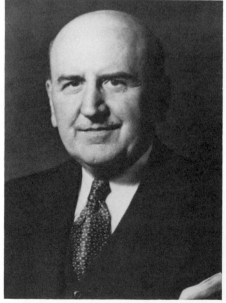

Chapter Eleven

The Nation Makes a Choice

No one thought President Harry S. Truman had a chance to win the 1948 election. Many Southerners, angered by a strong civil rights plank adopted at the Democratic Party Convention, broke away to form a States Rights Party headed by Strom Thurmond. Henry A. Wallace, President Roosevelt's first Secretary of Agriculture and his Vice President from 1940 to 1944, threatened to siphon off liberal votes with his new Progressive Party. But the main factor in the pre-election evaluations, in the experts' opinion, was that few people considered Truman anything but an interim president. The Republican ticket, headed by Thomas E. Dewey and Earl Warren, was regarded as a shoo-in by virtually every poll and politician.

Refusing to accept the early verdicts, Truman stubbornly climbed aboard his private railroad car, the Ferdinand Magellan, and whistle-stopped across the country, denouncing with masterful demagoguery the record of what he labeled the "do nothing" Republican Congress elected in 1946. He urged everyone to "go out and vote yourself a Fair Deal," a package of social benefits that included a program of compulsory national health insurance.

What happened, of course, was the most spectacular political upset in United States history. And it was regarded in some quarters as something more than that. Conservatives and many moderates had expected a broad disavowal of the leftward trend that United States domestic policy had taken after 1932. Now the possibility arose that a doctrine of expanding federal powers might be permanently in place. In its 1948 Man of the Year cover story—the subject was Truman—the politically moderate *Time* magazine described the federal government as "a modern, bureaucratic Great White Father," protecting the helpless, regulating business, guaranteeing full employment, and bringing security to the farmer and the worker, the old and the sick. According to the analysis in the cover story, in 1948, "the United States wanted a man who believed in [that] doctrine. It rejected the party which it suspected of wanting to change it."[1]

If the 1948 election surprised the media, it stunned the AMA. Along with a Democratic Congress once more, the country now had a president elected to office after committing himself to a compulsory national health insurance plan. Overnight, a threat that the AMA thought it had safely bottled two years earlier had burst loose again.

As the delegates assembled in St. Louis late that November, only three weeks after the fateful election, a sense of cheerless resolve hung over the meeting. The speaker, F.F. Borzell, M.D., took the occasion in his opening remarks to say, "I approach this, the third interim session...with prayerful contemplation." The Board of Trustees in a mood of backs-to-the-wall defiance volunteered "the expenditure of the AMA's total funds if need be to oppose the enslavement of the medical profession."[2]

Swinging into action, the House of Delegates began by adopting a platform for the AMA counterattack. Proposed by E. Vincent Askey, M.D., a California delegate, and approved by the house, a statement of policy reaffirmed the AMA's position. It stressed the association's belief in "the principle of medical care insurance on a voluntary basis" and described how the AMA had "encouraged and assisted the development of voluntary prepayment plans." It referred to the high quality of American medicine, the high level of health enjoyed by Americans, attributing those conditions to "a free profession working under a free system." It firmly rejected compulsory national health insurance as "a variety of socialized medicine."[3]

Looking specifically to the battle ahead, the house voted to expand the AMA Washington office, to assess each member $25 in 1949, and to engage the services of an outside public relations firm to help devise and execute a political strategy. Ernest B. Howard, M.D., who was present as the AMA assistant secretary-general manager, recalled thirty years later, "That was the year we went to war with Truman."[4]

As a figure of speech, the metaphor is not entirely wide of the mark. On both sides, the commitments ran deep. The emotional intensity of the disagreement had reached an uncomfortable high. The language, already tough, had grown harsh. Worse, each side nursed an unyielding suspicion as to the motives of the other. In a revealing moment, Senator Claude D. Pepper (D.-Florida), addressing a medical audience in Jacksonville, Florida, said, "I will not accuse you of being selfish and acting out of pecuniary motives if you will not accuse me of being a socialist and acting out of sheer political motives."[5]

Ranged against the AMA was an assortment of antagonists. Of these, the weakest, at least in terms of numbers, were two physician groups: the Physicians Forum with maybe 1,000 members, and the Committee of Physicians for the Improvement of Medical Care, with fewer than 100 members.[6] Yet both had their uses, for they represented an influential body of opinion in the Eastern medical teaching establishment, and they enabled the advocates of compulsory national health insurance to say, "Not all doctors agree with the AMA. Physicians are divided on the issue." The existence of the two groups constituted a burr under the AMA's saddle, for the AMA placed great emphasis on a united front.

The organization that was big and powerful and well-financed— the organization that led the public battle for the Wagner-Murray-Dingell bills—was the Committee for the Nation's Health. It was headed by an energetic staff director, Michael M. Davis, Ph.D., and drew much of its financial support from Mrs. Albert D. (Mary) Lasker, whose husband had accumulated a fortune as owner of the advertising agency that exists today as Foote, Cone & Belding. Both the Congress of Industrial Organizations and the American Federation of Labor (they had not yet combined) energetically supported the Committee for the Nation's Health. The American Federation of Labor's director of social insurance, Nelson H. Cruikshank, was especially active.

But the real push came from the federal government, specifically from the Federal Security Agency (forerunner of the Department of Health, Education, and Welfare) and its chief, Oscar R. Ewing. Both Ewing and his agency were committed to compulsory national health insurance, and in pursuit of that goal their zeal outmatched anything that came from the White House.[7] Federal Security Agency staff members helped draft the legislation and create the congressional testimony; they developed the arguments and they wrote the resource document—the major propaganda instrument—stating the case for a national compulsory health insurance bill. This took the form of a 186-page report, "The Nation's Health—A Ten-Year Program," issued in September 1948 and known as the Ewing report. Prepared at the President's request, it stated that the United States suffered from a shortage of doctors, that few Americans had the ability to pay for needed care, and that Congress must enact a system of compulsory prepayment health insurance to finance the care needed.

It was, in the understated phrase of Frank G. Dickinson, Ph.D., the then recently appointed director of the AMA's reconstituted Bureau of Medical Economic Research, "a semantic document." In congressional testimony later, Lowell S. Goin, M.D., representing the California Physicians Service, questioned the most sweeping claim in the Ewing report—that new health policies could save 325,000 lives a year.[8] He told the Senate Committee on Labor and Public Welfare, "Mr. Ewing begins with a dramatic statement." But, he argued, the figure seems to be chosen at random, with "no documentation offered." He went on to point out that actually 40,000 fewer Americans had died of communicable diseases in 1947 than in 1945, a statistical oversight that he regarded as not entirely accidental. Dickinson, a long-time economist at the University of Illinois, wrote a friend, "In all my twenty-five years of teaching, I have never had a sophomore student make a poorer case than did Mr. Ewing on the question of the shortage of physicians."[9]

But Ewing had powerful channels open to him. His office alone gave him a platform for frequent speeches, and he used it aggressively. At a convention of state health officers, for example, he asked representatives from across the nation to get behind the administration plan for national health insurance. He said, "Every community must organize its own committees to analyze the plan in relation to its own community resources and community needs. The committees must establish liaison with similarly organized state groups under your leadership charged with coordinating these resources and meeting demonstrated needs in a statewide program.

"Equally important is the need to start, now, a state and local campaign of education to explain the scope and purpose of the plan..."[10]

At the time, much was said about the money that the National Physicians' Committee and the AMA were spending in the publicity fight against the Truman plan—how much was being lavished on pamphlets, speakers bureaus, and newspaper advertisements. Compared to what the Committee for the Nation's Health spent, organized medicine's budget was indeed massive. But it should be emphasized that the AMA was contending with a far more formidable adversary, namely the propaganda capability of a large agency of the federal government. Much criticism was leveled at the AMA for its "swollen" war chest, its "power" as a lobby. Only rarely was attention focused on what it was up against. In an unusual editorial, the *St. Louis Globe-Democrat* made the point, calling the Federal Security Agency to account for using taxpayer money and taxpayer resources to sell the public on an unmistakably partisan proposition. Said the editorial:

> Ewing has gone all out on a lobbying expedition against the lobbying plans of the AMA against socialized medicine. Though the ethics would seem to decree that he stick to his legal chores, he is feverishly denouncing the AMA's frantic taxation of the members to finance the greatest lobbying effort in history. Curiously, he is condemning others for the kind of congressional pressure for which his and other social reform departments have long been noted...
>
> This appears to be the beginning of a gigantic compulsory health insurance campaign which Ewing is reported coordinating...But won't such a campaign be expensive? If so, whose slush fund is Ewing coordinating? Or will the work be done by regular FSA and Public Health Service employees whose salaries are paid by taxpayers who oppose as well as favor socialized medicine?[11]

In a situation of this sort, where private and governmental forces oppose each other, the government has an edge that is not always acknowledged. In making its case before the public, a private organization has to raise funds, hire people, generate publicity, take out advertisements. It becomes conspicuous as it develops and operates what its opponents invariably attack as a "slush fund" to finance a propaganda drive. The government, on the other hand, can avoid such adverse publicity. The people it needs for an opinion battle are already at work in the appropriate governmental agencies: the researchers, the statisticians, the writers, the polemicists, the public opinion experts.[12] What's more, the spokesmen for the government position, already occupying public office, can use their office to attract news coverage; they enjoy an *ex officio* assurance of audiences and attention.

Moreover, the pre-Viet Nam, pre-Watergate press especially would often concede the government a *pro bono publico* motivation almost as a matter of course. Because we had a government "of" the people, the argument went, how could we have anything but a government "for" the people? The press had (and still has) an in-built suspicion of the motives of a trade association, a corporation, or any other sort of private group with an interest in legislation. The government, by contrast, often enjoys the benefit of the doubt, at least initially. And almost invariably, those organizations that choose to battle out a public issue of which the government takes the opposing side come away from the fight with their credibility sharply questioned and, at times, damaged by the media's inclination to be more trusting of the governmental statements and more suspicious of the private, or "interest group," viewpoint.

The instrument chosen by the AMA to organize its opposition to compulsory national health insurance came tailormade. Not only had the San Franciso-based political public relations firm of Whitaker and Baxter worked successfully with the California Medical Association in 1945 to turn back Governor Warren's proposal for statewide compulsory health insurance; its principals, Clem Whitaker and his wife, Leone Baxter, were shrewd enough to see beyond the labels that were being flung about and to identify the political factors that would ultimately mean votes.

At first Whitaker and Baxter refused the assignment.[13] For one thing it would mean moving their operation to Chicago; for another, it would disrupt their immediate plans for a trip to Bermuda. But in New York a telephone call from one of the trustees, John W. Cline, M.D., caught up to them. Cline, who as a delegate had urged the resignation of Morris Fishbein, was a friend from the days when the California Medical Association used Whitaker and Baxter to fight Governor Warren's bill, and he was now a member of the recently appointed ten-man AMA Coordinating Committee for a National Education Campaign on National Health Insurance. "You've got to take this job," Cline insisted. "It's the same as if a patient asked me for treatment in an emergency and I said no." Leone Baxter said, "We couldn't turn him down after that." The AMA paid Whitaker and Baxter an annual fee of $100,000. Expenditures for the National Education Campaign (which included the fee) amounted to $1.6 million in 1949, $2.6 million in 1950, $530,000 in 1951, and $255,000 in 1952.*

Whitaker and Baxter had a fifteen-year record in California political campaigning that could be matched by no one else: fifty-eight

*In 1950, it might be noted, the AMA started a fund to aid the medical schools. The AMA voted $500,000 from the money raised by the 1949 assessment—just under 20 percent of the total—to this fund, following up the initial gift with half million dollar donations to the medical schools in each of the following three years.

wins to five losses. They had helped Earl Warren into the Governor's Mansion in Sacramento in 1942 and then turned around and beat him on his health bill in 1945. Whitaker and Baxter obviously had a special talent, embracing some political theories that are widely accepted today but ahead of their time in the 1940s.

As a reporter covering the state legislature in Sacramento after World War I, Whitaker could study the political process as it really worked. "His acid observation on the quality of the California Assemblyman," writes the political expert Theodore H. White, "led him to think that, on the whole, it would be cheaper to influence politics by mobilization at the grass roots than by buying votes retail, one by one, as was then the practice of California state lobbyists…" Carey McWilliams, another political analyst, said the same thing in a slightly different way. He wrote, "In the book of Whitaker and Baxter, it says that lobbying is a waste of time and money because it is inconclusive. Not only is the composition of the legislature always changing, but legislatures are like women—you have to keep buying them candy and flowers. But a campaign won as a public issue will stay won—for some years at least."[14] Whitaker and Baxter were early believers in direct democracy; they felt that if you could sway the opinions of the electorate you could command the votes you needed in a legislature. Lobbying in the ordinary sense was not for them; marshaling public opinion was.

The battle lines came down sharply in early 1949. In January, President Truman proclaimed, "In a nation as rich as ours, it is a shocking fact that tens of millions lack adequate medical care. We need— and we must have without further delay—a system of prepaid medical insurance." The system must be national and compulsory, he added, and it must be financed through Social Security taxes. Two or three weeks later, in early February, addressing a meeting of AMA and state medical society leaders in Chicago, Clem Whitaker stated the position of the physicians. "The doctors of this country are in the front lines today of a basic struggle…between socialism and private initiative…Oscar Ewing, the great patent medicine man…apparently is grimly determined to bring socialized medicine from sick England to healthy America."

Though it had fueled countless demagogic fires during the early decades of the twentieth century, the word socialism carried a particularly high octane rating in the late 1940s, for this was when

McCarthyism began. It was a time of suspicion and fear, when foreign agents were stealing America's atomic secrets, when American Communist Party leaders were charged with conspiring to overthrow the government, when magazine editor Whittaker Chambers accused a former high State Department officer, Alger Hiss, of having given secret documents to Soviet agents.

During the 1947 hearings on national health insurance, Marjorie Shearon, Ph.D., a former employee in the Public Health Service and the Federal Security Agency who had turned health consultant to the Republicans, unleashed a stream of charges accusing her former employers, particularly the Federal Security Agency's Isidore S. Falk, of a conspiracy to nationalize American medicine. It was headline material that intensified the emotional heat surrounding the health insurance issue, and it even caused the Congress to set up a subcommittee under Republican Congressman Forest A. Harness of Indiana to investigate lobbying, subversion, and propagandizing conducted by the executive branch of the federal government.

Ewing, the Federal Security Administrator, found the charge of socialism especially irritating. When an AMA president in a *JAMA* article accused his agency of favoring socialism, Ewing hit the roof and demanded evidence. Citing a government pamphlet, "Common Human Needs," issued over his name, the AMA directed his attention to the statement: "Social security and public assistance programs are a basic essential for attainment of the socialized state envisaged in a democratic ideology, a way of life which so far has been realized only in slight measure." Ewing bit his tongue and ordered the pamphlet withdrawn.[15] The tag socialized medicine was an old one and, as a propaganda weapon, an effective one. But while Whitaker and Baxter intended to take full advantage of it, an attack on "socialism" constituted only one element of their overall strategy.

With cool efficiency, Whitaker and Baxter made the necessary moves. They transferred their San Francisco headquarters into rented space at 1 South LaSalle Street, Chicago, a fifteen-minute walk from the AMA offices, and engaged a staff that grew to thirty-five people. They developed hard-hitting campaign literature. "Words that lean on the mind are no good," Whitaker used to explain, "They must *dent* it." Whitaker and Baxter made sure that the whole county-state-national structure of the AMA entered the fight, noting, "People are more interested in politics than ever before, but their interest is an after hours interest...To attract their attention you must put on a fight or a show or both."

Whitaker and Baxter revived the famous Fildes painting, "The Doctor," the one showing the deeply worried physician hunched over the seriously ill child. In the background of the dimly-lit scene in a modest cottage, the emotionally torn father stands beside the grief-stricken mother. Carrying the same sort of emotional punch that a Norman Rockwell *Saturday Evening Post* illustration could generate, "The Doctor" adorned pamphlets and booklets; it was distributed as a poster for display in 65,000 physician reception rooms; it was reproduced on a gigantic banner and displayed at AMA meetings.* And across it ran the urgent charge, "Keep politics out of this picture!"

Whitaker and Baxter had no gift of humor, little appreciation for subtlety. As a matter of professional conviction, they dealt in hammer blows, repeated hammer blows. Hard-sell marked their ads, the pamphlets they prepared, the speeches they wrote. They simplified the issues; they emotionalized them; often they exaggerated and overstated them.

The typical Whitaker and Baxter touch can be seen in the inaugural address given by AMA President Elmer L. Henderson, M.D., on June 27, 1950. First of all, to get the AMA message to the public—at the very least to the physician public—Whitaker and Baxter alertly bought time on two national radio hookups and then scheduled the speech (the annual meeting was in San Francisco that year) for 6 p.m. Pacific Coast Time—drive-time in the West, prime listening time in the Midwest and East. The cost, $16,500, was a bargain.[16] Much of what Henderson had to say about medical progress was believable and effective. But the speech was laced with the sort of language that brought the performance down to the pitchman's level. Henderson said, "American medicine has become the blazing focal point in a fundamental struggle which may determine whether America remains free or whether we are to become a socialist state...Never will our people accept the socialist program that grasping men in our government have planned for them."[17]

That sort of language is, at best, pompous overstatement, a rhetorical pitfall that Whitaker and Baxter appeared to seek rather than avoid. They liked to claim that government health insurance bills constituted a first step toward totalitarianism. They did not hesitate to decorate their pamphlets with pealing Liberty Bells, to wrap their arguments in the flag, to threaten that President Truman

*In 1981 the AMA was still receiving two or three requests a year for the picture.

was going to bring the unpleasantness of the Army's "sick call" to the whole population and put a politician "between you and your doctor."

But the misdeeds of Whitaker and Baxter, their claims and exaggerations, did not go beyond the bounds of acceptable political hyperbole. Certainly they did no worse than President Truman, who fallaciously made political hay out of the rates with which draftees were found medically unfit for service in World War II, or those of Oscar Ewing, the Federal Security Administrator, who claimed that new legislation could prevent 325,000 deaths every year. Whitaker and Baxter avoided the viciousness that characterized the material generated by the National Physicians' Committee. The Whitaker and Baxter campaign probably had the intended effect on the public. But unfortunately for the AMA, it antagonized the press and affronted important segments of medical academia.

Whitaker and Baxter were careful to heed Rule Number Eight on their list of fifty campaign dicta: "You can't beat something with nothing." At the kickoff of their campaign in Chicago in February 1949, Whitaker came down hard on the need for private, voluntary health insurance—Blue Cross and Blue Shield—as an alternative to compulsory national health insurance. "We want everybody in the health insurance field selling insurance as he never sold it before," he told the medical leaders. "If we can get ten million more people insured in the next year and ten million more in the next year, the threat of socialized medicine in this country will be over."[18] Sales did not move quite that briskly. But a trend was unmistakable; the number of persons covered by Blue Cross/Blue Shield and medical society plans more than doubled, from 18,899,000 to 38,822,000, between year-end 1945 and year-end 1950.[19] The Whitaker and Baxter slogan, "The Voluntary Way Is the American Way," proved to be less of a claim than a statement of what was actually taking place.

But the key to Whitaker and Baxter's strategy was their endorsement campaign, conducted with breath-taking speed and unflagging energy. The point was to convince lawmakers as quickly as possible that many groups and many political constituencies besides the AMA thought that the voluntary approach to health insurance was more desirable than a governmental, compulsory approach. What persuaded Whitaker and Baxter to pursue this aspect of their campaign was a simple fact of legislative life, interest group politics. Then (and before and after) American political theory perceived the electorate to be multi-group in nature, with the major

groups easily identifiable: union members, farmers, small businessmen, property owners, young parents, senior citizens, veterans, ethnic groups, and so on. The way to govern, went the theory, was to
accommodate the various claims of the interest groups in as fric-
tionless, painless, and unobtrusive a manner as possible. The legitimacy of the claims could be largely ignored; what counted was the
potential impact at the polls. "Politics," observed Sidney Hillman,
who founded the political arm of the Congress of Industrial Organizations not long before, "is the science of how who gets what, when
and why."

Fully understanding the game, Whitaker and Baxter played their
cards like masters. At the AMA's meeting in June 1949, as their
campaign was moving into high gear, the House of Delegates received a report that their firm had contacted:

    12,000 trade associations
     2,700 chambers of commerce
       500 civic clubs
       120 advertising clubs
     1,500 Kiwanis clubs
     4,500 Lions clubs
     2,300 Rotary clubs
     1,300 Carnegie libraries
       900 college libraries
     8,000 public libraries
    14,000 school principals and superintendents
     9,000 YMCA city associations
       200 YWCA city associations
   130,000 dentists and druggists

Speaking to the House of Delegates, Whitaker could legitimately
claim, "Medicine isn't fighting alone now. This is rapidly becoming
a great public crusade and a fundamental fight for freedom. The
American Farm Bureau Federation, the American Legion, and the
American Bar Association, the National Grange, the National Association of Small Businessmen, the National Fraternal Congress with
its hundreds of lodges, and the General Federation of Women's
Clubs with its five million members—these are just a few of the
powerful public organizations which have taken their stand beside
American medicine in this battle."[20] As they usually did after the
spell-binding oratory of Whitaker (or his stunningly beautiful wife)

the delegates rose to their feet and cheered.* At the same time, congressmen were impressed. The alignment of major groups behind national compulsory health insurance legislation seemed to be thinner and thinner.

The endorsement strategy of Whitaker and Baxter was something that Fishbein probably never understood, for he was a crusader at heart rather than a pragmatist. That is to say, he would have kept on making his "socialism" arguments (which were effective), content to pit the "justice" of the physicians' case against the "justice" of the claims advanced by various interest groups for govenment-paid medical care. Fishbein's approach made for fiery editorials; it created a glowing aura for a righteous crusade. But it was not realistic politics.

In retrospect, it probably made little difference who conducted the AMA campaign in 1949 or whose strategy was followed. The truth of the matter—in the perspective of thirty years' hindsight, to be sure—is that the 1949-50 AMA effort was an exercise in overkill. Ernest B. Howard, M.D., the number two staff man at the time and later the executive vice president, felt that the board was stampeded. "It overreacted to Harry Truman's election," he said in a 1979 interview. "The votes for a compulsory health insurance bill were never there. There was no chance that Congress would ever have adopted the proposal...Given the job they were given, Whitaker and Baxter did a superb job. They collected hundreds of resolutions from all over the country. They killed any possibility of legislation."[21]

Especially now, it is hard to reconcile the forlorn prospects for passage of the bill with the ongoing enthusiasm of its adherents and the unrelenting opposition of its adversaries. Like its predecessors in 1943, 1945, and 1947, this proposal for compulsory health insurance didn't even generate enough backing to be reported out by a Senate or House committee. It wasn't just the AMA that opposed the bill, or those solicited by Whitaker and Baxter for endorsement of the AMA position. Most of the press opposed the bill, including the *New York Times*. The Brookings Institution, less liberal then than now but equally influential, thought it would introduce politics into

---

*Hugh H. Hussey, M.D., then a delegate, said in a 1979 interview, "Those standing ovations in the house did not reflect what Whitaker and Baxter did so much as their ability to give an overwhelmingly dramatic speech. They really were the type who could sell refrigerators to Eskimos."

medicine and raise costs. A Gallup poll indicated that the public preferred other solutions to the problem.[22] And even President Truman neglected to give it highest priority. The national health insurance bill, S. 1679, was ticketed as a bill with which the President was "generally in accord." But it did not bear the stamp of an administration bill.

And there was disagreement within the Senate Labor and Public Welfare Committee, lots of it. In addition to Senator Taft's conservative proposal, there were two middle-of-the-road bills, the Flanders-Ives proposal and the Hill-Aiken bill. With the loyalties of the committee members distributed among all four, Senator Murray was never close to having the votes to get his bill reported out by the committee. Actually, the legislation that stood the best chance of all was the Hill-Aiken bill, which had the support of the American Hospital Association and proposed subsidies to states so that they might help pay the premiums for private insurance plans (like Blue Cross) for the indigent. One authority speculates that if Truman had been willing to settle his differences with Southern congressmen (a softer line on civil rights?) and shift his backing to the Hill-Aiken bill, he might indeed have achieved a significant extension of medical care to the population of the United States during his administration.[23] But, presumably, Truman's commitment to labor and other segments of the liberal constituency that had elected him permitted no retreat from his position in favor of a national compulsory health insurance bill.

Nevertheless, for reasons of ideology and doctrine, of sincerity and zeal, a highly emotional brawl between voluntary and compulsory health insurance advocates extended from early 1949 through most of 1950, moderating after the outbreak of the Korean War on June 25. Whitaker and Baxter plunged ahead with their well-financed, hard-nosed campaign. The Federal Security Agency, the Committee for the Nation's Health, and labor fought back.

One night in February 1949 someone broke into the deserted AMA building in Chicago at the time of the trustees' meeting, rifled the trustees' briefcases and searched the board files but took nothing. No one was caught, though the AMA considered "labor" the culprit.

In the fall of 1949, J. Howard McGrath, the United States Attorney General and a supporter of the Wagner-Murray-Dingell bill, decided to contribute a little muscle. He notified the AMA through an assistant, "In connection with an investigation by this Department of

Justice of alleged violations of the antitrust laws in the medical field, it is requested that you make available for examination by the bearer, an agent of the Federal Bureau of Investigation, such of your files as he may request." It was revealed that fourteen county or state medical societies were also under investigation for antitrust violations, along with Michigan Blue Shield.

Thus, beginning in October 1949 and extending into April 1950, peak months in the AMA's campaign against the administration's compulsory national health insurance proposal—FBI agents prowled through the AMA, pulling documents from the files and selecting some 14,000 for microfilming. Since nothing further ever came of this investigation of alleged antitrust violations, it is hard to characterize it as anything but an attempt to intimidate.[24]

While the propaganda battle raged—and it was a noisy one—scarcely anyone noticed that the legislation itself was dying a slow death. The wounds were multiple. There was a damaging split within the Senate Labor and Public Welfare Committee, nearly fatal by itself. There was the thinness of public support. There was the opposition of the AMA and its allies.

The fatal stab came in the form of congressional opposition to Oscar R. Ewing, mainly because he had established himself as the administration's flugelman for the forces for compulsory health insurance. In August 1949 the Senate voted down 60-32 a governmental reorganization plan which would have elevated the Federal Security Agency to departmental status, on a par with the Departments of Agriculture, State, Justice, the Treasury, and so forth. In speaking against the reorganization plan, Senator John McClellan (D.-Arkansas), said that if it were not defeated the Federal Security Agency's elevation would "lend impetus to and greatly augment efforts of high government officials to force acceptance of [socialized medicine] through the prestige and power of a cabinet office." Just about a year later, in July 1950, the House of Representatives considered the question of promoting the Federal Security Agency to departmental status, and the House voted against it, 249-71. As in the Senate, the debate focused on the possible dangers of Oscar R. Ewing's promotion to cabinet rank.[25]

The issue of national compulsory health insurance lingered on through the last of the Truman administration, entirely dependent on respiratory machines and other artificial support measures. It is difficult to pinpoint the actual moment of death. Possibly it took place in Springfield, Illinois, one day in August 1952 when Governor Adlai E. Stevenson, the newly nominated Democratic candidate for the presidency, held his first major press conference following his nomination. The Washington and New York reporters crowded him, trying to discover where he stood vis a vis General Eisenhower, the newly nominated Republican candidate, and President Truman, the retiring Democratic President. Would he continue the New Deal? Did he represent a different philosophy? Would he put his own personal stamp on his presidency if elected? The reporters reached out in all directions. "Did he favor the Truman national health program?" one of them asked. "No," Stevenson said, and that seemed to be the end of it. There weren't even any follow-up questions.[26]

Some of those who write popular books about the AMA emphasize a negative picture of the organization, accusing it of acting contrary to the majority opinion of the profession and thwarting the will of the public. Authors who are themselves convinced that a nation's health problems will yield only to compulsory government health insurance are particularly wedded to this viewpoint. In tones that range from scorn to disbelief, such authors point out, correctly, that the United States is the only industrialized nation in the world without some form of national compulsory health insurance, attributing this lapse in our otherwise praiseworthy social development to the unfairly concentrated power of the medical profession rather than the public's wishes as expressed through Congress. It may therefore be useful to restate briefly the major medical decisions of the 1940-50 decade and appraise the role the AMA played in them.

On the matter of facilities—the post-World War II expansion and modernization of our medical care plant—the AMA backed the Hill-Burton legislation that financed new hospitals and clinics through federal assistance to the states. A massive refurbishing was badly needed, for little had been built throughout the pinched years of the Depression or during the war years when national priorities lay elsewhere. On the expansion of federally financed biomedical research—the start of the National Science Foundation, the additional National Institutes of Health, government support for scientific study done at the medical schools, hospitals, and foundations—the AMA again took a positive position, once its early fears about control by political figures were allayed.[27] The AMA gave its blessing to the new emphasis on more extended graduate medical education while continuing its traditional insistence on the highest standards of medical training. (The increase in the number of medical schools and the number of physicians are more issues of the 1950s, and they are dealt with in the following chapter.)

The AMA cannot and does not claim to have designed or created the system by which Americans receive and finance their medical care. No one can make that claim, largely because the system is so diverse, so pluralistic. Within it, for example, is a state-run medical system, the Veterans Administration, which is about the size of Sweden's entire medical system, and just about every other kind of medical system you can name. There is no denying that in the 1930s the AMA, often in conjunction with county or state medical societies, adopted attitudes that ranged from skepticism to opposition to various forms of group practice and voluntary health insurance. But that stand, as we have seen, had moderated at least by 1942 and probably well before that.

In concentrating on the AMA opposition to the Wagner-Murray-Dingell proposals for national compulsory health insurance, it is all too easy to exclude from the mind everything but the negative position of the association and the negative actions of the various congressional committees—or, more accurately, their non-actions. What is easily overlooked in the congressional unwillingness to enact national health insurance legislation is that sometime between 1945 and 1950 the United States, in effect, *did* come to a basic consensus as to the way it preferred to finance medical care. Americans decided that in future years they wanted to finance medical costs, at least for the employed, self-supporting population, through private insurance rather than through out-of-pocket payments, which had been the practice. They decided further that they wanted a method of financing that insofar as possible would remain under private, rather than federal, control.

Because of its opposition to the Wagner-Murray-Dingell bills and its role in developing and promoting non-profit, voluntary medical and hospital insurance, organized medicine exerted an unmistakable influence on the direction in which the system developed. But while the AMA influence was strong, it was by no means exclusive. The hospitals and the medical schools, the unions and industry, the government and insurance companies (profit and non-profit), all contributed.

The public's decision on the type of medical care system it preferred was not the sort of decision that falls into the classic mold. That is to say, it did not have the "decisiveness" of General Eisenhower going with the temporary break in the weather and launching the D-Day invasion, or of President Kennedy weighing his options and then telling Khrushchev to take his missiles out of Cuba.

The character of our medical care system was, rather, created by a marketing decision—the ultimate effect of millions and millions of individual preferences. It was, in fact, the kind of decision that has determined many of the characteristics of the American way of life: our reliance on the personal automobile, for instance, or our preference for shopping in supermarkets, or our inclination to read morning rather than afternoon newspapers.

Although the AMA was more vociferous than anyone else on the question, few groups or individuals really wanted the Wagner-Murray-Dingell bills. The exceptions were a hard core of adherents, many of them leaders in organized labor. In its protest against the legislation, the AMA neither contravened the wishes of the profession (Table 1) nor frustrated the wishes of the public (Table 2).

Opinion polls and politics aside, what were the key arguments made for and against the Wagner-Murray-Dingell bills? How valid was the logic underlying the cases developed by the opposing sides?

The major document of the Truman administration was the Ewing report, prepared within the Federal Security Agency. This report was released just two months before the 1948 elections, and it suffered from the weaknesses of any political campaign document. It made three major points: (1) by the better application of existing medical science, 325,000 deaths per year were currently "preventable"; "GOAL: KEEP THEM LIVING," urged the headline; (2) there was a shortage of doctors; (3) only a system of compulsory government health insurance could eliminate the economic barriers between the sick and medical care, could provide the sort of access that would eradicate national health problems.

The Ewing report was long on claims and packed with figures, but its authors often failed in their attempts to connect the two. Talking, for example, about the number of accidental deaths per year, then 100,000, the report claimed that 40,000 could be prevented. But just how this 40 percent drop was to be accomplished through changes in the medical system was not clearly explained. As for the 325,000 "preventable" deaths, the report severely hedged its own claim. Read the report, "It is, of course, impossible to arrive at any precise estimate of the exact number of people whose lives we could save every year." To support its most dramatic claim, the Ewing report offered no scientific documentation.[28]

Those advocating the Wagner-Murray-Dingell bill argued that the wider availability of medical services offered a direct route to improved health. They chose not to consider other and often more im-

TABLE 1
Survey of Opinions of Physicians on the Wagner-Murray-Dingell Bill, 1945 and 1947

Are you familiar with the Wagner-Murray-Dingell Bill which proposes to set up a federal medical care program to be paid for out of increased social security payroll deductions?

	1945	1947
Yes, am familiar	86%	91%
No, am not.........................	14	9

From the standpoint of the general public, do you think passage of this bill or some similar bill will be a good thing or bad thing?

	1945	1947
Good thing for the public	13%	11%
Bad thing.........................	75	78
Some ways good, some ways bad....	10	10
No opinion........................	2	1

From the standpoint of the doctors of the country, do you think passage of this bill or some similar bill would be a good or bad thing?

	1945	1947
Good thing for doctors	13%	9%
Bad thing.........................	76	81
Some ways good, some ways bad....	9	3
No opinion........................	3	3

Source: *Opinions of the Public and of Physicians*, a report prepared for the Medical Services Foundation based on data from nationwide surveys done by the Opinion Research Corporation of Princeton, New Jersey, and submitted to the Centennial Assembly of the AMA House of Delegates, June, 1947.

TABLE 2
Surveys of Opinions of the Public on the Financing of Medical Care, 1943, 1945, 1947

Do you think anything might be done to make it easier for people to pay doctor or hospital bills?

	Something might be done	No	Don't know
Total 1943	63%	11%	26%
Total 1945	71	12	17
Total 1947	70	9	21

What especially (do you think might be done)?

Respondents who think something might be done to make payment of doctor bills easier:	1943	1945	1947
Number	3238	1142	1402
Percent of total...................	63%	71%	70%
Prepaid medical care or hospitalization or insurance of some kind	39%	41%	44%
Compulsory government insurance, deducted from wages so everyone will be covered.................	8	3	8
Monthly payments; doctors and hospitals should use installment plan	6	8	5
Prices doctors charge should be controlled; should be ceiling prices............................	3	3	5
Welfare or charity agencies should take care of those who can't afford it......................	2	3	3
Teach people to save for a "rainy day"........................	2	2	2
Raise wages.........................	*	*	1
Borrowing plan.......................	*	*	1
Other ways	1	4	3
Could give no way....................	4	4	3

*Not mentioned, or mentioned too few times to warrant separate category. Percentages add to more than totals shown because of multiple answers.

Source: See Table 1.

portant factors that affect health: diet, sanitation, housing, genetics, environment, economic well-being, health habits, and so on. In his pleas for the legislation, President Truman kept referring to the high rejection rates for men drafted for service in World War II as proof that a new system of medical care was needed. It was an argument with a certain demogogic appeal but decided flaws in logic.

At the 1946 hearings, which began in April, Senator Pepper (D.-Florida), a member of the Senate Education and Labor Committee (which then had jurisdiction), made a forceful case for the Wagner-Murray-Dingell bill. He followed Senator Wagner (D.-New York), who was mainly concerned with making the point that the bill was not "socialistic," and Representative Dingell (D.-Michigan), who used his time to rant against the AMA. Like Truman, Pepper argued that the problem was access—economic barriers between a person who was sick and the medical care needed. Here lay the cause of the nation's poor health, he said, and its cure was enactment of compulsory national health insurance. "Most people in Florida no more expect hospital care during a serious illness than a trip to Europe in the summertime," he said. "Can it be said that farmers with mouths to feed, clothes to buy and insurance to pay can afford the $100 a year or so it costs on the average to purchase even minimum adequate medical care under our present system? They cannot and they do not...They and their wives and children go without instead."

Finishing up, Pepper enumerated the shortcomings in voluntary or private insurance (limits on coverage, restrictions on eligibility, etc.) Arguing that the burden of sickness and medical care payment should be distributed throughout the population, he said that only compulsory national health insurance could accomplish that goal. He offered no specific cost figures for the proposed program, but he did promise that the expense "will not be greater than that of our present inefficient and wasteful fee-for-service system."[29]

The AMA counterattack took sharp issue, first, with the accusations that the health of United States citizens had fallen to the shameful levels suggested by President Truman and Senator Pepper. Life expectancy at birth, the association stated, had risen from 49 years in 1900 to 59.5 in 1930; to 63.8 in 1940; to something like 68 in 1949. Roscoe L. Sensenich, M.D., chairman of the AMA Board of Trustees, testified a few days after Senator Pepper's testimony in 1946 that the United States' death rate was lower than England's, Germany's, and Sweden's.[30]

At the 1949 hearings, Lowell S. Goin, M.D., argued that nationalized medical systems do not necessarily provide the public with better care than private systems. "Do you know," he asked the committee, "that the American death rate for diphtheria is about half that of Great Britain or pre-war Germany? Diphtheria is an excellent indicator [of how well a medical system works] since it is one of the few diseases for which we have specific preventive and curative measures, and, since there being no secrets involved, the German and British physicians know as well how to treat it as do Americans."[31]

The AMA rested its case on voluntary, private health insurance plans, pointing out in its rebuttal to the Ewing report that "A family may purchase a typical Blue Cross-Blue Shield membership which will pay the bulk of its...medical bills for about 20 cents a day ... the price of a package of cigarettes or a bottle of beer or a gallon of gasoline."[32]

The chairman of the Senate Committee that conducted the hearings and, of course, one of the sponsors of the bill, Senator James E. Murray (D.-Montana), started out convinced that there was only one way to go with health insurance. "I am satisfied," he announced at an early session, "when the committee hears all the evidence that they will agree with me that it is impossible under any voluntary system in the United States to furnish the American people with a system of prepaid medical care and hospitalization." Nothing was said at the 1946 hearings (where he made that statement) or at the hearings in 1947 or 1949 to change his mind. He was, of course, wrong in his forecast of what the other members of his committee would conclude.

For its part, the AMA remained equally adamant in believing that a compulsory government health plan could only lower the high standards of medical care that the AMA had spent a century trying to establish. The voluntary approach to health insurance continued to gather momentum, and the AMA argued that was the best way to go.

A political collision as uncompromising, as forceful, and as highly emotional as this one always leaves behind some breakage. And the fight over the Wagner-Murray-Dingell bills, which occupied the AMA so intensively from 1943 into the 1950s, caused its share of damage. The physicians won their battle over the legislation, but they suffered casualties both inside and outside their organization.

The levy of a $25 assessment on all members in the year 1949, followed by the institution of annual dues in a similar amount in 1950—the first general membership dues since 1911[33]—underscored a sharp change in the character of the organization. To decide how to meet the new societal demands, the AMA now had to debate new and emotionally charged issues. No longer could the delegates simply chew over the topics that physicians traditionally felt comfortable with: medical education, ethics, the impact of new technology. Moreover, the AMA now found itself having to deal more frequently with unfamiliar institutions, with the Congress, the press, the public itself—and public opinion.

For a few physicians the $25 assessment symbolized a departure they could not accept. The reason was less a disagreement over policy than a divergence over the basic function of a medical society. Here can be heard an echo of Olin West's speech to the executive session in 1943, the one in which he said, "I maintain that the AMA has no excuse for existence except as a scientific and educational institution."

Despite the political heat from the Truman administration, some physicians retained their purist stance. In *JAMA*, February 19, 1949, there appeared a letter signed by 148 doctors stating their opposition to the new direction and declaring their belief that a large segment of the profession was "likewise not in sympathy." Without saying how they might meet the new challenges, they announced their refusal to pay the assessment and their distaste for funds raised for "propaganda and legislative lobbying." The Medical Society of the County of New York (Manhattan) rejected the AMA policy and said it would not collect the assessment from its members. Bernard DeVoto in his *Harper's* magazine column, "The Easy Chair," called the language used in the AMA's public relations material "feculent" and told of deducting 25¢ from a recent $15 payment to his own physician in order to notify his doctor that he (DeVoto) was not going to have anything to do with financing the AMA's efforts.[34] At the annual meeting in 1950, one state medical society, Nevada, entered a resolution objecting to the Whitaker and Baxter $1 million advertising plan that had been authorized for the coming year.

Carol Brierly Golin, an assistant managing editor of the *AMNews* in 1984 but a young newcomer to the AMA in 1950, recalls the meeting of the house that fall. "There was that impressive troop from California, Whitaker and Baxter," she remembers, "and the big backdrop with the doctor painting. The house, I'd say, generally thought that it was about time the AMA was doing something like this. Yet there were an awful lot of reluctant bridegrooms in that House of Delegates who stood up and said the AMA should not be getting itself involved in political activity, that it should remain a basically scientific organization."[35]

By the time the assessment had fallen due, it was clearly apparent that physicians who belonged to their state and county societies by and large supported the AMA. Something like 65 percent of those eligible to pay the 1949 assessment did so. And the next year 77 percent of the state-county members became regular, dues-paying AMA members.* The figures represented a strong endorsement of the leadership and policies of the organization.[36]

Yet there was no denying that the issue was controversial, and distasteful enough to some physicians that they dropped out. Aggravating those difficulties was what often happens to an organization as the result of a public row with the government: destructive criticism in the press of its motivations, principles, and general credibilty. The AMA had gone along for years, regarded as virtually sacrosanct. But now, here it was, charging dues, raising funds for a public relations-advertising campaign, mounting legislative assaults in Congress, and behaving for all the world like organized labor or a political lobby. To the press, to the public, and to many physicians, the AMA was not the same organization it had been, and it began losing the immunity it had enjoyed from all but the most carefully considered outside criticism. At the same time, physicians felt a different relationship between themselves and the AMA, and some of them even sensed a different relationship between themselves and their patients.

The 1940s left a deep mark on the AMA. Liberal elements within the Democratic party, led by Senators Wagner, Murray, and Pepper and joined by President Truman, had, for the first time, placed broad medical issues on the nation's political agenda for public debate and legislative resolution. Given the choice between staying aloof from the new decision-making process or becoming actively engaged in it, the AMA—over the sharp resistance of a few members and the reluctance of many—decided that it should be the

---

*The assessment brought in $2,289,956 in 1949 with $70,284 additional in late payments in 1950. Dues revenue in 1950 amounted to $2,839,402. AMA membership rose from 140,260 in 1948, to 145,036 in 1949, and to 147,725 in 1950.

organization to represent the medical profession publicly, legislatively, and politically. The AMA of 1950 thus became a far different organization from the AMA of 1940, and the transition was understandably turbulent.

Chapter Twelve

The Not-So-Quiet 1950s

Although the proposals for compulsory national health insurance lay buried in a congressional committee, an expanse of difficult terrain still stretched before the AMA of early 1950s. To be sure, the nation was apparently in agreement with the association that private health insurance would be the basic financing method for medical care in the future. Yet private insurance did not address the medical needs of the welfare population or the elderly indigent. Traditionally dependent on charity or on municipal, county, or state programs, those who were not self-supporting felt they were getting second-class care, and they became more and more insistent on being included in the mainstream of American medicine. As the decade progressed, the matter of financing medical care for the poor and the elderly started to become a significant political issue.

At the same time, many professional issues demanded attention. Organized medicine increasingly felt the impact of scientific progress. As knowledge and technology expanded, so did the specialization of the profession. As research grants and Hill-Burton assistance to affiliated teaching hospitals became more available, the medical schools started to transform themselves into the giant medical centers we know today.[1] In many communities, this led to a rankling conflict between the traditional, individual practitioner and what he regarded as unfair competition from the new, tax-supported hospital across the street that siphoned off potential patients.

Meanwhile, the AMA was experiencing internal pains. These were brought on by the need to respond to a wide range of new problems, such as more urgent socioeconomic issues, changes in the way care was being financed and delivered, and new public expectations from the new medicines and surgical techniques. Dynamic new forces began to affect medicine in the 1950s, extending some of the old conflicts, intensifying others, and creating new ones.

Of all the friction points that developed in the 1950s none generated greater heat than the question: Do we have enough doctors? The topic reached the public agenda following two events in the fall of 1948. The first was the release of the Ewing report, prepared by the Federal Security Agency; the other was a bill, introduced by Senator Claude D. Pepper (D.-Florida) and passed by the Senate, calling for a five-year program of broad federal aid to medical schools.[2] According to the Ewing report and underlying Senator Pepper's rationale, there would be a shortage of 42,000 physicians by 1960 if the rate at which the United States was adding to the pool of physician manpower remained unchanged.*

Little argument was heard against the need for additional financial support for the nation's medical schools. The chairman of the AMA Council on Medical Education, Herman G. Weiskotten, M.D., was among those who said so: "The American people should realize that the first and most important step in improving the health and medical care of our people is the more adequate support of more than half of the medical schools of this country."[3]

But the action proposed by Senator Pepper went beyond that. He wanted federal subsidies to expand medical education quickly and substantially. At this the AMA bridled. Having just waged a strenuous campaign to block the entrance of the federal government into nationalized health insurance, the AMA could not consistently sanction the federal government's broad intrusion into medical education. Physicians were especially concerned about protecting the criteria for admission to medical schools and the scientific integrity of the curricula. The AMA said no to the idea of subsidies unless there could be guarantees of academic freedom.[4]

Throughout 1949 and 1950 a sullen impasse prevailed, with charges in the press that the AMA was trying to keep the supply of physicians down in order to keep fees up. The standoff was all the more unyielding because the antagonists perceived the central issue so differently. The government focused on its perception of a physician manpower shortage; the AMA, which rejected the reasoning

*No one has been able to state precisely and authoritatively what constitutes a physician shortage or a physician sufficiency. According to Frank G. Dickinson in his "An Analysis of the Ewing Report" (*Bulletin 69*, Bureau of Economic Research, AMA, August 1949, pages 8-9), those who developed the Ewing report averaged the physician to population ratios of twelve states, most of them states with high levels of prosperity and physicians. Applying this supposedly "ideal" ratio to the entire United States population, they calculated what they defined as a nationwide "shortage."

used in the Ewing report to establish a physician shortage, was concerned over the threat to academic freedom. What the government subsidized, the AMA was convinced, the government would control.

The AMA was not alone in its concern. The Commission on Financing Higher Education, which included the presidents of Brown, Stanford, Johns Hopkins, Cal Tech, and Missouri, plus the provost of Harvard and the acting president of Columbia, also thought subsidies "dangerous to the intellectual heritage of freedom and the diversity which characterizes American higher education." Direct federal subsidies to education were regarded as "innovative" at that time, and both the AMA and the educators thought that subsidies should be considered only after it was certain that private sources of support were inadequate to the task.[5]

A bit ingenuously, the AMA created the American Medical Education Fund (AMEF) in 1950 to raise money from business, medical society, and physician sources to support the medical schools. It was an extension of the AMA's belief in the private solution of public problems. In announcing the board's decision to start the fund and an initial AMA contribution of $500,000, the fund chairman, Louis H. Bauer, M.D., said, "If all other organizations and individuals will render support of this worthy cause in accordance with their financial ability, not only will the financial security of the medical schools be assured but their freedom will be protected."[6]

The schools had immediate needs, however, and with pressures for their expansion mounting, the AMA gave ground, adopting a resolution endorsing the principle of a one-time federal grant-in-aid on a matching basis, based on the Hill-Burton formula and administrative machinery, for construction, equipment, and renovation of the physical plants of the medical schools.[7]

But the action of the house in June 1951 giving approval to bricks and mortar support was far from unanimous, and the delegates opposed to it refused to let the issue die. A culminating debate took place at the 1956 annual meeting. The forces that advocated the reversal of policy were led by an ultra-conservative Texas delegate, Milford O. Rouse, M.D., who numbered among his patients the billionaire oilman, Haroldson L. Hunt. To applause from the house, Rouse emphasized, "We say repeatedly, we don't want the government to be monkeying in our business."

But the vote went against him. Delegate John W. Green, M.D., of California made a telling point. He said,

I have been chairman of the California delegates for their AMEF efforts ever since it started. I have been very disappointed by the results of our efforts...You said this morning that you didn't want any more dues attached to you for AMEF. On the other hand, you want to expand your medical school programs, the number of students who matriculate. You want to have the necessary professors to carry out the program. You want to have new laboratories, more equipment...Every member of this house would say, "We want to be independent. We want to keep Uncle Sam from digging into us and influencing our schools and our method of teaching and one thing and another."

Let's put up $1,000 apiece and stop it there. Then we would be talking.

He sat down to applause too.

Louis H. Bauer, M.D., the former chairman of the Board of Trustees and the man who had headed the educational fund drives, then ended the discussion.

I don't think there's a Chinaman's chance of our getting enough money to give to the schools to extend their facilities from the bricks and mortar standpoint or to build additional schools. That is going to have to come from somewhere, and unless, as Dr. Green brought out, every doctor is willing to kick in $1,000, we are not going to get it. If we don't, not only will the government come in and give money to build medical schools, but they will come in and give money to control the academic curricula of our schools. And that, God knows, is something that we must prevent at all costs.

His statement was the clincher, and the AMA, though clearly reluctant, stayed with its position of approval for federal bricks and mortar grants to expand medical schools.[8]

In terms of what the medical schools actually received, the federal support programs proved inconsistent. The construction grants, for example, did not rise to significant amounts until near the end of the decade. On the other hand, the research and training grants grew steadily from $12.2 million in 1950 to $147.9 million in 1960. By the end of the decade roughly 40 percent of medical school expenditures derived from funds granted by the federal government.[9] The ratio of physicians to population remained constant at 144 per 100,000 through the 1950s, higher than the ratio in 1940 (133 per 100,000) and higher than that of virtually all other industrialized nations.[10]

Nevertheless, for opposing the arguments in the Ewing report that a physician shortage was in the making and for opposing Senator Pepper's expansive legislation, the AMA found itself accused of restricting the output of physicians for selfish reasons. In response, the Council on Medical Education developed a thoughtful, careful statement on educational policy and submitted it to the house in June 1951 over the signature of its chairman, Herman G. Weiskotten, M.D., dean of the Syracuse University College of Medicine and a respected educator. Below are excerpts from the statement, which was adopted by the house:

Discussions of the supply of physicians...in recent years have sometimes implied that the AMA seeks to limit the supply of physicians ... by limiting the number of medical schools it approves, by curtailing enrollments in schools it approves, or by otherwise preventing expansion of the nation's facilities for the training of physicians...

The AMA has no desire to limit the production of properly trained physicians...The policy of the Association is to assist and encourage any responsible group or institution endeavoring to create new facilities or expand existing facilities for the training of physicians.

The number of medical schools approved is determined entirely by the ability of schools to meet acceptable educational standards...

The Association does not attempt to regulate the size of the national student body in medicine. The number of students admitted to individual schools is determined by the faculties, administrative officers and governing boards of each school, in accordance with the school's educational philosophy and its own judgment of its educational resources...

The number of medical students in approved schools has been steadily increasing. In 1910 there were 12,530 students in approved schools; today there are more than 26,000...In the last ten years the number of medical students increased by almost 5,000. This is the equivalent of creating at least 15 new schools of average size...

Still further increases in the production of physicians are in prospect. The present freshman class numbers more than 7,100 students, the largest on record. It is 23% larger than the freshman class entering medical schools in 1940...Physicians have increased in numbers more rapidly than has the population at large for more than 20 years...

By 1960 the production of physicians will be at least 30 percent greater than in 1950, a rate of expansion that promises to exceed that of any other major profession, and will greatly exceed the general population increase.

The AMA also facilitated the entrance into practice in this country of physicians educated abroad. After due study, it has recommended to the state licensing boards that the graduates of 48 foreign medical schools be accorded the same opportunities for licensure as graduates of approved medical schools in the U.S...

The AMA is duty bound to protest exaggerated estimates of the need for additional physicians that can only be met by debasing the quality of medical education...[11]

In retrospect, it is fair to say that the AMA failed to anticipate a rise in public expectations relating to medical care. It underestimated, as did many others, the increased demand for medical services in the 1950s that followed the postwar return of prosperity and the rapid spread of medical and hospitalization insurance. Neither the AMA nor anyone else had any evidence that patient utilization of medical services was any different from the pattern of the 1930s. The AMA disagreed sharply with the dubious polemics of the Ewing report, which was what Senator Pepper was going on, and said so forthrightly, advancing the careful arguments of its staff economist, Frank G. Dickinson, Ph.D., the director of its Bureau of Medical Economic Research.

Because accusations have repeatedly been made that the AMA has sought to maintain a scarcity of physicians for economic reasons, this is an appropriate point to examine the origins and validity of the charge. There are two periods in recent history during which the annual number of medical school graduates has significantly declined, the first between 1904 and 1920, the second between 1937 and 1943. (See Charts 2 and 3 and Appendix B). Two questions have to be asked. One, did AMA policies immediately before those periods of decline contribute to the drop? And two, if AMA policies did contribute, were the decisions behind those policies motivated by economics or something else?

In the first instance, there can be no question that AMA policy decisions led to a long and substantial decline in the number of medical school graduates in the United States, from a high of 5,747 in 1904 to a low of 2,658 in 1919. After the AMA began its campaign for higher standards of medical education—tougher entrance requirements, more sophisticated clinical facilities, better qualified teachers, more exacting curricula—there followed a 40 percent

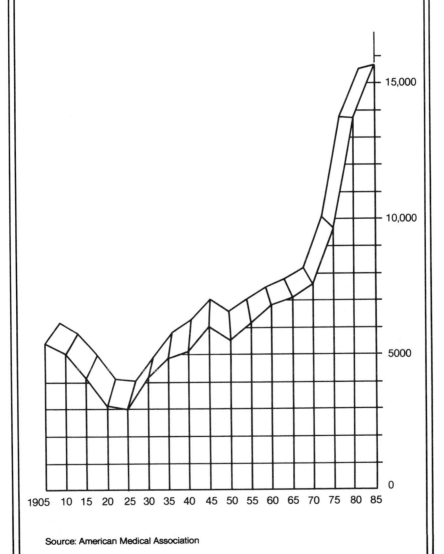

CHART 2

U.S. Medical School Graduates by Year

(Points on the chart represent the average
number of graduates during the preceding
five years. Year by year figures in Appendix B.)

Source: American Medical Association

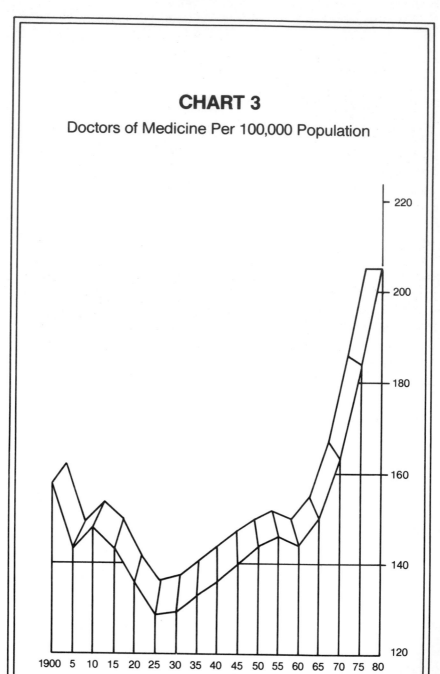

CHART 3

Doctors of Medicine Per 100,000 Population

Source: American Medical Association

drop in the number of medical schools in the next fifteen years. After the AMA recommended that more college preparation be required for admission, students found it increasingly difficult, academically, to gain admission to those that did survive.[12]

As to motivation, however, it is difficult to establish that the AMA wanted anything other than the end to a professional disgrace—the diploma mills, the cram schools, the "colleges" that existed primarily for the financial benefit of their proprietors. What little evidence there is that the AMA sought economic advantage for its members consists of assumptions relying for support on occasional references by AMA officials to "overcrowding" in the profession. One instance sometimes cited is the 1903 presidential address of Frank Billings, M.D., in which he denounced both the shameful conditions in the schools and "the evils of an overcrowded profession, which reduced the opportunities of those already in the profession to acquire a livelihood." However, Billings, a noted educator who built the University of Chicago medical school into a first rate institution, was more interested in spurring the AMA's interest in better medical education. On balance, his speech was idealistic, reflecting an educator's quest for higher standards rather than a practitioner's complaint about competition.[13]

The "overcrowding" matter also turns up in a speech by George H. Simmons, M.D., who became the editor of *JAMA* in 1899 and was one of those within the AMA who fought hardest for educational reform. Dedicating a new building for the Drake University medical department in Des Moines on January 29, 1904, Simmons stated early in his speech, "Our profession is enormously overcrowded... We have twice as many physicians, in proportion to the population, as England, four times as many as France, five times as many as Germany and six times as many as Italy." But Simmons was not pleading for a reduction in the size of the profession so much as he was attempting to allay fears that the reform measures then being talked about might bring on a physician shortage. He mentioned the surfeit of American physicians to argue that reform would not mean hardship.[14]

The evidence of another motivation—the desire to upgrade medical education—is overwhelming. The reform movement launched by the AMA won the applause of the educational community, of the public, and of the major educational foundations, which soon began to fund the new, reformed medical schools with major donations. This was a reform-minded era with a reform-minded press, and it is doubtful that the AMA could have accomplished what it did had its motives been as self-serving as sometimes portrayed later.

What about the late 1930s? The annual number of medical graduates again declined, but this time only slightly, from 5,377 in 1937 to a low of 5,089 in 1939. The number did not climb to where it had been until 1944.[15] Compared to what had happened three decades earlier, this was not a dramatic change. However, the decline did follow actions by the Council on Medical Education.

During the Depression, the AMA became concerned about its effect on the quality of medical education. To conduct another Flexner-like study, the Council on Medical Education asked Herman G. Weiskotten, M.D., then dean of the Syracuse University College of Medicine, to make a survey of all eighty-nine schools in the United States and Canada, including two unapproved schools.[16] As was done at the time of Flexner's survey, someone from the Council on Medical Education accompanied him. The Weiskotten survey confirmed suspicions that some of the financially weaker schools, having found their sources of outside support drying up as a result of the Depression, were inflating enrollments to boost tuition income without a compensating expansion in facilities, equipment, and faculty. The AMA issued warnings, which were accepted as constructive criticism by the affected schools. Corrective action was undertaken, but it was necessary in some schools to reduce temporarily the number of entering first year students until the facilities and faculty could be expanded. The result in the number of graduating students showed up in 1938-43.

Although little evidence exists that the Council on Medical Education sought to do anything other than maintain the standards of medical education, the air was full of restrictive demands. As the Depression worsened, the millions of unemployed were not the only ones having a difficult time. The average annual income for non-salaried physicians dipped below $3,000 one year.[17] There were, many people thought, "too many" physicians, just as there were too many lawyers, too many business executives, too many accountants, engineers, skilled and unskilled laborers. In an editorial in *JAMA* on August 27, 1932, Morris Fishbein noted a report elsewhere in the same issue that the number of medical school graduates had for ten years exceeded the annual number of physician deaths by 50 percent. "Perhaps," he observed, "there is need for professional birth control."

That same year, a Commission on Medical Education, which was organized in 1925 by the Association of American Medical Colleges and received financial support from the medical schools, the AMA, and the Rockefeller, Carnegie, and Macy Foundations, announced, "There are more physicians in the United States than are needed to provide an adequate medical service for the country." According to its study director, Willard C. Rappleye, M.D., later dean of the Columbia University College of Physicians and Surgeons, the number of "excess" physicians was 25,000.

But if pressures were put on the House of Delegates to take what might be considered restrictive action, it stood its ground. In 1933 it did warn that "the profession is overcrowded," but asked only that steps be taken to insure that high school and college students knew that before making choices of a career.[18]

In both 1933 and 1934 the incoming presidents of the AMA discussed the overproduction of physicians in their addresses to the house. Walter L. Bierring, M.D., spoke more bluntly than his predecessor:

> When considered in the light of present acute problems of the practitioner and the facts concerned with the future practice of medicine, one is forced to the conviction that more doctors are being turned out than society needs and can comfortably reward...It is only natural to place the responsibility with the medical schools, in that they hold in their hands the power to control the supply of physicians for the future, but the time has arrived for the AMA to take the initiative and point the way...A fine piece of educational work could well be done if we were to use only half of the seventy-odd medical schools in the United States.[19]

However, the medical schools, the Council on Medical Education and the House of Delegates felt differently. The number of graduating students increased steadily from 1930 through 1937. Despite the declines in 1938 and 1939, the medical schools were graduating nearly 15 percent more physicians per year near the end of the Depression (5,097 in 1940) than they were near the beginning (4,565 in 1930).[20]

Unlike Harry Truman, President Dwight D. Eisenhower presented the AMA with few proposals that made front-page headlines. The association and the administration were philosophically in tune, and the American public, overjoyed at the end of the Korean fighting, desired nothing so much as a rest from controversy and struggle. But the presidential aura of tranquility did not settle on the internal concerns that the AMA had to deal with. The spread of group health insurance, the progress of science, the growth of specialization, and the gravitation of medical care toward the hospital all were beginning to pose policy questions of mounting urgency. Like any traditional organization, the AMA was having to examine a number of old decisions in the light of new realities.

Among the delegates' more prickly tasks in the mid-1950s was the job of developing an updated, workable definition of something called the corporate practice of medicine. A lawyer would describe this as the employment of a physician by a lay-controlled corporation that sells the services of the physician for a profit. The practice first gained attention in the early part of the century when medical corporations recruited physicians and then contracted with mining, lumber, and railroad companies to provide care for their employees in remote areas.[21] In 1912 the AMA tried to discourage the practice by adding to its Principles of Medical Ethics a statement that it was "unprofessional for a physician to dispose of his services under conditions that make it impossible for him to render adequate service to his patient."

What the AMA was referring to here was a conflict of interest. To whom was the corporate physician loyal? The medical needs of his patient? Or the profit-making demands of his employer? In the 1920s, as complaints grew more numerous, the problem of medical care provided by lay organizations, including fraternal lodges, became more acute, causing the AMA's Judicial Council to brand the practice "destructive of that personal responsibility and relationship which is essential to the best interest of the patient." In 1934 the AMA Principles of Medical Ethics were amended to define the corporate practice of medicine more precisely, and, for the first time, to state that the patient should have a "free choice of physician."

Organized medicine found that corporate practice violated the Principles of Medical Ethics on a number of counts. It compromised the physician's allegiance to his patient, that is, his obligation to make medical decisions solely in the patient's interest. Furthermore, it denied the patient's freedom to choose his physician, important in establishing a mutually rewarding physician-patient relationship. Corporate practice, repugnant to doctors and contrary to patient interests, was outlawed in many states.

Almost no one defended corporate medicine as described above, but in the 1950s the issue came up in a different context. Questions were being asked with growing heat about the increasing provision of patient medical services in hospitals by salaried doctors, in pre-paid group insurance clinics by salaried doctors, and in teaching hospitals by residents and full-time, salaried faculty members. A trend was clearly underway toward care delivered by institutions.

One survey found that in 1958, in addition to residents, an estimated 15 percent of active, fully trained physicians were in some form of full-time hospital employment.[22] Between 1951 and 1960 the number of faculty members engaged full-time in medical school clinical departments rose 214 percent, from 2,069 to 6,487. The number of residents in graduate training programs run by medical schools rose from 4,259 to 12,504, a jump of 193 percent.[23] A key part of the clinical curriculum, the practical teaching and learning process, was involving the treatment of more and more patients in the teaching hospitals. One AMA executive who joined the staff in the 1950s likens the growth of institutional care in this period to "a beginning of an industrial revolution in medicine."

The looming competitive threat of the hospitals, especially the university teaching hospitals, angered many AMA delegates. What was the difference, they asked, between a doctor salaried by a hospital corporation and a doctor salaried by a regular corporation? Didn't the physician's allegiance to the patient become weakened in either case?

A resolution introduced by Delegate J.P. Culpepper, M.D., of Mississippi at the December 1954 meeting of the house reflects the resentment that many private, solo practitioners felt at that time. Though not adopted, it triggered a series of studies of care provided by institutions and group insurance plans. Culpepper's resolution cited the threat posed by "a tax-supported medical school that is engaged in the practice of medicine in which fees are levied and collected under a policy allowing this practice to employed physicians." It also called upon the AMA to reaffirm "its unalterable opposition to socialized and state subsidized medicine regardless of the form it may assume."[24] Another delegate, Eustace A. Allen, M.D., was drawing flak from his colleagues back home. "We in Georgia are in almost as bad a fix as Culpepper says he's in in

Mississippi," he told the house. "The dean of the medical school of the University of Georgia told our council that 85 percent of the teaching institutions of the United States were circumventing the state [corporate practice] laws...If they are going into the practice of medicine, I don't see that they can ask doctors to subscribe through the AMEF to those schools that are practicing medicine against them."[25]

Other delegates applied the brakes to the discussion, emphasizing the complexities of the corporate practice issue. Finally, the resolution was referred to the Council on Medical Service for more thorough consideration.

Meanwhile, legal decisions regarding institutional practice were running against the Allens and the Culpeppers. These arose as attempts were made to enforce the corporate practice statutes in respect to hospitals. Originally, the courts had upheld the statutes forbidding corporate medicine on the basis that only a natural person could be licensed to practice medicine; since corporations were "artificial persons," they could not qualify for licensure. And if they sold the professional services of a licensee, they would be engaged in illegal corporate practice of medicine.

But when the cases of not-for-profit hospitals came up, the courts found that their employment of physicians did not constitute the illegal corporate practice of medicine. The courts construed physician employment by hospitals to be an independent contractor arrangement, with the doctor free of hospital control over his medical decisions. Because the hospitals did not attempt to control medical policy, but merely made certain that medical services were provided, the courts held that the salaried physicians were not engaged in illegal corporate practice.

By the end of the decade the issue was also resolved insofar as AMA ethical principles were concerned. The key paragraph in the Principles of Medical Ethics was amended to read, "...a physician should not dispose of his services under terms or conditions which tend to interfere with or impair the free and complete exercise of his medical judgement..."[26] In other words, as long as physicians had unrestricted control over their medical decisions, they were practicing ethically, salaried or not.

A ninety-six-page report on the varieties of medical insurance plans was issued in 1959 by an AMA commission headed by Leonard W. Larson, M.D., a trustee who became president in 1961. This further clarified the association's position on corporate medicine, particularly in regard to closed panel, direct service, clinic-type plans. During the early 1930s these had drawn strident opposition, moving Morris Fishbein to brand them as "medical soviets."[27] Because they relied on salaried staff physicians and because patients were often directed to whoever was on duty, the subscribers usually did not have a physician they regarded as "theirs." The AMA's ethical principle regarding free choice of physician was aimed at just this type of medical practice.

Now, however, the Larson report, as adopted by the house, took a substantially different position. The new policy read: "The AMA believes that free choice of physician is the right of every individual and one which he should be free to exercise as he chooses. Each individual should be accorded the privilege to select and change his physician at will *or to select his preferred system of medical care,** and the AMA vigorously supports the right of the individual to choose between these alternatives."[28]

Commenting soon after the annual meeting at which the new policy was adopted, the president, Louis M. Orr, M.D., wrote, "That, as I interpret it, reaffirms our fundamental faith in the principle of freedom of choice, but it also recognizes the patient's right to select the type of medical care plan he wants—including a closed panel plan."[29]

Thus the ethical constraints on institutional medicine were eased. From the vantage point of the 1980s, it is easy to say that the step was inevitable, an instance of policy simply catching up with reality. Nevertheless, it would take several more years before many private, solo practitioners and county medical societies would stop looking upon institutional medicine with a resentful eye.

Although the issue of institutional medicine touched the tenderest spots, an exhaustive review of many other ethical questions engaged the House of Delegates during the 1950s. An examination of the rules against rebates, commissions, and fee splitting was made. But with prohibitions already in effect and administration of them at the county level, little direct action seemed feasible. The house argued at great length about the ethics of a physician admitting a patient to a hospital he owned, or selling appliances, drugs, or eyeglasses he prescribed. Such conflicting interests were obviously unethical.

---

*emphasis added

But what about the exceptions? What about the physician who started a hospital in a remote area where otherwise no hospital facilities would exist? Or rural physicians who kept commonly needed drugs on hand and sold them to patients to save them a long trip to a pharmacy? Were such practices entirely unethical, though clearly done in the patient's interest? The house seemed to wrangle endlessly with what the Principles of Medical Ethics had to say on such matters.[30]

The problem was that the ethical code at that time was a long, tangled document of 5,000 words, a hodge-podge. Some of the language derived from the Hippocratic Oath; some of it derived from renaissance England, with roots reaching back to the medieval guilds. Many of the sections dealt more with matters of custom and etiquette than morality. If you wanted to label another physician unethical so colleagues would shun him, it was easy because "unethical" could cover so many things—not conforming to medical customs, for example, or doing something that was no worse than unrefined. You could be a perfectly moral person and still violate the Principles.

Cumbersome as they were and difficult as it was to apply them in the exceptional circumstances that could be cited, the house considered revision only with great reluctance. No one wanted to eliminate much from the existing code. The delegates' sentiment for something close to the original is indicated by the title of an intermediate revision that was proposed but not accepted, "Principles of Medical Ethics and Precepts of Manners."[31]

In time, ten general precepts were extracted from the old hodge-podge and advanced as the preferred version. This one consisted of 500 words versus the old code with its 5,000. What was finally done, at the June 1957 meeting, was to persuade the house that adoption of the new Principles did not necessarily invalidate the old. When the new, shorter, more flexible Principles were presented to the house, the chairman of the Council on Constitution and Bylaws said, "The fear has been expressed that...the profession will somehow lose the benefit of the valuable explanatory reports and opinions published by the Judicial Council during the last fifty years. This fear is groundless."[32] A complete annotation was prepared by the Judicial Council, incorporating the major decisions and precedents established in the past. With that proviso, the new Principles of Medical Ethics were adopted. Though they were modified later, the new Principles together with the opinions and reports of the

Judicial Council, redefined the ethical basis of American medicine. Here is a sampling of the sort of things they cover:

- physicians should not practice under conditions that prevent the free and complete exercise of their medical judgment
- physicians are required to increase their knowledge and skills
- they must follow methods of healing founded on a scientific basis
- they may not neglect a patient or discontinue services without giving due notice
- they may not solicit patients
- they should limit their source of professional income to services rendered to patients; that is, no fee splitting, rebates and so forth
- drugs, remedies, and appliances may be dispensed if in the patient's best interest
- physicians must respect the confidentiality of relationships with patients
- they must seek consultation upon request or in difficult cases

In an even more agonized exercise that arose from the same need to adapt to altered conditions, the house reversed its long-standing ethical objections to the practice of osteopathy. Started in 1874 by a physician named Andrew T. Still, M.D., osteopathy held that the normal body produces forces able to fight most diseases and that ailments are caused by various derangements in the musculoskeletal system. The first osteopathic school opened in Kirksville, Missouri, in 1894, and its teachings were rejected by allopathic (conventional) physicians. Throughout the first part of this century, the AMA's ethical strictures applied to osteopaths because their healing methods were considered not to rest on a scientific foundation. Physicians conforming strictly to the AMA code could have no professional association with them.

But in the late 1930s, about the time the first antibiotics were introduced, osteopathic schools started emphasizing conventional medical science. In his address to the AMA's June 1952 meeting President John W. Cline, M.D., the same Californian who had earlier sought Fishbein's ouster in part because of his views on osteopathy, said that "modern osteopathic schools now are patterned largely after...schools of medicine...In thirty-odd states the licenses granted to osteopathic physicians approach or approximate, for legal purposes, those granted to doctors of medicine...It is my considered opinion that the Council on Medical Education should be permitted to aid and advise schools of osteopathy...[we should] remove any barrier of unethical conduct on the part of doctors of medicine who may teach in those schools."[33]

A committee to study the relations between osteopathy and medicine was created, and it proposed that the AMA conduct on-site studies of the osteopathic schools before making a final recommendation. At the June 1955 meeting the committee reported favorably on visits to five of the schools. The sixth osteopathic school refused to participate. Those surveyed expressed a desire for the assistance of medical physicians on their faculties, and all said they would welcome residency opportunities for Doctors of Osteopathy (D.O.s) in conventional medical institutions. Furthermore, the committee could find "no evidence persisting in the teaching of the narrow, cultist doctrine of Andrew T. Still that all disease was due to abnormalities in or about joints." The committee recommended that the house declare a policy to encourage M.D.s to assist in osteopathic teaching programs and remove the cultist stigma from osteopathic education.[34]

But in 1955 the house was not ready for such a proposal. Though the reference committee that June accepted the study committee's recommendations, a minority report was submitted by Texan Milford O. Rouse, M.D. Arguing in the house that osteopathy was still a cult, Rouse met past-president Cline head on.[35] Rouse cited the current catalog of the Still College of Osteopathy in Des Moines, quoting a passage that "the college strove to teach the fundamental tenets of osteopathic medicine as stated by Dr. Andrew T. Still." Rouse wanted further evidence that the cultist aspects of osteopathic medicine were gone. Cline fumed. Rouse's minority report he said, was "unrealistic...limited by emotion, by prejudice. It does not represent a progressive, forward-looking point of view where we can do something to benefit the health of the American people." But when the votes were counted, Rouse carried the day.

In 1958, however, the American Osteopathic Association adopted a crucial amendment to its constitution. Its statement of objectives, which formerly spoke of promoting "the public health and the art and science of the osteopathic school of practice of the healing art," now spoke of objectives "to incorporate scientific research and to maintain and improve high standards of medical education in osteopathic colleges." No more mention of the "osteopathic school." Noting the change, the AMA modified its position in June 1959, rescinding its former view that the training in osteopathic schools lacked a scientific foundation and agreeing that AMA members could now ethically take part in the education of osteopathic students.[36] In 1968 osteopaths were declared eligible for AMA membership.

As more and more medical questions became subject to public review and determination, the AMA found its scope of activity broadened. It started to represent the profession in areas where previously little representation had been needed at all. As a result, the organization grew in size, its annual budgets now headed on a steeper upward path. Non-publication expenses grew from $5.5 million in 1950 to $15.3 million in 1959, an increase close to a factor of three. On a percentage basis, the growth in the money spent to finance the work of the councils, committees, and staff was far more dramatic in the 1950s than it was in the 1960s or 1970s. If adjustment is made for the inflation that began to afflict the economy in the late 1960s, the expansion of the 1950s appears all the more dramatic.

The number of employees changed moderately, from around 800 in 1950 to around 650 in 1960. But that difference is deceptive because in 1956 the AMA closed its printing plant in the headquarters building, entering into contracts with outside suppliers for the production of its journals and eliminating some 230 staff jobs. The difference, and a bit more, was made up in a number of ways: an expansion of economic research activities under Frank G. Dickinson, Ph.D., public relations (from six people in 1950 to sixty ten years later) under Leo E. Brown; and the legislative staff under C. Joseph Stetler. At the same time, the Student American Medical Association was launched, and the AMA, along with the American Hospital Association and the American College of Physicians, joined the American College of Surgeons in forming the Joint Commission on Accreditation of Hospitals.

More significant, however, was a sharp upsurge in the number of AMA councils and committees.[37] By 1957 the AMA had mushroomed into a structure of twelve councils, sixty-four committees, and one commission. Most of these groups had ten to twelve members. They had budgets; they traveled; they met, four times a year for the more active groups; and they required staff support to carry out studies, develop information, write newsletters and brochures, and assist with reports for the board and the house. Some of the councils displayed a bureaucratic gift for spawning subsidiary bodies. The Council on Occupational Health oversaw no fewer than eighteen committees; the Council of Foods and Nutrition had ten.

The Council on Medical Service had seven committees under its jurisdiction and the full attention of the house whenever it felt the need for additional staff or increased budgets. Its power continued to challenge that of the board, with the board reluctant to take full charge of the organization. The board and the house frequently feuded, and the Council on Medical Service was often in the eye of the storm. There was jealousy, a testiness about prerogatives, a wasteful maneuvering for position. At times, the AMA seemed to be a system of satellites in search of a planet.

Joe D. Miller, a new employee in 1957 but an experienced administrator, and in the 1970s and early 1980s the AMA's number two staff executive, was disturbed by the way the AMA was then managed. "There was no cohesion," he recalls, "no one to give the organization form or substance so that it could be run in a business-like way."

The roots of the problem were not hard to find. One factor was the heavy reliance on the council-committee system itself. Over the years, whenever a new challenge or opportunity presented itself, the AMA instinctively responded by creating a committee to handle it. In time, the number of councils and committees grew, each oriented to a particular aspect of medicine or an interrelated set of issues. The inevitable result was a system of almost autonomous, isolated bodies, each dedicated to objectives of its own and only minimally committed to the central interests of the parent organization.

The other problem was leadership. The two forces that could have imposed or induced unity were weak. The Board of Trustees, which had statutory powers translatable into a leadership role, found itself hamstrung by the house, usually through the house's sponsorship of the Council on Medical Service. The other deficiency could be charged to the leadership of the staff.

This rested in the amiable, gentle person of a man who was graduated from medical school before World War I. Not an aggressive personality to begin with, George F. Lull, M.D., became the secretary-general manager of the AMA in 1946 after his retirement as a Major General in the Army Medical Corps. He was acutely conscious of Morris Fishbein's mistakes. After Fishbein's downfall, Ernest B. Howard, M.D., recalls, "The role of the staff was subdued.

Lull was profoundly disturbed by the overt, policy-making activities of a full-time staff man—Fishbein—and he carefully avoided that role. Lull was not overly quick, but you would have to say that he was a highly intelligent man, whose intelligence was masked by gentleness, sweetness of character."[38]

F. J. L. Blasingame, M.D., a member of the board from 1949 to 1958 and the man who succeeded Lull, uses the word "lovable" to describe him. Blasingame remembers that Lull preferred to solve problems in the simplest way possible and that he "did not feel it was his responsibility to make any major changes during his tenure of office." In 1956, as Lull neared his seventieth birthday, he spoke of retiring voluntarily. But when he delayed, the board called in a management consulting firm, and his retirement soon became involuntary.[39]

Given its growing pains, its expanded public activities, the rising influence of the specialty societies, and increasing criticism from the public, which was something new then, it is not surprising that the AMA indulged in some serious self-examination in the middle of the decade. The first rumble of the staff upheaval that was to come took the form of an innocent-sounding resolution introduced in the November-December 1954 meeting. It called for a committee to see if the association's administrative facilities needed expansion. The reference committee amended that slightly, and a committee was formed to determine if there was "a need for a survey of the administrative organization of the AMA." Reporting back in June 1955, the committee reviewed the major areas of concern—press relations, the public's perception of the AMA, the antiquated printing plant, the need for more office space, the need for additional personnel, and the expensive proliferation of AMA committees. But to hire a firm of management consultants to analyze the AMA's problems was, in the opinion of the committee, "foolish."

Nevertheless the board remained uneasy. It authorized a job evaluation study to be done by the board's executive committee in 1955 and engaged an outside firm specializing in executive compensation in 1956. Finally, in February 1957, it did what the house had agreed earlier was "foolish" by bringing in the management consulting firm of Robert Heller and Associates of Cleveland.

In the meantime, the board had authorized the staff to engage Ben Gaffin and Associates of Chicago to survey public attitudes toward physicians and physician attitudes toward the AMA. The results were reassuring to the AMA leaders, a high percentage (86 percent) of the public saying they had a family doctor and voicing warm, confident feelings toward him.[40] Then, as now, the man in the street expressed positive feelings toward his own doctor, but somewhat less positive attitudes about other doctors. The generally good findings ran counter to the frequently critical coverage of medicine in the press, coverage that physicians found highly irritating. (They also looked to the AMA public relations department to either stop the flow of negative stories or counteract it.) As for the AMA itself, neither the public nor physicians were markedly critical of the AMA's political activities; this too had been a source of concern to AMA leaders.

By the spring of 1957 the report from the Heller organization was finished, with copies going to the board right away and to the delegates at the annual meeting in June. In keeping with custom, the speaker appointed a committee to study the sixty-three-page document. The committee chairman, William A. Hyland, M.D., a delegate from Michigan, made its recommendations at the December 1957 meeting. Again as customary, these received consideration in a reference committee hearing, and the house then voted on the reference committee report. Since the actions of the house entailed changes in the Constitution and Bylaws, the appropriate amendments were drafted and then formalized at the annual meeting in June 1958.

In reporting its conclusions, the Heller organization delivered its opinions with the bark off. Though the language of the report was civil, the findings and criticisms were brutal. The authors, for example, went directly into the problem caused by the way the house undercut the authority of the board by having its own councils and committees, for example, the Council on Medical Service and the Council on Medical Education. "Because the house made these councils responsible to itself, it restricted the authority of its own elected administrative body, the Board of Trustees, and created a source of conflict between the two. This," the report said, "weakens the overall effectiveness of the association's work." Making these two councils responsible to the board was recommended strongly.

As for the staff organization and performance, the report was devastating. It described an operation marked by duplication, over-staffing, unclear authority, outdated procedures, and widespread uncoordination. It pictured a staff that was often passive and deferential "with a general belief, built on experience over the years, that employees are expected by members of councils and committees to do what they are told, to carry out instructions, and not to make too many suggestions." Even the janitorial services in the headquarters building, according to the Heller report, fell short of the mark.

The AMA took the report equably, rejecting parts of it and accepting others. The house decided that it wanted to keep its relationship to the board just as it was and therefore did not act on the Heller recommendation that the Council on Medical Service be shifted to the jurisdiction of the board. The Council on Medical Education also stayed where it was. The wasteful, unproductive games that the house and board had been playing with each other would continue. A Heller proposal that trustees be elected from defined geographical areas was rejected, as was a suggestion that the more or less redundant office of vice president be abolished.

On a more positive note, the house agreed that the editor of *JAMA*, heretofore responsible directly to the board, should now report to the chief executive officer. The Washington office, which had also been dealing directly with the board, was similarly placed under the jurisdiction of the head staff man in Chicago. The house agreed to a number of other proposals, among them the formation of a committee to redefine the association's central objectives, an exercise in what would now be called long range planning. To the criticism that the staff had to toady to council and committee members, the house reacted tartly, stating that the remarks in the report were unnecessary and based on insufficient evidence.

The major accomplishment of the Heller study was, however, the recommendation to create a chief executive officer with more clearly defined powers. Accordingly, the dual position of secretary-general manager, which had been Olin West's and George Lull's title, was changed. A new one, executive vice president, was created with clear lines of authority to the Board of Trustees. The title of secretary, for many years a staff job filled by an annual appointment by the House of Delegates, was combined with the title of treasurer, the new secretary-treasurer to be an AMA officer elected by the trustees from among their own members.

Implicit in the creation of the office of executive vice president was the understanding that when formally authorized by the Constitution and Bylaws it would be filled by a new, vigorous administrator, and that once in office he would deal with the operational deficiencies identified in the Heller report.

Actually, as soon as the house indicated what parts of the Heller report it would accept,[41] the board started moving. It relieved George Lull as general manager, something it could do without consultation with the house, and gave the job to Blasingame in early 1958 so that he could get a headstart on a restructuring of the AMA staff. Until the changes in the constitution and bylaws were made official in June, Lull retained his office as secretary. But it was clear to all that once the office of executive vice president was established, Francis James Levi Blasingame, M.D., would be the first one to fill it.

The man the AMA chose to take over the staff operation was in most respects a reverse image of his predecessor. Where Lull had been a public health administrator, Blasingame had been a practitioner, a surgeon in group practice in Wharton, Texas. Lull came to the AMA at the age of fifty-nine, a major career achievement (Deputy Surgeon General of the U.S. Army) already attained; Blasingame's ambitions still lay ahead of him. More significant, Lull, though popular and respected, was something of an outsider to organized medicine; Blasingame, by contrast, had moved through the chairs. He had been president of the Texas Medical Association, an AMA delegate, a trustee, and vice chairman of the board. Lull, albeit an ex-Major General, did not have a take-charge personality; Blasingame did.

As a member of the board that originally decided the AMA's problems needed the attention of a management expert, Blasingame was fully aware of what had to be done. His first step, following recommendations in the Heller report, imposed a new organizational form on the staff, with lines of authority and responsibility clearly laid out where everyone could see them.[42] Instead of nineteen people reporting to the chief staff executive, now there was only a handful. Five of these were the directors of newly created operational divisions: legal affairs and legislation, business operations, communications, publications, and field work; that is, liaison activities with the state and county organizations.

Ernest B. Howard, M.D., who had been the assistant secretary-general manager under Lull, stayed on as the newly titled assistant executive vice president, with two additional operating divisions, socioeconomic activities and scientific activities, to be developed under his direction. To correct the more egregious deficiencies identified in the Heller report, a new, tough-minded business manager, Russell H. Clark, was brought in to take charge of such activities as advertising sales, physician records, circulation fulfillment, purchasing, printing, and housekeeping operations.

It was a complete overhaul, and no one admired it more than Joe D. Miller. Though he and Blasingame were to have a major collision ten years later, Miller applauded the new administrative moves. "Looked at purely from the management standpoint," Miller says, "Bing [Blasingame] was the guy who moved this organization into the twentieth century."[43]

Substantial as his administrative improvements were, Blasingame's contribution went beyond the creation of new boxes and lines on a sensibly drawn organization chart. He had done a great deal of thinking about the relationship between board and staff, and he was forthright in putting his ideas before the trustees. In a full-dress presentation to the board on August 1-2, 1958, he reviewed the personnel and organizational changes he had made and then defined new roles for both the board and the staff. "As I envision the major responsiblity of management," he said, "it is to free the board of administrative detail and give you the time and opportunity to consider higher level policy and program planning."

For years the board had frequently bogged itself down in operational detail, sometimes considering details as small as a $300 annual raise for an employee. John Ballin, Ph.D., who joined the AMA in 1955 as assistant secretary to the Council on Pharmacy and Chemistry (later Drugs), can remember taking the departmental budget to the board in the pre-Blasingame days. "You had to defend it all," he says, "everyone's salary. The number of secretaries, all the minutiae. It was incredible."

Blasingame drew a new line of demarcation between the responsibilities of the board and those of the staff, making a rousing case for an enlarged staff role. He told the trustees:

Medicine must offer aggressive leadership in the health field, develop clearer concepts of its philosophy, and carry its story to the profession and the public. I am convinced that a strong and vigorous staff is necessary. We must think big; our responsibilities and opportunities are big. The stakes are high...It is the responsibility of the house and the board to set policy. The staff must not and cannot do so. But I hope you will agree that a stout, thoughtful and experienced staff... should be given the opportunity to recommend policy to you...subject to your vote, your rejection if you disagree. If a staff works with you on this basis, a healthier and more stimulating atmosphere obtains; and the life of the association is invigorated and will be more productive.[44]

Though he argued for a new and upgraded function for the staff as a whole, it was clear that Blasingame also foresaw a stronger leadership role for himself.

For the new executive vice president, the transition period was made more difficult by national political fires that once again started to smoke. Late in the 1957 Congressional session two executives of the AFL-CIO in Washington, Nelson H. Cruikshank, director of social security, and Andrew J. Biemiller, director of legislation, had prevailed upon Representative Aime Forand (D.-Rhode Island) to introduce a bill that would provide hospital, nursing home, and medical benefits to retirees through Social Security. Though the bill attracted only modest support, concern for medical care of the elderly and the indigent was increasing. No one could say that another 1949 lay ahead, but nevertheless the pressures were building within the AMA in anticipation of another public confrontation, this time over national health insurance for the elderly.

These, in turn, raised a number of internal questions for the AMA. First of all, was this sort of legislative advocacy—as in 1949—what the members as a whole sincerely wanted? Was representation on socioeconomic issues widely supported as a proper association activity? And, if indeed it was, how well equipped was the AMA to carry out such a mission?

In developing an answer to the first question, the AMA acted on a recommendation in the Heller report that it undertake a broad examination of its central objectives and programs. A committee under Lewis A. Alesen, M.D., was appointed by the house in December 1957 and conducted extensive survey research in pursuit of objective findings. Feeling that the activists in organized medicine—the trustees, the delegates, the council/committee members, and the state/county executives—might feel one way and the profession as a whole another, the survey questionnaire was distributed separately, first to what could be called an insider list and then to a probability sample of all physicians, including both members and non-members.

The results, when tabulated, indicated no great disagreement between the two groups, only an overwhelming affirmation of the AMA's involvement in the socioeconomics of medicine. At the same time, the poll results stressed the need for better relations with specialty societies and for better ways to carry out scientific programs. Possibly the most interesting section of the Alesen report is its appraisal of the milieu in which the AMA then found itself. Said the report:

> If it can be said that these many and varied criticisms point in any central direction, it would be that the central problem of our association in the year 1958 is "splintering"—the dynamics of medicine are driving us in so many directions simultaneously. The result is more and ever more divisions and subdivisions in the practice of medicine. One may justly ask, is medicine organized or disorganized? The central imperative for our association is to re-establish its leadership, and unify the fragments into a cohesive entity under one umbrella."[45]

Aware that many of the specialty societies were spinning off into a more distant orbit, the AMA sought to strengthen itself internally for the legislative struggle that loomed on the horizon. First of all, the board, without forewarning or later explanation, peremptorily dismissed most of the members of the Committee on Legislation, appointed replacements, elevated it to council status, gave it a big budget, and assigned it wider responsibilities. Besides reviewing all legislation and initiating field action, the new council was charged with overall responsibility for legislative and political activities.[46]

Another focus of attention was the AMA's Washington office. A worry spot for years, the operation was at times the victim of unclear direction, at other times guilty of overly independent action. Now firmly placed under the control of the executive vice president in Chicago, it had a need, as the Heller report put it, "for some persons with sufficient stature to develop close relationships with legislators themselves." Heretofore, it had confined its contacts largely to congressional staff members. The board authorized Blasingame to recruit the people he needed, something he proceeded to do. "But one of the problems," he recalls, "was to make them realize they had to work through my office. I had to roll over three heads down there before I got one who would believe me."[47]

To take fuller advantage of the AMA's nationally distributed membership and its nation-wide federation of county and state organizations, the AMA widened its internal communications channels. A fortnightly membership newspaper was started, the *American Medical Association News (AMNews)*.* Originally, it made little

---

*Weekly since 1962.

effort to cover anything except from a policy standpoint. At that time, the AMA had no convenient way to communicate with its membership regularly other than *JAMA*, which was, after all, a scientific journal. Some other medium was badly needed as a platform to state policy positions, to keep the membership informed on socioeconomic issues, and to cover the legislative front in Washington.

To create grassroots strength—and make that strength visible to legislators in Washington—the board authorized the expansion of a skimpy state-county liaison operation into a field service division. To be its director, Blasingame appointed Aubrey D. Gates, a former agricultural extension agent in Arkansas who had joined the AMA as secretary to the Council on Rural Health in 1952. A Texan like Blasingame, Gates had in the course of his early experience formed a close friendship with Arkansas Congressman Wilbur Mills, who had just become the Chairman of the Ways and Means Committee of the House of Representatives. Because this committee had jurisdiction over tax legislation, it had jurisdiction over amendments to the Social Security Act and therefore most health legislation.

Gates built up a staff of savvy, experienced field representatives who developed closer ties between the AMA and the state medical associations and, at the same time, made Washington aware that the influence of the AMA extended into all corners of the country. Gates' field service division grew quickly into an essential part of AMA's legislative operation, and Gates himself became a power within the organization.

With its operational structure modernized and many key policies updated, the AMA neared the end of the 1950s a far stronger organization than it was at the start of the decade. Thanks to the institution of dues, its financial base had broadened. And thanks to the findings of its survey research, it was confident now of wide physician backing for its socioeconomic activities. It represented a profession grown diversified in terms of medical specialization but drawn together by the fear that professional integrity might be lost to the power of the federal government. Politicized by external events, it was better prepared than it had been ten years before to deal with non-scientific issues. Yet it would be some time still before the AMA's elected leadership understood how the American political process really worked.

EARLY ACTIVISTS in the American Medical Political Action Committee include (starting below and moving counter-clockwise) Frank E. Coleman, chairman in 1964; Joe D. Miller, AMPAC's first executive director; Donald E. Wood, chairman in 1962; Ernest B. Howard, the assistant executive vice president at the time AMPAC was started; and (top) Blair Henningsgaard, chairman in 1968. At right, a design used to decorate the program of one of the AMPAC workshops periodically held for physicians and their spouses in Washington.

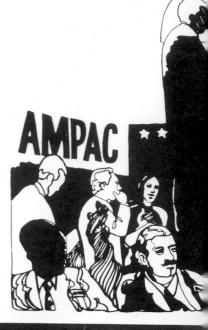

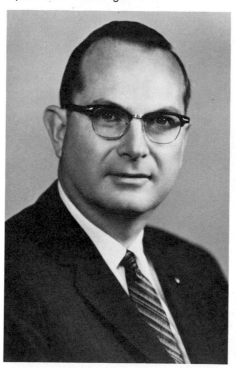

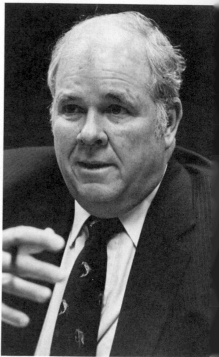

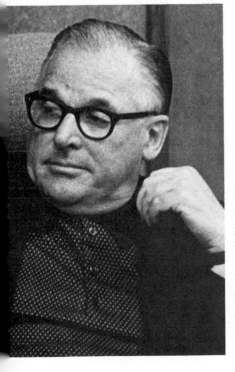
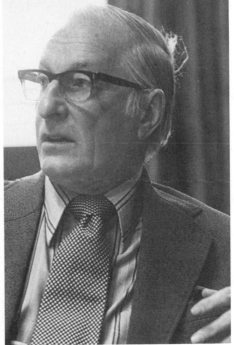
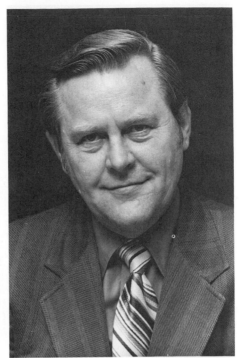
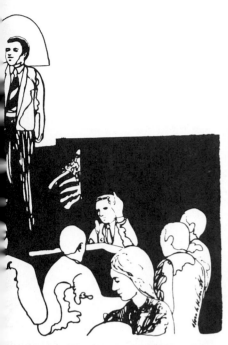

Chapter Thirteen

A Careful Plunge into Political Action

When an organization decides that it must intervene in the public policy decisions that are affecting its future, it has three broad strategies to consider. One, it can engage in the legislative process directly by lobbying. This calls for the employment of people who know their way about the legislative and executive branches of government, who are skilled at marshaling facts and developing allies, and who know how to get their arguments before the key decision-makers. Two, it can take its case to the public. This usually requires the services of public relations and advertising agencies and an effort to create such a groundswell of favorable public opinion that no governmental body dares challenge it. Three, it can undertake a program of political action. This entails an involvement in the elective process and support for candidates who are philosophically in harmony with the organization's objectives. The three strategies do not exclude each other; they are, in fact, mutually reinforcing, and many private efforts to affect public decisions rely on a mixture of all three.

In 1948, when everyone was expecting that President Truman would try to make good on his campaign promises for a health bill, those were the three options the AMA theoretically had. Strategy number one offered little hope, mainly because the AMA Washington operation was weak, a victim of the association's lingering uncertainty that lobbying was a proper activity for a scientific organization. Strategy number two was selected as the medication of choice, and it was administered generously. Strategy number three was ignored, partly out of a vague fear that the AMA might lose its tax-exempt status, partly out of the fear that it might violate the Federal Corrupt Practices Act.

At that time, although the AMA as an organization stayed away from the election process, individual physicians did not. Acting outside the regular medical organizational structure, they plunged right in, many of them starting local election committees, often in the form of healing arts committees that included dentists, pharmacists, and other health personnel.[1] During the elections of 1950 such activities were credited with bringing on the defeat of Senator Claude D. Pepper in Florida, Senator Elbert D. Thomas in Utah, and Representative Andrew J. Biemiller in Wisconsin.*

Late in 1957 the AMA sensed a new threat in the form of the Forand bill, which proposed hospitalization insurance for the retired population through Social Security. It seemed like the 1940s all over again. The immediate objective, as the AMA leaders viewed events, might be hospital insurance for the over sixty-five population, but the ultimate goal was something else: compulsory national health insurance for everyone. Convinced that all-inclusive, government-run health insurance was the final aim of a tireless coalition of Democratic party liberals, career officials in the Social Security Administration, and labor leaders, medicine regarded the Forand bill as the thin edge of the wedge.

The AMA felt almost as beleaguered as it had in 1948, and it was just as determined to resist with every available weapon. In searching for ways to strengthen its effectiveness, the AMA began taking a fresh interest in strategy number three, the use of political action committees, or PACs. Although a 1925 federal law forbids a corporation from making contributions to or expenditures on behalf of candidates for federal office, the prohibition does not apply to unincorporated committees, which may accept gifts from corporations for political education purposes and voluntary gifts from individuals for use in elections.

In 1943 American labor noted the distinction and established the first political action committees, using them successfully to elect candidates to office, attain legislative objectives in Congress, and secure a seat near the head of the table at Democratic party councils. So highly regarded was labor's political arm as early as 1944 that President Franklin D. Roosevelt deferred decisions on his running mate that year to Sidney Hillman, the chairman of the CIO-PAC, thus conferring fame on his instructions, "Clear everything with Sidney."

*Pepper returned in 1962 as a congressman to serve for many years in the House. Biemiller became the AFL-CIO chief lobbyist and a bitter AMA critic.

After the American Federation of Labor and the Congress of Industrial Organizations merged in the mid-1950s to form the AFL-CIO, the Committee on Political Education (COPE) became labor's operative political body, keeping an alert eye on congressmen's voting records, endorsing candidates, marking others for defeat, purchasing pre-election air time, and coordinating the work of local organizations, which rang the doorbells, furnished the campaign workers, and got the right-minded people to the polls on election day. Though COPE's perceived power may well have exceeded what its actual performance merited, it has long been—and still is—a force to be reckoned with.

During the 1950s physicians in a few states expanded the healing arts concept into coalition-style political action organizations—in Florida and Iowa, for example, and the Indiana Health Organization for Political Education (I-HOPE). The earliest of all such organizations, California's Public Health League, dates from the 1930s. But at the national level, labor had the field to itself. There were no other political action committees.

It is difficult to say exactly where the American Medical Political Action Committee began or who began it. Probably the first person to appreciate the need for it was Ernest B. Howard, M.D., then the assistant executive vice president of the AMA. From his frequent contact with Clem Whitaker and Leone Baxter* in 1949 and the early 1950s he developed a sophistication about how the political process worked and how it could be made to respond. Their National Education Campaign for the AMA demonstrated to him an alternative to the traditional strategy of lobbying, suggesting that the levers of political power worked not only in legislatures but also in hometown election districts.

Moves within the AMA to start a political action committee were afoot as early as October 1958, evident in a memo from the director of the AMA law department to George M. Fister, M.D., then a trustee and chairman of the Council on Legislative Activities, later (1962) an AMA president. The memo said, yes, the AMA could legally set up a political action committee. This indicated that the legislative council at least was thinking about the idea. In response to an informal request from one of the delegates during the December 1958 meeting, the board sought an opinion from AMA lawyers on the legality of various forms of political activity.[2]

*They are generally regarded as the first professional political consultants in the United States.

While the house, the board, and the Council on Legislative Activities were inching forward, Howard was moving ahead of the official actions. Sometime that winter, in the early part of 1959, he called Joe D. Miller, then a field service staff man under Aubrey Gates, and invited him to lunch. Seated at Ireland's, a seafood restaurant not far from the AMA headquarters, Howard, out of the blue, asked Miller if he thought the AMA should have a political action committee. "My reaction," says Miller, "was immediate and positive."[3] Howard obviously liked the response, and told Miller that the house and board would soon be establishing a political arm and that he, Miller, would be a likely candidate to be its director. Miller left the lunch with an informal in-addition-to-other-duties assignment to spend some time in Washington learning how other organizations, both liberal and conservative, were approaching the question of political participation. "It was clear at the time," says Howard, "that the AMA could not make contributions or take other actions that were quote political unquote without grave danger of government action against the AMA. The question was: how could physicians use their resources to help elect people to Congress?"[4]

Though the idea of a political action committee had backers in many places, the events of 1959 failed to surround the proposals with any sense of urgency. The Forand bill won the endorsement of the young Democratic senator from Massachusetts, John F. Kennedy, and a Senate Subcommittee on the Problems of the Aged and Aging staged road-show hearings in seven cities, a form of political theater that is invariably good for press coverage and thus a way of generating support for a piece of legislation that otherwise seems stalled. But the bill itself stayed penned up in the Ways and Means Committee, whose conservative new chairman, Representative Wilbur Mills (D.-Arkansas), was working with Senator Robert Kerr (D.-Oklahoma) on a different kind of solution to the health needs of the elderly indigent. This was the Kerr-Mills bill, supported by the AMA, passed by Congress, and signed into law by President Eisenhower in late 1960. The legislation authorized federal grants to states to support state-run medical assistance programs for elderly persons who could establish a need for it.

For the AMA it seemed to be almost a time for second thoughts about starting a political action committee. Present as always was the inertial weight of those who never did think the AMA should soil its hands with politics. Some trustees asked the lawyers if political activities might not cause the AMA to lose its tax status under the Internal Revenue Code. Not entirely without reason, others wondered about the establishment of a new AMA body that would have to have a large degree of autonomy. Would the political action committee turn into a tail that would start wagging the AMA dog? The director of the AMA's law division and secretary to the Council on Legislative Activities at that time, C. Joseph Stetler, remembers a year of heavy discussion over whether the AMA should supplement its legislative capabilities with a political action committee. "Physicians were hesitant, to say the least," he says. "I can remember arguing the idea at a number of meetings. Since I was a proponent, I kept saying we were like a boxer going into the ring with one arm tied behind his back. Until we developed our political potential, we really weren't using our maximum talents."[5] Frank C. Coleman, M.D., then a member of the Council on Legislative Activities, a member of a three-man subcommittee of the council appointed to explore the pros and cons of political action, and a physician with many years of experience with political action in Iowa, remembers "difficulty in coming to a conclusion in that study as to whether we should have a political action committee." In October 1959, the subcommittee actually voted not to take the step, and at the December 1959 meeting of the house, the AMA president, Louis M. Orr, M.D., urged physicians merely to participate "as citizens" in political action committees "on a local basis."

Nevertheless, the idea was beginning to take a deeper hold. In several parts of the country a new generation of physicians, impatient and politically oriented, was supplying the initiative to get statewide political action committees launched. A survey done by the AMA in February 1960 revealed eight states with political action committees in functional condition, three more with "organized forms" of political action programs, and sixteen indicating that there were physicians politically active on an individual basis. In April 1960 the board voted $7,500 to the Council on Legislative Activities to underwrite three regional meetings that summer to educate physicians in political techniques. In effect, it was a series of how-to meetings on creating political action committees. Helping with the programs were Clifford White, a professional political consultant, and Richard Armstrong, a public affairs expert.

At the three regional meetings—in Salt Lake City, French Lick, Indiana, and Hershey, Pennsylvania, Howard was the lead-off speaker, presenting a review of the bills that had been before the eighty-sixth Congress. But he concluded his remarks with a reference to the sort of political pressure that was behind the Forand bill. "We cannot win this fight," he said, "unless lawmakers are elected who agree with our point of view...There is no point to electing men whom you control. Elect men like yourselves, who have the same philosophic point of view, who, when they go to Congress, will vote for conservative principles." In his opinion, the decisive encounters would take place at the polling places, not in the lobbies of the Capitol building. It was a call for grassroots action.

William L. Watson, then a staff member of the Pennsylvania Medical Society in the legislative department, later field man for the AMA's political action committee and its executive director (1968-81), remembers attending the meeting at Hershey that August. "At first," he says, "it was just another meeting. But after a few hours I really became intrigued. We had a pseudo-PAC in Pennsylvania then, $25, $50 contributions to various state races, activities like that. Nothing very sophisticated. Among our doctors there was a lot of nay-saying. But I got fired up, and I remember a doctor who was considered to be the real comer in PMS saying, 'We've go to do this.'"[6]

Back in Chicago the Board of Trustees still needed convincing, and the executive vice president, Blasingame, became active in the evangelizing. At one point, a day or so before a board session that fall, he asked Joe Stetler, recently promoted to be director of the AMA's legal and socioeconomic division, to give him a list of reasons to start a political action committee. In his memo, Stetler mentioned the widespread sentiment in favor of the idea, "the endorsement and interest being demonstrated at the state and local level." He thought that the regional conferences had indicated a need for a full-time organization and expressed the thought that a political action organization might get underway even without the AMA's blessing. There is no record that Blasingame passed on Stetler's thoughts to the board, though that is likely.

At the October meeting of the Council on Legislative Activities, Stetler staged a powerful presentation in favor of starting a political action committee that took the form of a debate (later repeated for the board) between himself and a new lawyer in the AMA Washington office, Paul R. M. Donelan. Following the formal rules for parliamentary debate, with provisions for rebuttals and so forth, Stetler outlined the handicaps the AMA suffered because it did not have a political arm, while Donelan stressed the local aspect of politics, arguing that a national organization should await the formation of a full complement of state committees. The council was almost persuaded, approving something it called the National Physicians Committee for Good Government, but it postponed final action until January, so that the state medical associations could be polled on their attitudes toward a national political action committee.[7]

However, that became unnecessary, as did further debate, when John F. Kennedy, a friend of labor and a supporter of sweeping health legislation, won the presidential election less than a month later. Early in 1961, with an eye on the new administration, the council recommended and the board approved the formation of the American Medical Political Action Committee (AMPAC).

Though Kennedy's election, like Truman's twelve years earlier, triggered an immediate action within the AMA, the rationale underlying the start of AMPAC should be considered in more long range terms. Though the timing makes it appear that way, AMPAC was not a simple, tactical countermeasure but part of a coherent strategy, here summarized by David G. Baldwin, who joined the AMPAC staff in 1961. From 1968 until his retirement in 1980 he headed communications in AMA's Washington office where, among other things, he proved to be a shrewd analyst of the political scene. He begins,

> Let's go back for a minute to the Truman health bill and start with that. What options were open to the AMA then? You could not very well send in the lobbyists and hope that on the basis of sheer logic and persuasion your case would prevail. The lobbyists would have been going to congressmen and, in effect, saying, "Here's our position. You can see it is right. Now forget all the political considerations and vote for it."
>
> That's a pretty dangerous way to go about any legislative effort. You just can't expect a congressman to die as a martyr to your convictions. If you can't go that route, what's left for you? You can, of course, go to the country with a vast public relations program, and the Whitaker and Baxter thing was a brilliant campaign. But you can't do that too often. For one thing, you start to bore people to death. Big public relations campaigns, even when you win them, create enemies. And after a while, the number of enemies grows.
>
> By 1960 the AMA simply couldn't appeal to the public every time it had to go to the mat with the federal government. We couldn't go back and do Whitaker and Baxter over and over again. What we had to do circa 1960 was develop political allies in Congress. But as you

do that, you have to be conscious of the terms of your welcome. After so many trips to the well a congressman will turn to you and say, "You guys are the first ones to ask me to put my head on the chopping block for your program. But where are you when I need you? I could have used a lot of help in my last election. I didn't see any interest from your organization either in terms of a dollar contribution or volunteer help."

If your organization is not doing things like that, you get to the point where your lobbyists are not going to be listened to very carefully. And the reason for that is you haven't got any political participation. Your effectiveness in a legislative program is geared to your commitment to a political program.

That was the basic thinking behind AMPAC.[8]

At its May 1961 meeting the Board of Trustees formally created AMPAC,* approving bylaws for a non-profit, voluntary, bipartisan, unincorporated political action committee, with emphasis on the bipartisanship.[9] Membership was open to physicians, wives, families, and others. The governing body was to consist of seven directors, six of them doctors and one a member of the Woman's Auxiliary of the AMA, all appointed for one year terms (with a maximum of five) by the AMA Board of Trustees. (The number of physician directors was later raised to nine). Among the first appointees were Frank C. Coleman, M.D., who had been active in an Iowa political action group, and a fellow member of the Council on Legislative Activities, Donald E. Wood, M.D., who had been active in I-HOPE. The first AMPAC chairman was Gunnar Gundersen, M.D., a former AMA president (1958) and board chairman (1955-57). "He was not in love with politics," Baldwin says. "But within the AMA he was a symbol of decency and rectitude. His choice said to the membership that we weren't going to be dominated by power brokers or runaway right-wingers or whatever." Coleman says much the same thing. "We had great trouble with credibility at the start. Gunnar's personal prestige had a lot to do with getting AMPAC underway."

Though he clearly had the backing of the top AMA staff executives, notably Howard, Joe Miller still had to be chosen by the new AMPAC board as the executive director, and there were other candidates. At the first meeting of the board at the Drake Hotel in

*The action was contingent on the Department of Justice reaction to the bylaws. When no objections were raised, the board gave the final okay at its June meeting.

Chicago on August 10, 1961, the candidates went in for their interviews. Miller recalls being down in the lobby after his interview, "biting his nails," when Dick Flynn, the longtime manager of convention services at the Drake, walked by and casually said, "Congratulations, Joe." To this day, says Miller, he does not know how Flynn got the word.

In AMPAC's formative stage, a question that bothered the AMA board and the association's director of the law division, Joe Stetler, was the matter of separateness. How much distance did there have to be, legally, between the unincorporated political action committee and the incorporated professional association that was, in effect, its parent? There was only one existing precedent that might help define the proper relationship, that between the AFL-CIO and COPE. But since those two organizations lived in a warm symbiosis with the Democratic party, Stetler did not want to rely on that as his guide. "I was supersensitive," he says. "I was insistent that the AMPAC board be a totally separate entity. The bank accounts had to be separate. The two staffs had to be located separately. There had to be a complete division. Blasingame did not think all that was necessary, and Howard thought that AMPAC should be more under AMA control, more than I thought it could have legally. I always felt that there were people in the Justice Department in Washington just standing in line waiting for us to break the law."

To be sure, the AMA board appointed the members of the AMPAC board; the terms were only for one year; and AMPAC was dependent on the AMA for most of its non-political operating funds. Yet largely because of the way the AMA lawyers interpreted the Federal Corrupt Practices Act, AMPAC was launched as a highly autonomous organization. Symbolizing the separateness, AMPAC's offices were located three blocks East of the AMA headquarters, at 520 North Michigan Avenue.

Being that independent of the AMA, the new AMPAC board and its new executive director had, in effect, the large and challenging assignment of starting a whole new national medical organization. At the age of thirty-seven, Joe Miller had already built a reputation as a good organizer and administrator. Before joining the AMA he had served as the executive director of the Kentucky Tuberculosis Hospital Commission, a point of frequent interface between medicine and politics. Now another quality of Miller's would become visible. "Joe Miller," says Baldwin, who worked with him closely for AMPAC's first seven years, "had a marvelous understanding of physicians, of just how much and just how fast doctors could be led. That was a quality that was very much needed. Remember, politics was a new world for most of them."

Even though the major commitment had been made, the Board of Trustees submitted its action establishing AMPAC to the House of Delegates at the November 1961 meeting, seeking an endorsement and laying the groundwork for financial support. The delegates showed a rare enthusiasm. An Illinois delegate who characterized himself as "hard to get money from" announced he had already given $99* to become a sustaining member of AMPAC and told the assembly, "Go home and organize your family and neighbors. Be sure they are registered...Get these people to organize the town." Malcolm C. Todd, M.D., soon to join the AMPAC board and later (1974) to become an AMA president, waved aloft checks for $2,500 that he had collected from his fellow California delegates and urged everyone "to take the message of AMPAC back home." Others spoke with similar fervor. Finally, the speaker, Norman A. Welch, M.D., of Massachusetts, gaveled for quiet and declared the board report describing the creation of AMPAC adopted, "heartily, unanimously and enthusiastically."[10]

Now that the AMA had a political action committee, what sort of organization should it be? What should it be modeled after? Says Coleman,

> Nobody had much feel for how to go about this. We looked at what California had done with its Public Health League. It was a collaborative committee, doctors, nurses, dentists, and, I think, some hospital people. And we looked at COPE. The longer we looked, the less we liked the collaborative type of set-up. It was complicated; we might be together on some issues and then apart on others. So we looked more closely at COPE. But they established policy at the national level and sent the word down. Doctors, it was obvious to us, would not take that. The AMA couldn't control its members the way the AFL-CIO controlled theirs. In the end, we decided against using either for a model, and we came to the view that we would have to have state PACs and work through them.

*There are several reasons why $99 was chosen as dues for a year's sustaining membership in AMPAC. First of all, it was catchy, a figure more likely to arouse curiosity than $100 and thus more likely to attract attention. Also, contributions of $100 or more had to be reported; the use of $99 served to eliminate paperwork. Active membership cost only $10 ($20 after 1980), and the average contribution to AMPAC during its early years ranged between $10 and $20.

From the start AMPAC stressed the dual nature of its organization. Instead of recruiting members and raising funds on a national basis unilaterally, AMPAC focused on joint efforts—the establishment of state committees where they did not exist and the strengthening of state committees where they did. Once that was done, membership and fund-raising could proceed on a joint basis. From the national viewpoint, the idea had the virtue of spreading the support base and providing local identification for AMPAC. People at the state level benefited from the expertise of the full-time Chicago staff and felt a sense of involvement, of participation, in a coordinated national effort.

Equally significant was AMPAC's early decision to stay out of presidential campaigns. Besides reflecting AMPAC's policy of bipartisanship—its goal being a strong conservative coalition in Congress that would include both Democrats and Republicans—there were practical considerations as well. "For an organization like AMPAC to be successful," notes Miller, "you have to keep your lines of communication open with the leadership of both parties. When you get into a one-party alignment, which you do when you start endorsing presidential candidates, then you lose the opportunity to communicate with the leadership of the other party. Now, labor can pull it off because its membership is so big and its resources are so large that even the opposition party has to listen. But we just weren't big enough to meet those conditions, and we aren't today."[11]

Considering the novelty of the concept and physicians' distrust of anything not proven, it is astonishing how quickly AMPAC sprung to life. During his first few months on the job, Miller traveled tirelessly, as did many members of the AMPAC board, explaining to the state organizations what the AMA had done, what the legal ramifications were, and urging states to join in. "The profession was thoroughly ready to go for this," says Miller. "There were dozens, hundreds, of men and women just waiting to get involved." Almost everywhere AMPAC was finding ready-made missionaries already in the field, younger physicians at that stage where they might be expected to begin their traditional move through the chairs of organized medicine. But before them now was an exciting new interest, a different channel for their energies, a new, shorter and more dramatic route to the top elective positions. "It was a group that was young, energetic, ready to go 110 percent in creating a strong political action arm for the AMA," says Miller.

Though it was not quite so close to the surface as the overall enthusiasm, the potential financing for AMPAC was there too. The AMA, together with a few of the larger pharmaceutical manufacturing companies,* volunteered "soft" dollar support (the income that could be used for everything *except* candidate contributions) to the extent of nearly $1 million annually in the first three years. Through AMPAC's own efforts and those of the state committees, the "hard" dollars (individual donations and membership dues that could be used in elections) also started flowing: $201,240 in 1961-62 from 13,416 individual members.** Most significant of all for the long term, AMPAC could, after its first fifteen months of operation, point to forty-five states with organized, working political action committees.

So began a highly successful effort to give a political education to American physicians. Trained in the scientific method, with its emphasis on hypothesis, experiment, and objective proof, physicians at first had difficulty with the trade-offs and compromises that often characterize the political process. Frank C. Coleman, M.D., who talked political action to doctors for twenty-five years, found them naive politically. "At the local level they don't grasp the relationship between getting involved in a candidate's campaign early on—with financial support and volunteer work—and the chips you develop that you can cash at a subsequent time."

Physicians also tended to choose candidates solely on the basis of ideology, unaware of the sometimes more important considerations of practical politics. Part of AMPAC's first educational job was to get doctors, as Baldwin put it, "to behave in a schizophrenic fashion." He adds:

> Sometimes they just had to bite the bullet and support a candidate in the other party because that is what the political realities called for. Say, for example, you're up against a congressional committee chairman you know you can't beat. Say furthermore that your people in Washington can usually get his vote on about 40 percent of the bills you really care about. Well, the realities of political life tell you that it's better to contribute your money to that incumbent with the hope of improving communications in the future than to back a hopelessly outclassed opponent, even though you might be much closer to him ideologically. It was a grueling process.

*AMPAC accepted no more outside support after 1972.
**In 1979-80 the equivalents for the two-year period were 126,220 members and $1,890,300.

Physicians also had to learn that AMPAC's endorsement and support were by no means automatic for physician candidates for office. AMPAC often had to go to great pains to explain that it applied the same criteria to physician candidates as it used in evaluating all candidates.

To gather in and organize the enthusiasm it was finding, the AMPAC staff concentrated heavily on building its communications. A monthly newsletter, *Political Stethoscope*, informed members of the growth of AMPAC itself, reported developments, tracked the start-up of political action committees in various parts of the country, and encouraged present members to bring in new ones. Speakers fanned out across the country to propagate the faith at meetings of county and state medical societies. At the twice-a-year AMA conventions, AMPAC put on big dinners with speakers and slide presentations afterward to describe its work.

In the 1960s those conventions attracted as many as 60,000 persons, and booths in the convention halls manned by AMPAC staff members answering questions and distributing pamphlets reached a wide geographical cross-section of the profession. At the meetings of the house, the AMPAC board chairman was accorded a speaker's spot on the opening program, used to intensify interest and visibility. More and more of the officials and visitors who flooded the hotel corridors and lobbies at the conventions sported the "99" lapel button of the AMPAC sustaining member or the red-white-and-blue AMPAC membership ribbon on the convention identification badge. Some of the state committees started coming through for AMPAC in a big way. Probably because of Coleman's long interest, half the physicians in Iowa enrolled in the Iowa Physicians Political League and voted a sizeable proportion of its dues to AMPAC. In Wood's Indiana, I-HOPE signed up 1,000 doctors, who contributed heavily to AMPAC. A fund-raising dinner in Texas netted $18,000.

Simultaneously, a well thought-out training program was developed to turn the enthusiastic political amateurs into savvy political workers, into people who knew the ropes and could set up effective candidate support committees at the local level. Through workshops, training films,* pamphlets, even a lending library of books on politics, physicians and especially physicians' wives—through the Woman's Auxiliary to the AMA—received a grounding in basic political campaign techniques. A three-hour "barnstormer course"

*Two titles: "The Fable of the Foiled Physician," and "How the Opinion Maker Makes Opinion in Politics."

was offered that covered such fundamentals as political party structure, precinct organization, and voter registration.

As such ventures go, AMPAC's education and training program was well ahead of its time. The use of survey research, demographic data, and attitudinal studies in political campaigns was not especially common at that time; political analysis was largely (though not entirely) a seat-of-the-pants business. But to physicians, with their scientific training, the application of research methods to political action had immediate appeal, far more, for example, than the doorbell-ringing aspects of campaign politics. Thus AMPAC sponsored several of the pioneering studies in the field of political analysis; almost from the start, AMPAC was a state-of-the-art operation.

Of the many research organizations employed over the years by AMPAC, one of the earliest used was the California firm, Spencer/Roberts*. This firm offered expertise in attitudinal research and the use of that discipline in campaign strategy. What emerged from that early association was something called PIPS, for Precinct Index Priority System. Basically, it was a method by which a candidate could decide the most efficient way to deploy his campaign resources, including his own time. Starting with a precinct voter list and a survey of a small percentage of the people on it, the PIPS program could tell a campaign support committee a great deal about a precinct, especially in terms of the attitudinal differences from one section to another. By extending the study to a whole Congressional district (without necessarily surveying every precinct), PIPS could indicate to a candidate which sections of his district merited the most intensive efforts. "In effect," says William Watson, the former AMPAC chief, "PIPS could show him which trees to shake in order to yield the maximum number of apples."

Other nationally known political experts engaged in AMPAC's political education program in the early days include Roy Pfautch of St. Louis, whose firm, Civic Service, Inc., offered campaign management, polling services, and post-election analysis; John Kraft & Associates, whose polling organization was widely used by Democratic candidates; and Vincent P. Barabba, who left Spencer/Roberts to start his own firm, DMI (for Decision Making Information), and later (in 1973) became the Director of the United States Bureau of

---

*Stuart Spencer was President Ford's political campaign consultant in 1976 and was called in on the Reagan campaign when he appeared to be faltering in the fall of 1980. Bill Roberts remains active, especially in California political campaigns.

the Census. "We got into research early," Watson says, "certainly ahead of COPE. The things we were doing back in 1964 and 1965 are the things now being taught at all the political campaign schools."

To broaden the educational process and to help get locally organized candidate support committees going, AMPAC had a field staff of four people in 1962 and added four more in 1963. Located around the country, each had a territory and an assignment to service the needs of six to eight states. With few exceptions the state medical societies were not prepared, from a personnel standpoint, to meet the commitments of a political effort. AMPAC field personnel often had to take up the slack. They provided continuity, helped out with the management process, and maintained the liaison between Chicago and the state organizations.

From the start the idea of an AMPAC field staff caused problems.[12] Both Blasingame and Aubrey Gates foresaw a conflict with the AMA Field Service Division. Gates had distinct and important legislative responsibilities, and his field staff was charged with keeping the state medical societies involved with the AMA's efforts in Washington. In fact, a large part of AMA's effectiveness on Capitol Hill depended then (as now) upon reminders that organized medicine was not only the AMA in Chicago but also medical organizations back home in the election districts.

After first opposing an AMA annual grant large enough to finance an AMPAC field staff, Blasingame reluctantly gave in. But the overlapping nature of the two field staffs was to create growing friction, not so much between the field men themselves as between Gates and Blasingame on the one hand and AMPAC on the other.* There is a distinction between a political effort, which was AMPAC's job, and a legislative effort, which was the AMA's. But at the end of the political lines, back in the congressional election districts, jurisdictions have a way of getting blurred.

The only other cloud on AMPAC's horizon came in the form of a tape sent in by a field man working for the state political action committee in Pennsylvania. He believed it was a recording of a United Steelworkers official urging a group of fellow unionists to use their muscle to elect liberal candidates for Congress. The field man said he heard about the recording through a tip and bought it for $20 on a street corner one night from a man named Cousin. AMPAC distributed 5,000 copies of the recording in 1963, hoping it

---

* On even-numbered years, i.e. election years, after 1966, AMA field service personnel went off the AMA payroll to work as AMPAC field staff.

would arouse listeners and generate membership contributions. However, the recording was exposed as a fake. The AMA had to apologize and settle a lawsuit for libel filed by the labor leader for $25,000. The mystery as to the source of the recording has never been unearthed. Some AMPAC staff members think it was a plant—what became known in the Watergate era as "dirty tricks." But there are others who argue that it was the work of an overzealous supporter, someone a bit immature and dangerously ignorant of the libel laws.

Embarrassing as the incident was to a group that prided itself on its political sophistication, it could not derail the momentum that AMPAC was gathering. Its purposes were clear and easily stated, probably never with more clarity than in Frank Coleman's address to the house as AMPAC chairman in 1965. He told the delegates, "The solution to the problem of keeping politics out of medicine no longer lies in asking Congress to act wisely; the solution lies in helping to elect a wise Congress."[13] From 13,416 members in 1961-62, the total of AMPAC members rose to 33,663 two years later and to 81,950 at the end of the decade. Membership dollars, hard dollars, which amounted to $201,240 during the first two-year period, jumped to over $1 million by 1969-70.

In considering such figures, it is important to understand that medicine's total political activity operates at three levels. First, there are local candidate support committees, which may consist of physicians and their spouses in a congressional district who decide on their own to raise money and go to work for a candidate they like. Second, there is the state political action committee, which acts quite often at the invitation of the candidate support committee. It might contribute $5,000 to the campaign, or a lesser amount. Third, of course, were the financial resources of the national organization, AMPAC.

Often, all three organizations agreed on their evaluation of a candidate, and in such instances they worked in concert. Thus the amount of AMPAC hard dollars indicated only a fraction of what organized medicine spent altogether on political activities. After enactment of the Federal Election Campaign Act of 1971 and subsequent rulings by the Federal Election Commission, AMPAC and the state committees were judged to be parts of the same organization. This meant that *combined* state-AMPAC contributions were limited to $5,000 per candidate per election. One effect, in the late 1970s, was to shift AMPAC dollars into providing in-kind services to candidates (e.g., bench mark surveys) and into independent expenditures (e.g., paid advertising done without the candidate's knowledge, consent, or awareness).

At the same time, it should be recognized that the national, state, and local decisions as to whom to support are made independently. AMPAC does not necessarily do what the state committees do, and the states do not necessarily march in step with the local candidate support committees.

During its first years, as many had predicted, AMPAC did stir resentment in the House of Delegates. "We were the new chicken in the yard," Donald Wood recalled. "Some of the delegates and a part of the membership felt that AMPAC was a rump organization that was coming on with a cause and was going to take over and be the new policy-making body of the AMA. It did create problems." Wood, who was the AMPAC chairman in 1964, became aware of them when he entered the race for AMA president-elect that November* and lost 131-94. Because his opponent, James Z. Appel, M.D., was unusually well-respected and had made major contributions to the AMA over many years, it is unfair to conclude that Wood was defeated by an anti-AMPAC vote. It is fair to say, however, that AMPAC certainly did not dominate the house, as many physicians had feared that it would. It was not until 1966, with the election of Max H. Parrott, M.D., of Oregon to the Board of Trustees, that the first physician generally considered to be an "AMPAC candidate" was elected to a major AMA office.

Actually, Parrott never served on the AMPAC Board of Directors, and he sometimes asked, not entirely seriously, how anyone could label him an AMPAC candidate. Though he did come up through the chairs—he was president of his state medical association, an AMA delegate, and a member of the Council on Legislative Activities—he had a great deal to do with getting the political action committee movement going, and he served as a trustee of the Oregon Medical Political Action Committee. Both by his outlook and his actions, Parrott was clearly one of those physicians ready to sign up and go enthusiastically to work the minute AMPAC began.

Measured by the standards of later election laws and the creation of the Federal Election Commission, the rules that applied to polit-

---

*After three months in office, President Norman A. Welch, M.D., died. The president-elect, Donovan F. Ward, M.D., succeeded to the office, creating a vacancy in the office of president-elect. It was in this election that Wood was defeated by Appel.

ical action in the 1960s were downright permissive. There was, for example, no limit on how much money a committee could donate to a campaign, so long as those dollars came from individuals and were clearly intended for political use, and so long as the amounts given were correctly reported, as appropriate, to the Clerk of the House of Representatives or the Secretary of the Senate. Because of that requirement, a limit of sorts was imposed, equal to the threshold of embarrassment of the contributing organization or the recipient congressman. AMPAC, as a rule, limited itself to contributions of $5,000 per candidate per election, the same limit as that imposed later by law. In addition to dollar contributions, a political action committee could also donate services—baby sitters and chauffeurs to get voters to polls on election day in the case of COPE, or research and campaign strategy, such as PIPS, in the case of AMPAC.

From the start it was apparent that AMPAC could not participate in every primary and every runoff. There would have to be some mechanism for deciding which races to enter and which to stay out of.[14] The job fell to a Congressional Review Committee, which consisted of the AMPAC chairman and two or three of the other directors, whom he named. One hard-headed decision, still followed with considerable consistency, was to concentrate resources on elections that were expected to be close, that is, where the margin between winner and loser might be no greater than 5 percent. What was the point of investing limited dollars on causes that were obviously hopeless, or on shoo-in candidates who really needed no help?

Once the Congressional Review Committee had determined that the election itself was one where AMPAC intervention might count for something, its members looked at the ideological posture of the candidate. This was done without reference to party label, since it was AMPAC's objective to build a bipartisan conservative coalition. For assistance with a question of general ideology, the Congressional Review Committee consulted with the state committees for their evaluation. The review committee sought help from local organizations on other questions, such as the amount of enthusiasm generated by a candidate in the local physician community, an estimate of general attractiveness and speaking ability, and the quality of the election organization he or she had been able to put together. After its screening, the review committee's recommendation went to the AMPAC board for final action, usually undertaken jointly with the local committee. Whenever possible, the actual check representing the AMPAC campaign contribution was presented to the candidate by a physician from the congressman's home district.

Quite often, especially where a decision had to be made about backing or opposing an incumbent, AMPAC sought advice in Washington. Here it often turned to the National Congressional Campaign Committees, of which there are four, one for each party in each chamber of Congress. The AMPAC directors, the top people in the AMA Washington office, and Joe Miller worked closely with these committees. Miller developed cordial relationships with their staff chiefs. Ken Harding, the head of the Democratic Congressional Campaign Committee in the 1960s, and Jack Mills, who held the same position in the Republican committee, were featured speakers at some of the AMPAC workshops. Wood can remember several times in the 1960s when the AMPAC board would take rooms at the Hay-Adams Hotel across Lafayette Park from the White House "where at some length we'd discuss our political concepts with the Democratic and the Republican leaders in Congress. We explained candidly that we wanted to support those individuals in their party who felt as we did about legislative issues. We were honest about it. These were eyeball-to-eyeball meetings with the leadership of both parties in Congress."

Referring to the same period, before the Federal Election Campaign Act of 1971, Coleman recalled,

> We wanted above everything else to establish our credibility as an organization. We had to watch out carefully for people on the far right and people on the far left. We wanted to make clear that we were people who could look candidly and objectively at candidates on both sides of the aisle. We wanted to establish ourselves as an organization which did not necessarily favor Republicans over Democrats or vice versa. We did not want to be known as people who would take AMPAC dollars and give them to our friends. That sort of credibility was a big problem for us in the early days, and we got around it through an intensive candidate review process.

The review process was impressively extensive and thorough. This is how it struck an Oregon physician, Blair Henningsgaard, M.D., in 1962, shortly before he became an AMPAC director (he later became AMPAC chairman). "I remember having a member of the Congressional Review Committee visiting me in Astoria. He'd come out so we could do some fishing on the Columbia River. One day he got a conference call from back East, and at his invitation I listened in. I sat quietly for two and a half hours, listening to a race-by-race analysis of where we were, who the candidates were, what their ideology was, who was supporting them at the local level, and whether AMPAC was going to put any money into the races. It was exciting stuff, and it made me realize that the congressional review process was the real guts of the AMPAC operation."[15]

Clearcut as the review criteria were, AMPAC occasionally had trouble applying them. From time to time a conflict would arise over which candidate to back in a certain district, the AMA Washington office insisting on one man, the local group arguing the cause of the other. The differences usually arose over the question of support for a key incumbent with whom the AMA lobbyists had established good relationships. More concerned with ideology, the local committee was inclined to argue for its candidate on the basis of principle. On the few occasions when the conflicts were battled out, the fighting was intense. Watson says,

> Probably the most agonizing moments I had as executive director of AMPAC came in the various skirmishes I had with the AMA Washington office. The feelings were sincere on both sides, the local PAC, the physicians in a community, feeling that a certain congressman just wasn't doing anything for medicine, the AMA Washington lobbyists feeling just as strongly that they were getting a good amount of time from the congressman and that he was important to them for that reason. It was especially tough if the congressman was in a leadership position. Many people in the PAC movement felt that since it was their dollars and their contributions of time, they ought to be able to call any particular shot as they wanted to. But it drove the lobbyists up the wall when a local PAC wanted to oppose someone they (the lobbyists) had developed a friendship and working relationship with.

But in overall terms, such conflicts were sufficiently rare, or at least well enough contained, that AMPAC operations expanded rapidly. In 1962, its first operational year, candidates regarded AMPAC with a degree of suspicion. "They didn't know what sort of animal they were dealing with," Baldwin says. "They had to be persuaded that this was a disciplined organization with some political couth. But by 1964 candidates were delighted to have AMPAC support." Coleman thinks AMPAC in 1962 was effective "only to a degree, because we didn't have enough money." AMPAC participated in some seventy elections its first year. Wood told the House of Delegates in his report at the November 1962 meeting that it was successful with about 70 percent of the candidates it backed. He was especially proud in describing how an AMPAC candidate had won out over a conspicuously backed COPE candidate. By 1966 AMPAC was able to increase its activities, participating in 131 House elections and fifteen Senate contests. But Coleman believes, "It was as late as 1968 before we were in a position to have a major impact." By the end of the 1970s, AMPAC was backing candidates in 220-240 congressional races every two years, of which thirty to forty were probably primary contests. AMPAC claimed that somewhere between 70 percent and 80 percent of the candidates it backed won their races.

What can be cited as AMPAC's major contributions? It is difficult to measure the success of any political action program in exact, specific terms. The conservative coalition in Congress, for which AMPAC worked so hard, actually attained majority status in 1981-82. But who can say with any precision how much AMPAC alone was responsible? Nevertheless, AMPAC did have something to do with that, and it is also possible to make some other generalizations.

Although it is widely considered to be the second political action committee with a national base and national goals (after COPE), AMPAC can claim status as a pioneer. At the time it began, a number of other organizations, especially in the business world, were considering forming political action committees, but they held back. Some were apprehensive about legal difficulties; others were unsure if they could accomplish much. For these organizations AMPAC showed the way.[16] It convincingly demonstrated that conservatively oriented political action committees could attract support and operate both legally and effectively. Moreover, AMPAC willingly shared its knowledge and experience with newcomers in the field.

The result—and this is a major contribution of AMPAC—was that labor's exclusive role in political action was effectively challenged. As the new, conservatively oriented political action committees gathered strength, they began to return an element of competition to the political marketplace. COPE had had the field to itself for a long time. After AMPAC started, that was no longer true. In 1982 there were some 3,000 political action committees.

Just as important are the internal ramifications of AMPAC's activities. What these come down to, in the last analysis, is a raised level of sophistication with which organized medicine has been able to conduct its business with state and federal governments. For years physicians thought of national health policy as something that lay almost exclusively in their realm of responsibility and authority. But after World War II, as more and more the health policy decisions moved into the public sector, physicians—the AMA—had increasing trouble dealing with them. What AMPAC did through the political education of a new generation of physician leaders was to make organized medicine understand the public nature of the policy-making process better and then to participate more completely in it.

To remain aloof from the political process, as physicians had tended to do, was to invite frustration and embarrassment, conditions in which the AMA continually found itself in the 1950s and 1960s. Those who fail to understand the interactive process by which much public policy is made, and the need to enter into the process, proceed at great peril. On this point both the scholar and the journalist agree. On the academic side is Arthur Bentley, author of the *The Process of Government: A Study of Social Pressures*:

> There is no political process that is not a balancing of quantity against quantity. There is no law that is passed that is not the expression of force and force in tension. There is not a court decision or an executive act that is not the result of the same process.[17]

Theodore H. White, the respected political journalist and author of the *Making of the President* books agrees. In *Breach of Faith*, in a chapter on what he calls the politics of manipulation, he describes Washington in these terms:

> Every group had to press its leverage in Washington by fair means or foul to survive. Money poured into national politics just to open doors. The airlines wheedled billions out of Washington and, for a while, thrived. The railroads could not learn the new language of politics and began to wither. The American shipbuilding industry learned the ways of Washington late—but when the Nixon shipbuilding subsidies began to flow from Washington, it rose from creeping decay to flourishing good health. Almost two million people worked in the American arms industry at its 1968 peak—their jobs dependent not only on the national defense program but also on the skill of their congressmen and lobbyists to keep Seattle or Fort Worth or Santa Monica or Long Island at the top of the Pentagon's procurement list. Scholarships and fellowships; symphony orchestras and art

museums; savings and loan societies; magazines with large or small circulations; private universities and public school systems; environmentalists and paper mills—all of them, and too many more to catalogue, depended for their well-being on the amount of pressure they could bring to bear in Washington.[18]

It is inaccurate to say that the AMA leaders of the 1950s and early 1960s were ignorant of the way things worked in Washington. They knew perfectly well what sort of pressures were brought to bear on legislation, and, as a matter of fact, the AMA seldom hesitated to exert pressures of its own. There was certainly no shyness about stating the AMA position on matters of policy either to the public or to congressional leaders.

The trouble was that AMA leaders, up until the late 1960s, came on as crusaders, as fierce, unyielding believers in principles that could not be compromised.[19] Admirable as such strength of conviction may be, it puts the holder at a disadvantage, especially where disputes are settled by parliamentary methods. The crusader is always throwing down the gauntlet and offering his adversary a hard choice: a fight to the death or unconditional surrender. The crusader makes it all but impossible for a legislature—especially a legislature responsive to a diversity of interests—to follow his lead.

But after 1965, when the AMA suffered a dramatic rout in the legislative struggle over Medicare, a new generation of leaders slowly came to power. Although these physicians held much the same beliefs as their predecessors, their style was different. They avoided getting locked into rigid positions, for they were not crusaders but pragmatists. They had a more realistic understanding of the political process; they were better equipped to operate within it. And, because AMPAC served as a training ground for many of these physicians, that may well be the most enduring of AMPAC's achievements.

Chapter Fourteen

A Liberalized Policy on Federal Aid to Education

Toward the end of 1957, for the annual education issue of *JAMA*, the secretary to the Council on Medical Education, Edward L. Turner, M.D., wrote a carefully worded editorial titled "Looking Ahead." Taking stock of the nation's medical education establishment and noting the estimates of population growth, Turner called for an effort by the AMA "to forecast objectively" the needs that lay ahead for "medical personnel as well as the faculty, facilities, and financing essential to their education and training."[1]

Although he did not mention the phenomenon by name, what underlay Turner's concern was the post-World War II baby boom. During the pessimism of the 1930s, births in the United States had hovered just under 2.5 million a year. With the boost in employment and wages brought on by the war (and the dynastic hopes of servicemen about to go overseas) the number rose to an average of about 2.9 million births per year. But in 1946 the number of newborns suddenly shot ahead to 3.4 million. It climbed to more than 4 million in 1954 and stayed there through 1964.[2] In those nineteen fecund years, 1946-1964, some 76,441,000 Americans were born,[3] the survivors making up approximately a third of our present population. More American babies were born in the year 1957—4,380,000—than in any year before or since.

Besides the surge in population, Turner touched on other "significant events" that he thought argued for increasing the rate at which the United States was producing physicians. At one end of the population span he foresaw a growing number of older people who, because of their age, would require more medical care; at the other, he foresaw an increasing number of college students clamoring for admission to medical school. Simultaneously, he observed that the trend to specialization, particularly in anesthesiology, pathology, and radiology, was taking physicians away from the routine care of patients.

The editorial marked a turning point in the AMA's thinking about the supply of physicians. During the late 1940s and early 1950s, Frank G. Dickinson, Ph.D., director of the AMA Bureau of Medical Economic Research, had argued that the 1950s physician had become more efficient than his 1930s and 1940s counterpart. Because of better roads and the wider ownership of automobiles, a physician could serve more patients over a larger geographical area. Because more people had telephones, physicians could follow the progress of patients with a smaller investment of time. Thanks to such improvements in transportation and communication, Dickinson argued, the modern doctor could deliver 33 percent more units of medical care per unit of time than possible heretofore. In other words, one 1950 physician should be considered substantially more than the equivalent of one 1940 physician. And, since the ratio of physicians to population had risen anyway, there was even less substance to the argument advanced in the 1948 Ewing report that a physician shortage was in the making.[4]

Turner acknowledged the validity of Dickinson's rationale, adding that progress in diagnostic techniques and the powerful new antibiotics were also making medical care more efficient. Because they could dramatically shorten the length of many illnesses, the new drugs could cut the duration of a physician's involvement in an episode of disease. But even so, Turner thought a careful assessment of future requirements should be made. He was looking uneasily at the surge in population and worrying about the trends in medical practice.

Since it is largely their number and the size of the classes they admit that determine the number of physicians, it is useful to examine briefly the condition of American medical schools in the 1950s. There were eighty-five of them in 1957. They produced 6,796 graduates that year and operated—most of them—under great financial strain. A medical education as conducted in the United States was and is an expensive proposition. Not only must a school maintain a large amount of costly scientific equipment; the nature of the clinical work demands a high student-teacher ratio. With medical knowledge becoming ever more specialized, medical schools today employ one full-time faculty member for every 1.2 students.[5] Including residency training, it takes several more years to educate a doctor than, say, a lawyer or someone with a master's degree in business administration. In addition, there is the considerable cost of the patient care and research activities that are considered necessary to the medical education process.

Financing for medical schools in the 1950s, other than student tuitions, came largely from three sources: federal research programs, private funding, and the state legislatures. Something under half of the schools were private (Yale, Northwestern, Stanford, etc.); more than half were part of state universities (Maryland, Texas, Kansas, etc.). The federal role was specific; it included generous grants for biomedical research, which often had the effect of subsidizing teachers engaged in research projects ($148 million in 1960), modest construction grants ($17.2 million in 1960), occasional help from federal housing agencies for the building of student dormitories, and Hill-Burton money for medical school affiliated hospitals.[6] Welcome as the grants were, they did not help the schools with recurring operating losses. There was no federal program for student assistance or for supporting the educational program.

Though it supported the idea of construction grants, the AMA warned against grants with incentives for expanding enrollment to the point where educational standards would suffer. Probably the fairest summary of the AMA position in the 1950s was executive vice president Blasingame's. He wrote to a congressional committee,

> Generally, the AMA is opposed to federal aid in those areas where the private citizens and the local communities are capable of providing for themselves. We believe federal aid to be a dangerous device because of the degree of control and regulation which must necessarily accompany federal funds. We believe, however, that there is sufficient need for assistance in the expansion, construction and remodeling of the physical facilities of medical schools to justify a one-time expenditure of federal funds, on a matching basis, provided, of course, that maximum freedom of the schools from federal controls is assured.[7]

Compared with what was to follow, there was little pressure to expand the schools to accommodate the number of student applicants. As a matter of fact, the number of applicants was actually dropping, and in some of the state university medical schools there were vacancies, generally attributable to the geographical restrictions on admissions. Many thought that the space program, then gathering momentum, was attracting some of the brainpower that might in other times have been attracted to medicine. But others related the fall-off in the number of applicants to the lowered birthrates during the depression twenty to twenty-five years earlier.

All that is not to say, however, that medical education had fallen into a backwater. Applications, though down, still outnumbered admissions, and six new medical schools were organized between 1950 and 1960, four of them state university schools. The ratio of physicians to population kept slightly ahead of the baby boom.

To those who ran the medical schools, the financial problems loomed larger and larger each year. Additional aid had to come from somewhere or the schools would be hard put to maintain standards or, in some cases, even stay open. C. H. William Ruhe, M.D., who joined the AMA staff in 1960 and later headed its medical education activities, saw the problem close-up. He was the associate dean of the University of Pittsburgh School of Medicine in the late 1950s and head of admissions. He says,

> The prospect for federal support was a wonderful prospect, and educators were anxious to get it even though some individuals feared federal controls.
>
> The Association of American Medical Colleges would get quite impatient with the AMA for not supporting its desire for federal support. It wasn't so much that the AAMC and the medical schools wanted to expand the physician population as they were anxious to get federal dollars to make ends meet. Many educators who had been AMA supporters resigned their memberships in the 1950s, resentful that the AMA opposed their opportunity to achieve financial solvency through the federal government. The policy difference widened the split between academia and the practitioner.[8]

To loosen the squeeze on medical school finances, the AMA still favored private initiatives. The American Medical Education Foundation, started in 1950, was trying its best, but it was able to raise only about $1 million a year (mostly from physicians); the National Fund for Medical Education, which solicited the business community, was raising about $3 million a year. Widening its efforts at the November 1959 meeting, the AMA board recommended and the house approved a special study committee under the Council on Medical Education to do several things: develop a medical student financial aid program; ascertain the maximum expansion of medical school student bodies that could be made without a loss in quality; and explore ways to draw more qualified college graduates into medical careers. A year later, preferring loans (which would, of course, be repayable) to outright gifts (i.e., scholarships, which are not repayable), the house adopted the special committee's proposal for the "principle of a security fund functioning as a co-signing agency to make available through community banks relatively large sums of credit at a low rate of interest to medical students."[9]

At the time, the board was thinking about a scholarship program that might cost $300,000 a year and a loan program that would cost $100,000 but generate $1,250,000 annually in guaranteed student loans. In endorsing the committee report, the board said its action was "based on the thought that there will be additional income because of the proposed increase in dues." In late 1961, the American Medical Research Foundation (which since 1957 had been making research grants from funds voluntarily given for that purpose) was merged with the American Medical Education Foundation to form the present AMA Education and Research Foundation. One of the designated functions of the new foundation was the administration of a loan guarantee fund. This commenced operation in March 1962 and in its first eighteen months guaranteed 12,000 loans to medical students, interns, and residents with a principal amount of $14 million.[10]

Meanwhile, the federal government was asking questions about the future supply of physicians. The Surgeon General of the United States, who heads the Public Health Service (then part of the Department of Health, Education, and Welfare, now part of the Department of Health and Human Services), appointed a consultant group on medical education, headed by Frank Bane, a recognized expert on public welfare with several years of Washington experience. The Association of American Medical Colleges was represented on the twenty-member panel; so was the AMA through Edward L. Turner, M.D., the author of the "Looking Ahead" editorial, and Julian Price, M.D., a member of the Board of Trustees.

The Bane report, issued in October 1959, gained wide acceptance and recognition. Unlike the Ewing report of 1948, which was released during Truman's whistlestop campaign for the presidency, the Bane report gave non-partisan consideration to the tough questions. Echoing Turner's editorial, the Bane group noted the rapid population growth and the impact of specialization on the number of physicians available for regular patient care. The Bane report recorded the overall growth in the number of physicians since 1930 and the rise in the ratio of active, non-federal physicians to population, observing, too, the annual addition to the supply of licensed physicians of about 750 foreign medical school graduates.

What had not appeared in Turner's analysis was a new and momentous fact: Whereas in 1930 the average American saw a doctor between two and three times a year, he now saw a physician nearly five times a year.[11] For a variety of reasons, among them the return of prosperity and the growth of private health insurance, the demand for medical care had at least doubled.

For all its careful, thoughtful work, the Bane group could not answer one question any better than similar committees before and after it: What constitutes the appropriate number of physicians? Just over a decade earlier, the Ewing report met the challenge apparently by averaging physician/population ratios in a few states, weighting the results on the side of the more prosperous ones, and declared that to be the ideal ratio for the whole country.[12] By this simplistic methodology, which was never clearly described in the report, Ewing argued that there would be a shortage of 42,000 physicians in 1960. In contrast, the Bane group frankly acknowledged the difficulties in quantifying future needs. What the Bane group finally did was to say, in effect, "Though we cannot assert with precision how many physicians the United States will require in 1975, let's at least make sure we have enough to maintain the physician/population ratio we have now." Working with the current population growth estimates and medical school expansion plans, the Bane report recommended that by 1975 the United States should have twenty to twenty-four additional four-year medical schools and an overall production of 11,000 medical school graduates annually.*

Within the AMA the realization was growing that private means could not furnish the level of support that the medical schools needed. The $1 million that the American Medical Education Foundation was distributing among the medical schools amounted to only about one half of the annual operating budget of one school. "From the time the Bane report was issued," Ruhe believes, "it was inevitable that the AMA would recognize the necessity for an expanded federal role in support of medical education." But the change was slow. "Almost invariably," Ruhe says, "there is a lag between the time when the people who are best informed in a given

---

*Both goals were exceeded. In 1975 there were 114 schools and 12,714 graduates. See *JAMA* 246 (1981): 2917.

field conduct their studies and the time when their conclusions are transformed into organizational policy. I've always believed that a staff should be well ahead of any committee which works on a subject, that the committee should be ahead of the council, the council ought to be ahead of the board, and that the board ought to be ahead of the house. By ahead, I mean farther along in their thinking, more conversant with the details of an issue, and consequently more likely to put forth proposals that are not consistent with current policy."

At the same time, federal policy-makers were re-examining their position. The Bane report found a receptive audience among President Kennedy's New Frontiersmen. While the federal priorities still included biomedical research, they now began to place a new emphasis on the education and training of medical personnel.[13] Legislatively, the Bane report developed into the Health Professions Educational Assistance Act of 1963. The original bill proposed a three-pronged program to expand the production of physicians in the United States. It called for: (1) matching grants for the construction, replacement, or rehabilitation of medical, dental, and osteopathic schools; (2) a loan fund for medical, dental, and osteopathic students; and (3) an expansion of the research facilities construction program. In testimony before the House of Representatives that February and before the Senate late in the fall,[14] the AMA gave its support to the construction programs, pointing out that it had favored such actions since 1951. However, it opposed the student loan provisions. AMA witnesses at the congressional hearings maintained that the AMA Education and Research Foundation loan program was meeting that need adequately; 93 percent of those applying for loans had received them; no one had been turned away for lack of money in the fund.[15] The AMA asserted that the federal loan program, because it was not self-supporting, called upon the taxpayer to subsidize the medical education of future doctors. It was not, for example, the sort of loan program that a well-run bank might set up on a non-profit basis. "Medical students and physicians in training have a responsibility to society," said a board report, "and should not expect the interest on their debts to be paid by a taxpayer's subsidization."[16]

The Student American Medical Association took a sharply different view. Addressing the House of Delegates in June 1963, medical student representative Robert O. Voy politely told the doctors that the students preferred the federal loans. The government, he said, was more generous—their program offered loans of $2,000 a year versus the $1,500 offered by the AMA's program plus easier interest and payback provisions.

Although Congress chose not to accept the AMA's arguments, it should be noted that the difference between the AMA and the government position was one of means rather than ends. Both agreed about the need for increasing the production of physicians; they disagreed over the best way to accomplish that goal. Two actions at the 1963 annual meeting confirm that view. First, a resolution to oppose the Health Professions Educational Act *in toto* was defeated. This left the board action favoring the construction grants alone and did not disturb the AMA Education and Research Foundation loan program to eliminate many financial barriers to a medical education. Second, the house adopted a Council on Medical Education report that forthrightly declared, "During the last decade the increase in number of medical school graduates has about kept pace with the growth of the population. This increase, together with the immigration of foreign-trained physicians, has resulted in a steady, slight increase in the ratio of physicians to population. However, to maintain and increase this ratio in the face of the expected growth of population will require a numerical increase of graduates far exceeding that of recent decades."[17]

Two years later the issue of medical education financing was back on the AMA's agenda. In the first part of 1965, Health Professions Educational Assistance Amendments were introduced in Congress, calling for the renewal of the expiring provisions of the 1963 Act—the construction grants and the student loan program. But the amendments bill also proposed something additional: basic improvement grants that could be used in the educational programs of the schools. This support for the operating budget was, of course, what the schools had wanted all along. The legislation also contained incentives for expansion; in order for a school to qualify for an improvement grant, the entering class had to be larger by either five students or 2.5 percent (whichever was larger) than any incoming class in the preceeding five years. Urging the deletion of these provisions from the bill, the AMA voiced its old concern. "It is our conviction that it is likely to lead to the federal domination of medical education."[18] The AMA did, however, support the construction grants again. As in 1963, the 1965 amendments passed very much as proposed, despite only partial endorsement by the AMA.

But dissatisfaction with the old position continued to mount. This surfaced at the June 1965 meeting in an odd manner, coming in a report from a previously appointed Committee to Review the Operations of the House of Delegates, chaired by Gunnar Gundersen, M.D. Commenting on the supply of physicians, the Gundersen Committee report said, "The AMA has not been successful in satisfying adequately the public demands." As for the financing of medical education, the report emphasized that funds should come from a variety of sources so that a school would not become entirely dependent on any of them. "Special thought should be given to tax funds," it added, "which presently represent by far the largest source." Action on the report was postponed.[19]

But it soon became academic, for a month later Congress passed the Medicare and Medicaid amendments to the Social Security Act. This changed everything. The new legislation, it was clear, would sluice new billions of dollars into the health care system, launch new demands for medical services, and raise new thoughts about the size of the medical education system and its financing.

Because no one, least of all the sponsors of Medicare and Medicaid, could predict how large the increase in demand might be, it was difficult to formulate a policy about supply. Everyone agreed that the number of physicians, as well as other medical personnel, would have to be increased. But by how much, and through what financing methods? The Council on Medical Service was struck by the scale of the problem. In a 1966 report the council said, "On top of an already over-extended health care system, we now find ourselves faced with the necessity of having to meet increased demands for medical service by 19-20 million people under [Medicare] and 35-50 million people under [Medicaid].* In addition, we are faced with the necessity of providing health manpower to support a major war in Viet Nam." The Council on Medical Education advocated an AMA joint committee to define the likely size of the shortages and future manpower goals. At the June 1966 meeting, the Board of Trustees announced that it had already done something like that through the appointment of a seven-member Committee (later Council) on Health Manpower.[20]

In the six years following the Bane report, a meaningful expansion of medical education had already begun. Seven new schools were organized in the 1960-65 period, with the number of graduates rising from 6,860 in 1959 to 7,409 in 1965.[21] Simultaneously, nearly 1,500 graduates of foreign medical schools were swelling the

---

*A better Medicaid estimate would have been 18-22 million.

ranks of licensed physicians each year. The physician/population ratio, which is not an ideal index of the sufficiency of physicians but is a simple, acceptable measure, grew from 144 to 150 per 100,000 population.[22] On the strength of the construction grant program, twelve institutions announced plans for new medical schools. In its statement on the 1965 amendments, the AMA added, "At least as many more institutions are seriously considering the establishment of new schools. In addition, many medical schools have made application for funds to assist in the replacement or rehabilitation of outmoded facilities, with the anticipation of expanding significantly the size of their present medical classes. It may, therefore, be concluded that the construction grants have been successful in implementing the program to increase the number of medical graduates."[23]

But with the passage of Medicare/Medicaid legislation the estimate for future needs had to be redrawn. "Notwithstanding the record production of physicians," said a Board of Trustees report sent to the house at the June 1966 meeting, "it is obvious that the pressure for health care will require an increasing number of physicians."[24] The reference committee that considered the report emphasized the "drastic shortage of health manpower" and recommended adoption of the report; the house did so.

At the November 1967 meeting, the AMA completed the policy change it began in 1957, withdrawing its objections to direct federal subsidies to support the educational curricula of medical schools. A Board of Trustees report recommended correcting the imbalance between biomedical research and educational support that was caused by the heavy (though desirable) federal funding of research. Specifically, it called for greatly increased support for the operational budgets of medical schools. It was, as the reference committee that conducted a hearing on the report made clear, a change in policy.[25]

But it was also an honest recognition that federal financing for educational programs was now accepted by the American medical schools. Testifying in favor of the Health Manpower Act of 1968 before the health subcommittee of the Senate Labor and Public Welfare Committee, William A. Sodeman, M.D., chairman of the Council on Medical Education, cited a recent joint statement by the AMA and the Association of American Medical Colleges that called for enough new schools to accommodate all "qualified" applicants and formally endorsed the concept of federal support for the operational costs of medical schools.[26]

If a heavier foot was needed on the accelerator, the Johnson administration was ready to apply one. Reflecting the exuberance of the President's Great Society program, the National Advisory Committee on Health Manpower declared "a crisis in American health care" due in part to a deficiency in the number of health care workers. In his annual health message of 1968, President Johnson proclaimed a shortage of 50,000 physicians, a tidy, headline-catching number that stood for years as a seemingly unchanging description of the American medical manpower situation.

Federal dollars soon began to wash over the medical education system in increasing waves. From $43 million during the 1960-61 school year direct federal support for education in the medical schools grew more than ninefold in the next fifteen years to $398 million in the 1975-76 school year and to $415 million in 1981-82. (See Table 1. Direct support for education falls in the "other federal"

TABLE 1
Trends in United States Medical School
Revenues (millions of dollars)

Revenue Source	1960-61	1965-66	1970-71	1975-76	1980-81	1981-82
Federal Research	133	350	438	823	1,446	1,578
Other Federal	43	118	322	398	396	415
State, Local Government	74	136	323	808	1,452	1,617
Tuition and Fees	28	46	63	156	346	413
Medical Services	28	49	209	609	1,850	2,140
Other Income	130	188	358	595	935	1,054
TOTAL	436	882	1,713	2,389	6,425	7,217

Source: *Medical Education: Institutions, Characteristics, and Programs* (Washington: Association of American Medical Colleges, 1983): 25.

category.) During the twelve years after 1968, the number of medical schools rose from ninety-four to 126, the size of the graduating class from 7,973 to 15,135,[27] and the physician/population ratio from 161 per 100,000 to 219.[28] The only qualification the AMA voiced in giving its blessing to the expanded federal role in the financing of medical education was a plea that the federal funds be accepted on a matching basis.[29] As long as the medical schools did that, the AMA believed, the schools could maintain a diversified financial base and therefore operate with a stronger degree of academic independence.

FERVENT STRUGGLE over enactment of the Medicare legislation gave the newspaper cartoonists lively material. Opposite, the AMA is shown in an almost equal contest with President Lyndon B. Johnson. But the portrayal below, picturing an AMA David hoping to stop a Medicare Goliath with its Eldercare bill projected a more accurate picture of the power line-up. The Democratic landslide in 1964 elections made enactment of Medicare inevitable.

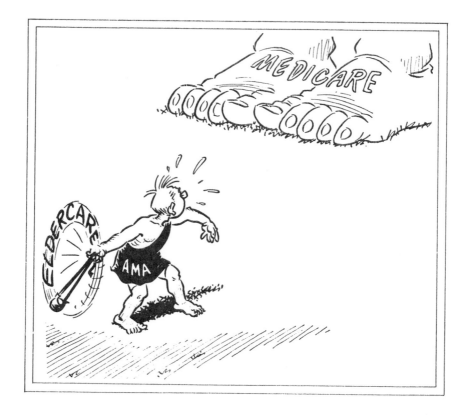

'Is There A Doctor In The House?'

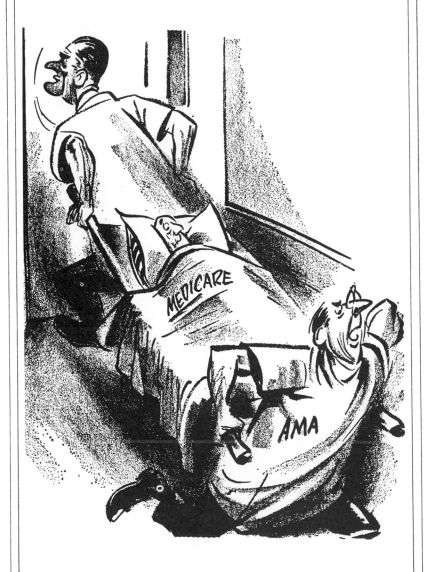

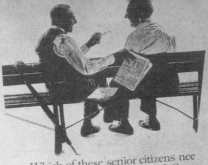

Which of these senior citizens nee
help to pay for his Medical Care

Citizen A is a well-to-do, retired executive. Citizen B is no longer employ
wealthy and is not protected by a private medical care plan. Both are ove

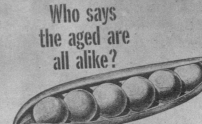

Who says the aged are all alike?

we oppose 'pea-pod' legislation drafting our senior
citizens into a federally-controlled system of

standardized medical care

But that's what the proposed King-Anderson Bill would do. It forgets that some of the aged
are rich, most are self-sufficient, and some are poor . . . that most are healthy . . .

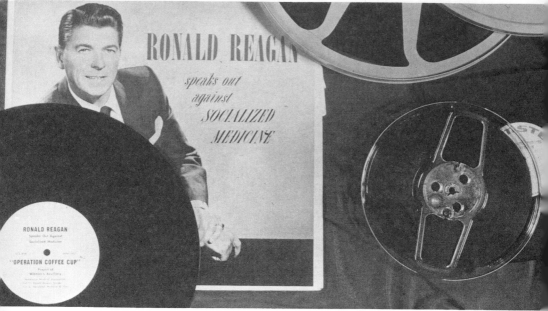

RONALD REAGAN

speaks out against SOCIALIZED MEDICINE

RONALD REAGAN
Speaks Out Against
Socialized Medicine

"OPERATION COFFEE CUP"

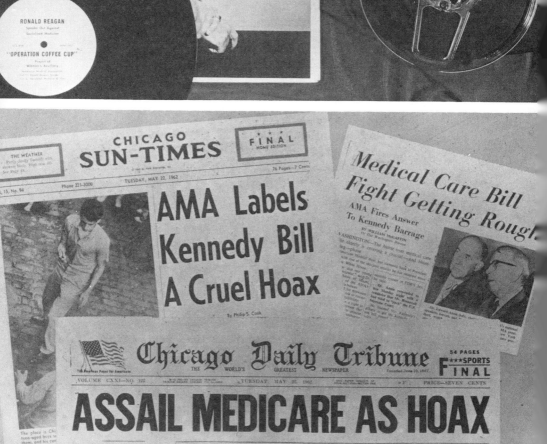

THE WEATHER

CHICAGO SUN-TIMES

FINAL HOME EDITION

TUESDAY, MAY 22, 1962   76 Pages—7 Cents

Phone 321-3000

Vol. 15, No. 94

AMA Labels Kennedy Bill A Cruel Hoax

By Philip S. Cook

Medical Care Bill Fight Getting Rough

AMA Fires Answer To Kennedy Barrage

BY WILLIAM McGAFFIN

WASHINGTON—The battle over medical care
to elderly . . .

Chicago Daily Tribune

THE WORLD'S GREATEST NEWSPAPER

Founded June 10, 1847

54 PAGES
***SPORTS
FINAL

VOLUME CXXI—NO. 122   TUESDAY, MAY 22, 1962   PRICE—SEVEN CENTS

ASSAIL MEDICARE AS HOAX

AMA ARGUMENTS against the King-Anderson bill, the original proposal for Medicare, ranged widely. Advertisements (opposite page, top) emphasized that the elderly population included people who did not need public assistance with medical bills as well as people who did. A 1963 campaign by the AMA Woman's Auxiliary (opposite, center) featured a well-known conservative speaking against socialized medicine. The AMA also made the point that the Medicare bill as originally drafted covered far fewer medical costs than most people thought (bottom). Too late as it turned out, the AMA promoted its own Eldercare bill (left) providing more generous benefits for the elderly who needed assistance, lesser coverage for those who did not.

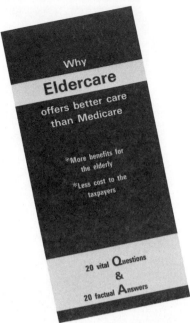

Why

Eldercare

offers better care than Medicare

*More benefits for the elderly

*Less cost to the taxpayers

20 vital **Q**uestions
&
20 factual **A**nswers

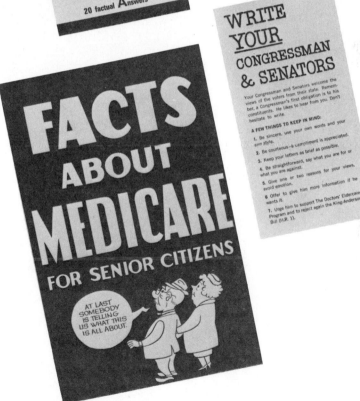

FACTS ABOUT MEDICARE FOR SENIOR CITIZENS

AT LAST SOMEBODY IS TELLING US WHAT THIS IS ALL ABOUT.

WRITE YOUR CONGRESSMAN & SENATORS

Your Congressman and Senators welcome the views of the voters from their state. Remember, a Congressman's first obligation is to his constituents. He likes to hear from you. Don't hesitate to write.

A FEW THINGS TO KEEP IN MIND:

1. Be sincere, use your own words and your own style.

2. Be courteous—a compliment is appreciated.

3. Keep your letters as brief as possible.

4. Be straightforward, say what you are for or what you are against.

5. Give one or two reasons for your views, avoid emotion.

6 Offer to give him more information if he wants it.

7. Urge him to support The Doctors' Eldercare Program and to reject again the King-Anderson Bill (H.R. 1).

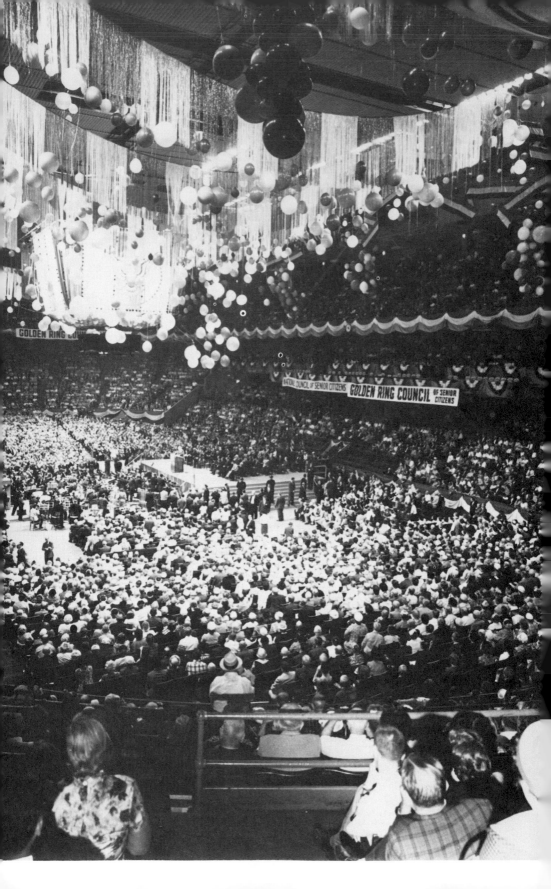

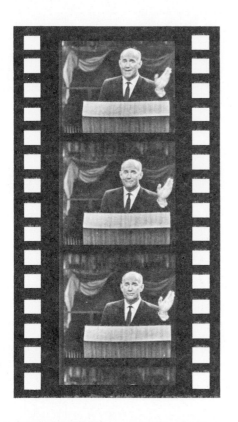

THEATRICAL CONTRAST marked a famous confrontation over Medicare in 1962. On Sunday afternoon, May 20, labor and labor-backed senior citizen groups packed Madison Square Garden (opposite) to hear President John F. Kennedy plump for the King-Anderson bill. His speech was carried on public service time by all three major television networks. Hours later, in a dramatic response, the AMA rented the Garden, empty except for the clutter left from the Kennedy rally, and filmed Edward R. Annis, M.D., (left and below) making a rebuttal. This was aired the following evening by the NBC-TV network on time purchased by the AMA.

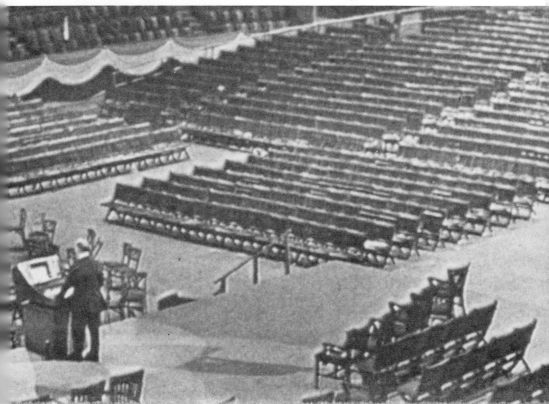

Chapter Fifteen

The Expansion of Access: Medicare & Medicaid

The political storms that engulfed medical policy-making in the early 1960s centered on the same issue that triggered the controversy in the late 1940s: access to care. Remember that the objective of the Wagner-Murray-Dingell bills was to make medical care more accessible, even "free," through a federally administered system financed by Social Security taxes. When President Truman, organized labor, and advocates within the Federal Security Agency failed to convince Congress that this was desirable policy, private, voluntary insurance continued to gain acceptance as the preferred means of easing access to medical care. With individual expenses distributed over a broad population base (and the premiums often paid in whole or in part by employers), insurance programs lowered the economic barriers to care for growing millions of working people and their families. By the late 1950s there was wide agreement that private health insurance was successfully meeting the needs of the employed population.

At the same time, it was apparent that private insurance often did not meet the needs of the non-employed, especially retired people. Health insurance for people over sixty-five was seldom an attractive proposition to the actuary, and companies that attempted to provide health insurance for the elderly risked seas of red ink.[1] A consensus began to grow that for at least *part* of the over-sixty-five population a program of governmental assistance was needed.

On the humanitarian principle involved in the issue there was no disagreement from the AMA. But over the means to the end, there was a great deal. As in the 1940s, an emotional political struggle erupted, and the resolution of the conflict came only after five years of contention and rancor.

It is not difficult to trace the ancestry of the health insurance proposals that launched the controversy. They derived from the Wagner-Murray-Dingell bills, and they were advanced by the same people. Toward the end of the Truman administration, those who had furnished so much of the initiative for the Wagner-Murray-Dingell legislation still occupied positions of power in the Social Security Administration, and they adopted a familiar political procedure. This is variously known as the politics of incrementalism or the strategy of gradualism. The terms mean the same thing. A bill that has run into opposition is stripped of objectionable provisions to the point where most of the objectors are mollified and a legislative majority becomes possible. With that in mind, Wilbur J. Cohen and Isidore S. Falk, the two men who did so much to develop the Wagner-Murray-Dingell bills from 1943 on, trimmed the old legislation into a new health insurance bill that would cover only hospitalization and apply only to the aged.[2] In 1951 Oscar R. Ewing, the administrator of the Federal Security Agency, which was the parent agency for Social Security, gave his blessing to a bill that provided sixty days of hospital care a year to Social Security retirees. "It is difficult for me to see," said Ewing, "how anyone with a heart can oppose this."[3] But as an issue, health insurance of any sort was dead for the rest of the Truman administration, and it lay dormant during most of Eisenhower's, surfacing only late in 1957 in modified form as the Forand bill.

The flame of national health insurance not only burned within the federal government—first in the Federal Security Agency, later in its successor organization, the Department of Health, Education, and Welfare—it was also kept alive within organized labor. And the proponents of health insurance legislation worked within their respective organizations in close collaboration with each other. Citing as sources several interviews in the Oral History Collection at Columbia University, Martha Derthick of the Brookings Institution describes in her book, *Policymaking for Social Security*, just how close that working relationship was.

> The constraints on official conduct meant that [Social Security] program executives needed a private collaborator, an unconstrained ally outside the government. They found one in organized labor—the AFL principally, as represented for years by Nelson Cruikshank. This outside ally could freely do things that they could not: sponsor bills that an incumbent administration opposed, openly lobby and engage

in propaganda contests, enter into campaign activity against program critics in Congress. However, the constraints on official conduct were never so rigid or so binding as to prevent program executives from collaborating very closely with this private ally, to whom they provided a steady stream of policy cues and usable information. Without this stream of official support and stimulation, the private ally would have been less active and less complaisant. With it, a close, mutually supportive relationship was formed.[4]

Derthick also gives her readers the following intimate glimpse of how some of the legislative work on health insurance for the elderly was accomplished. This excerpt is part of an interview in the Oral History Collection with Lisbeth Bamberger Schorr, a staff member in the AFL-CIO Industrial Union Department in Washington and an associate of Nelson H. Cruikshank, director of the union's Department of Social Security. Derthick, incidentally, describes Cruikshank in these terms. "A socialist in the 1930s with views so advanced that they were hard for the Methodist Church to tolerate in one of its ministers, Cruikshank was committed to the work of promoting social legislation, social insurance particularly."[5] From the Schorr interview:

> The AFL-CIO became a sort of headquarters offering at least logistical support—desks and mimeograph machines—for people who were trying to get something done about health insurance for the aged. I can remember the library in the IUD [Industrial Union Department] when we were assembling, cutting and pasting a bill... we were in a terrible rush for some reason, and I think it was Wilbur Cohen and Leonard Lesser of the IUD staff and Nelson Cruikshank and myself, and somebody had the stapler and somebody had the scotch tape...[6]

Late in 1957 a health insurance bill developed by Falk (who had left the government to work for the United Mine Workers), Cohen (who had left to teach at the University of Michigan), Robert M. Ball (a top career official in the Social Security Administration), and Cruikshank was ready. Cruikshank took it up to Capitol Hill to see if he and Andrew J. Biemiller, the AFL-CIO's chief lobbyist, could get action on it from someone on the House Ways and Means Committee. The chairman, Jere Cooper of Tennessee, turned them down. Wilbur Mills, the next ranking Democrat and the man who would soon succeed Cooper, wanted nothing to do with it, and they turned to Aime Forand, a Democratic congressman from Rhode Island.

Forand confessed that he would not have time to read the bill but said he would put it into the legislative process anyway.[7]

As noted, the Forand bill expired during the last of the Eisenhower administration. But soon after John F. Kennedy's election in 1960, what now might be called the Wagner-Murray-Dingell-Falk-Cohen-Ewing-Ball-Cruikshank-Biemiller-Forand bill took on yet another identity. This time (it was early 1961) the health proposal bore the names of Senator Clinton P. Anderson (D.-New Mexico), and Representative Cecil R. King (D.-California), a member of the Ways and Means Committee. It was addressed to the medical needs of retirees on Social Security pensions, providing them (in the original version) with ninety days of free hospital care, some nursing home care, but virtually no physician services. In view of what happened to it later on, the King-Anderson bill was a comparatively meager offering. In any event, it was introduced with aggressive support from the new administration, and the *New York Times* saluted it as "the greatest social innovation the government has undertaken in a generation."

The AMA thought otherwise. At its June 1961 meeting the House of Delegates adopted a statement that became known as the Bauer amendment. It said that the King-Anderson bill did not meet the needs of the situation and would lead inevitably to further government encroachments on medical care. In language interpreted by many King-Anderson supporters as a threat to boycott, the amendment said further, "The medical profession is the only group which can render medical care under any system...it will not be a willing party to implementing any system which we believe to be detrimental to the public welfare."[8]

Later in the year AMA President Leonard W. Larson, M.D., came closer to the philosophical heart of the matter. At the November meeting he told the House of Delegates, "We fight because the administration's medical care proposal, if enacted, would certainly represent the first major, irreversible step toward the complete socialization of medical care...Only in the case of the needy or medically needy should government intervene...The King-Anderson program does not provide insurance or prepayment of any type, but compels one segment of our population to underwrite a socialized program of health care for another, regardless of need."[9]

The Larson statement deserves emphasis, for it drew a distinction that was lost in the public debate that was to follow. The AMA did not object to the use of federal funds to help those elderly persons who genuinely needed assistance in meeting their medical expenses. What the AMA was objecting to was a new societal concept, a system to finance medical care for a category of the population that included people who needed assistance and people who were perfectly able to take care of themselves. Advanced as a plan to underwrite medical expenses for the elderly needy, the King-Anderson bill actually included medical benefits for all elderly people, needy or not.

The approach to the problem that the AMA preferred was already embodied in legislation, the Kerr-Mills bill, passed in 1960 at the end of the Eisenhower administration. Sponsored by Wilbur Mills, the ultra-cautious, Southern-conservative chairman of the Ways and Means Committee, and Senator Robert Kerr of Oklahoma, another conservative Democrat, who dominated the powerful Senate Finance Committee, the legislation served as an alternative solution to the medical care problems of the aged. Kerr-Mills authorized federal matching funds to support state administered programs to serve the needs of elderly people who were medically indigent, that is, those not so poor as to be welfare cases but not so well provided for that they could finance their own care. Its functioning demanded a determination by the states of an applicant's financial status (a means test). Medical Assistance for the Aged, as the operating program was called, reflected the AMA's traditional position: government assistance to those below certain income levels and the use of private resources for the self-supporting part of the population.

Initially, when Mills first started to develop the legislation in 1959, the AMA wrote him urging caution and further study. But as the bill progressed through a tangled process of compromise and revision to eventual enactment, the AMA supported it.[10]

Though the AMA position and the Kerr-Mills bill had strengths from a logical viewpoint, the stand was weak politically. In opposing the Wagner-Murray-Dingell bills in the 1940s, the AMA had private, voluntary insurance to offer as a functioning, attractive alternative. But, in the 1960s, as an alternative to more extensive legislation, the Kerr-Mills bill carried political liabilities. Because state governments are frequently stingy, when not genuinely strapped, Kerr-Mills was painfully slow in implementation; it grew into substantial programs in only a handful of states. Moreover, its dependence on a means test, on which American advocates of social legislation had always pronounced anathema, irritated the recipients and increased the vulnerability of the program.

Soon after the election of Kennedy and the introduction of the King-Anderson bill in February 1961, both sides commenced firing to open a bitter propaganda war. The AMA on one side and the labor-Social Security Administration-liberal Democratic coalition on the other, each hoped to create a wave of favorable public opinion tall enough to swamp the other's legislative hopes.

In the reporting of this contest it was popular to portray the AMA as the more powerful of the duelists, the adversary with the deeper pockets and the superior propaganda machinery. The case was superficially easy to make because the AMA's effort was easily visible and far from Lilliputian. The association staged an advertising campaign in April 1961, the first of three such efforts during the King-Anderson controversy, that relied primarily on a seven-column ad run in thirty-one major newspapers. The ad described the AMA position; that is, its preference for the Kerr-Mills bill over the King-Anderson proposal. The AMA also purchased time on FM radio stations in thirty-four cities to run six recorded messages over a five-week period. A two-day meeting of state and county medical society executives and officers was called to mobilize them for the campaign and distribute materials for use at the local level.

David G. Baldwin, who did much of the writing for the campaign, notably a ninety-one page elucidation of the association's position, recalls what it was like in 1961. "It was an allout effort," he says. "Pamphlets? We turned them out by the thousands. We wrote public service announcements and prepared newspaper mats for the local societies. The field service staff got to work on an endorsement campaign. We had speakers' bureaus. We had prepared speeches. We had canned radio talks. We had everything. We turned on every tap we could."[11]

But generous as the resources were that the AMA brought to this competition for public opinion, they did not match those marshaled by the opposition. While the AMA pushed its viewpoint in its publications, for example, it could not compete with the cumulative circulation of the union newspapers plugging for the swift passage of King-Anderson. COPE distributed a compilation of alleged AMA positions on sixteen historical issues from smallpox vaccinations to the Social Security Act, misrepresenting facts, taking statements out of context and distorting intentions.* It was a hatchet job, and it was

---

*See Appendix C for the COPE accusations and the AMA's response to them.

picked up and widely quoted by writers and speakers sympathetic to labor's cause. In 1961 labor helped organize and finance the National Council of Senior Citizens for Health Care through Social Security, a pressure group created to push for one specific piece of legislation, which in a few years grew to 2.5 million members. Aime Forand, who retired as a congressman in 1960, was the first chairman of the organization.

As Tables 1 and 2 show, the expenditures of the AMA for lobbying and for political campaigns during this period were considerably less than those of the AFL-CIO in most years.

TABLE 1.
Declared Lobbying Expenditures,[a]
1960-65

	AMA	AFL-CIO
1960	$ 72,635	$ 129,157
1961	163,405	139,919
1962	83,075	149,212
1963	74,457	145,636
1964	45,515	153,542
1965	1,165,935[b]	148,343 (national headquarters)
		60,143 (industrial union department)

[a] Organizations are required to report to the Clerk of the U.S. House of Representatives what they consider to be lobbying expenses each year, lobbying being defined as efforts to influence federal legislative proposals. Nevertheless, the reporting criteria are not necessarily consistent, organization by organization.

[b] In its declaration of lobbying expenses for 1965, the AMA included costs of its million dollar advertising campaign for the Eldercare bill.

Source: Congressional Quarterly Almanac.

TABLE 2.
Declared Expenditures on Political
Campaigns for Federal Offices, 1961-64

	AMPAC (AMA)	COPE (AFL-CIO)
1961	$ 26,759	$ 94,253
1962	248,484	761,468
1963	31,868	135,062
1964	402,052	988,810

Source: Congressional Quarterly Almanac.

Democratic Senator Pat McNamara of Michigan took a Special Senate Subcommittee on the Problems of the Aging around the country, conducting public hearings. When time would hang heavy at these hearings, Senator McNamara would give individuals the privilege of the microphone to tell their own medical case histories. Such anecdotal evidence did not really deepen the legislators' grasp of the problem, for often there was little proof that the stories were more than the emotional outpourings of people brought to the hearing by local labor organizations. That, of course, was not the point. The "horror" stories—isolated, unique, unrepresentative, or exaggerated—nevertheless made heart-rending newspaper copy, adding an emotional dimension to the drive for the King-Anderson bill.

At the same time, the secretary of Health, Education, and Welfare, Abraham Ribicoff, sought to weaken the AMA by attacking it as a coercive organization that habitually browbeat its members into obedience to policy decisions. He taunted the AMA president, E. Vincent Askey, M.D., calling him a "reluctant dragon." Askey was not a polished speaker and refused to accept Ribicoff's invitations to public debate. In November 1961 the White House staged twelve regional conferences on the health problems of the aged, featuring speeches by Cabinet members and other high administration officials. These served to create a sense of crisis and lent a feeling of urgency to the issue. Eventually, the AMA protested the improper use of federal employees and federal funds to promote a piece of partisan legislation, but the complaint fell on deaf ears in Robert Kennedy's Justice Department.

As for the press at that time, this editorial from the *New England Journal of Medicine* gives an idea of how the medical profession evaluated its objectivity.

> Literally and figuratively, the Administration has thrown down the gauntlet, challenging organized medicine to an all-out battle in 1962. A Boston television station, caught in the excitement of the pending campaign, introduced a program supporting H.R. 4222 [King-Anderson] with the words, "President Kennedy versus the AMA."
>
> It can be anticipated that political cartoonists will record the clash with sketches of the President fearlessly locking lances with what appears to be an overpowering, towering, glowering and evil Black Knight with AMA emblazoned on his shield. Cigar-smoking henchmen holding bags of money labeled "AMA lobby" will appear in the background giving support to the Black Knight. Sketches of lofty physicians blithely ignoring the pleas of the aged will be rife.[12]

At the end of 1961, however, neither the AMA nor the administration had won the propaganda battle. Public opinion toward a Social Security-financed program of limited hospital care for the aged had not swung decisively either way. In fact, the Kennedy campaign pledge to "get this country moving again" seemed to be mired in Congress. With an eye on the fall election, the administration began 1962 by unlimbering heavier artillery and announcing an offensive to bring the issue to a vote.

Through a mixup in the mailing list, the Massachusetts Medical Society received an invitation to attend a preliminary planning meeting on March 20 at the Hotel Bellevue in Boston.[13] Conducted by James C. O'Brien, a union representative assigned to the White House staff, the session presumably was typical of what went on in other areas where labor and the Democratic party were strong.

John D. Noonan, recently hired by the Massachusetts Medical Society and working on his master's thesis in public relations, attended the meeting for the state medical society and wrote a detailed account of it. He noted that the Democratic members of the Massachusetts state legislature had been caucused and told that the President was giving King-Anderson top priority. Every one of the 150 Democrats in the state legislature was pledged to speak for and support the campaign that was soon to be launched. Top lawyers, judges, physicians working for government agencies, and labor leaders heard O'Brien outline the build-up that would support the campaign. Over a seven-week period, nationwide, there would be 5,000 speeches given by at least 250 speakers. All the materials, trappings, and accouterments of a typical publicity drive were assembled, and a climactic series of rallies on May 20th in at least twenty key areas throughout the country was planned. The showcase rally would be staged by the National Council of Senior Citizens for Health Care through Social Security. It would be held in Madison Square Garden and addressed by President Kennedy himself. Rarely had a President of the United States committed himself so decisively to a piece of partisan legislation.

The response from the AMA covered a range of actions. Part of it encouraged the county medical societies to be a more effective force. A series of eighteen public service advertisements was prepared and distributed, devoted to such topics as the annual physical, choice of physician, grievances. Through the placement of these non-paid advertising messages (print and radio/television) it was hoped to gain more local visibility for the county societies.

The Woman's Auxiliary to the AMA, composed predominantly of physicians' wives, organized something called Operation Coffee Cup. It consisted of members giving daytime coffee receptions for friends and neighbors at which a recorded attack on socialized medicine by Ronald Reagan (not yet fully committed to a political career) was played. Address lists were passed out to the guests, along with urgings for them to write appropriate members of Congress stating opposition to the King-Anderson legislation.

William R. Ramsey, then the assistant director of the AMA field staff, recalls huddling with another field man, Harry R. Hinton, and developing other materials for the county societies. Kits containing detailed suggestions and instructions were sent out, typical enclosures beginning, "So, you have just been named the new publicity chairman for your county medical society..." or, "Now that you have been appointed to head the legislative committee..." What Ramsey and Hinton had in mind was a campaign that would generate mail to Congress and peak at just about the time of Kennedy's Madison Square Garden speech. "The strategy was to create action where the legislators were born," says Ramsey, "not where the legislation might be born."[14]

But how to respond to the Kennedy speech itself? A dramatic stroke was clearly needed. It was not easy to compete with the charisma of the President. Nor would the AMA membership, which would be angered by the President, be satisfied with a routine response.

Since the presidential address would be televised, that was the obvious medium to use for the response. Accordingly, much of the creative responsibility descended on the AMA's audio/visual director, Richard Reinauer. "It fell on me," he says, "to find some way by which we could create a show business presentation that would get at least the same amount of publicity. We all knew about Ed Annis at that time, a doctor from Miami who had become head of the speakers bureau and had a marvelous voice and who was an absolute master at grabbing an audience in ten seconds flat."[15]

With general approval for the idea that the response should somehow feature Edward R. Annis, M.D., rather than the AMA president or chairman, and Ed Annis somehow on television, Reinauer set out for New York to talk to commercial film producers. He went first to the Troy/Beaumont company, which had recently done some medically oriented films that attracted the AMA's attention. There, in a meeting that included a free lance writer named Harold Azine, who had written the scripts for many of the films,

Reinauer found the idea he had been looking for. Azine reminded the group of the Kennedy charisma. "The AMA was dead," Azine recalls saying, "unless it could somehow stage its show under the Kennedy marquee." Out of that meeting emerged the idea of having Ed Annis give his speech to a Madison Square Garden empty of everything except the political debris left by the Kennedy rally.

Back in Chicago there was a lot of conversation about Annis speaking to an empty Madison Square Garden, its floor still littered by the jetsam from the preceding occupants. The proposal was run by the board, and the chairman, Hugh H. Hussey, M.D., recalled a quick appreciation of the showmanship values of the proposal. Reinauer got his go-ahead.

On Sunday afternoon, May 20, as Kennedy's limousine sped him to his 4:00 o'clock date at the Garden, he became convinced that the speech that had been prepared for him was not right, and he started to scribble notes for an extemporaneous effort. According to Richard Harris's account in the *New Yorker*, "President Kennedy stood before a capacity audience of 20,000 old people, smilingly accepted their long and enthusiastic welcome, and then put aside his prepared text to deliver one of the worst speeches of his career." Harris, whose history of the Medicare legislation is marked by meticulous detail and an undeviating anti-AMA bias, quotes one of the AFL-CIO people who watched the telecast as saying, "...instead of steam for the Medicare piston we got a pail of cold water."[16]

About 10:30 that same night, Reinauer, Beaumont, and a camera crew, together with Ed Annis, AMA President Larson, and Leo Brown, the AMA's long-time communications director, marched into the empty Garden. Larson limped almost imperceptibly on a recently broken leg. Recalls Reinauer,

> The place was deserted. There wasn't even a sweeper around because we had specified we wanted the place just as it had been. In fact, I think we had to pay something extra not to have it cleaned up. Balloons were still hanging from the ceiling; coffee cups, cigarette butts and gum wrappers littered the floor; chairs were overturned. The bunting and banners still hung from the balcony railings. There were Welcome Kennedy signs all over the place. It was perfect.
>
> About midnight Beaumont had the cameras placed. Larson introduced Annis to the empty hall. And then on came Ed with a hellfire and brimstone speech that was just great.

Annis was good. As the camera panned around the littered hall in sync with the speech Azine had helped to draft, Annis underscored the opposition's power. "These people know how to rally votes, rally support, rally crowds and mass meetings. That's quite a bit of machinery to put behind something, isn't it?" Reminding viewers of Kerr-Mills, he warned, "The public is in danger of being blitzed, brainwashed and bandwagoned into swallowing the idea that the King-Anderson bill is the only program that offers medical care for the aged."

What was Annis feeling as he harangued an empty Madison Square Garden? "I felt like a ham actor," he says, "and I loved every minute of it."[17]

To get Annis' presentation of the AMA viewpoint before the public, the AMA not only had to produce its own show; it also had to purchase television time, which could be done then. (Soon afterward the network news departments insisted on policies that virtually forbade the airing of programming not produced by the news departments themselves.) At 8:00 p.m. on May 21, the day after the President spoke, the AMA program was telecast by NBC-TV and carried by all but two of its affiliated stations.

As the reviews came in, it was clear that the AMA had won this skirmish in the propaganda war. Even King-Anderson supporters conceded that Annis had outpointed the President, and more than 40,000 viewers wrote the AMA, 90 percent of them applauding Annis. With the press reaction split, Kennedy drew some rare criticism. To demonstrate how medical care for the elderly could bring hardship to even the affluent, he had cited in his speech the case of an unnamed congressman from Massachusetts. This man's father, said the President, had incurred such expenses during a two-year illness that the congressman was being forced to give up the idea of sending his daughter to boarding school.

To William Steif, a Scripps-Howard reporter, the story didn't quite ring true. Screening the Massachusetts congressional delegation, Steif found only one member who matched the President's description. He was Torbert H. Macdonald, a friend and Harvard classmate of the President's. The Macdonalds had a teenage daughter and a parent who had been recently hospitalized. But on checking with the family, Steif found discrepancies between the facts and the President's story. For one thing, the senior Macdonald had been ill for four months, not two years. For another, he had health insurance and was thus not a severe burden on the family. Moreover, the daughter was still planning to go to boarding school, and the Macdonald's son would remain in Andover. Asked about life on a congressional salary, Mrs. Macdonald told Steif, "I wouldn't call it a struggle."[18] If President Kennedy was referrring to some other Massachusetts congressman, he did not say who it was.

Though not alluding specifically to the Macdonald case, Arthur Krock of the *New York Times*, then generally considered the dean of the Washington press corps, observed, "President Kennedy complained that much of the opposition to the King-Anderson bill was created by 'misinformation.' But to his elderly audience....the President contributed to the misinformation he was attacking."[19]

But it was not an unrelieved public relations victory for the AMA, because charges were made that the AMA was simply outspending the National Council of Senior Citizens* and other pro-Medicare forces. In one of his four articles in the *New Yorker* covering the history of the Medicare legislation Richard Harris stated that the AMA "had bought a half hour of television time...and rented Madison Square Garden, too, at an estimated $100,000." The Senior Citizens, he added, "had paid for the Garden by charging $1 a seat."[20]

Harris, however, was not comparing like with like. His $100,000 figure is probably close as a statement of the AMA's overall cost—the air time on one network, the production of the film, and the $6,000 it actually cost the AMA to rent the Garden. (Charging $1 a ticket for approximately 20,000 seats in the old Garden presumably allowed the Senior Citizens to more than clear expenses.)

In dollars spent, the AMA was undoubtedly the leader on this occasion. Citing dollar outlays only, a writer can easily portray the AMA as the Goliath of the adversaries. But to arrive at an honest judgment of just who was out-propagandizing whom a number of other factors should be taken into consideration. For example, what value should be placed on the participation of the President of the United States and the public service time donated by the television networks, all three of which carried the speech live? (Annis appeared on NBC only.) A complete and objective accounting of the *value* of what each side employed on those two days, rather than what they spent, would modify, if not reverse, the David and Goliath roles.

*The Council has endured. In its "Keeping Up" column, December 13, 1982, *Fortune* called it "an organization of professional complainers that gets funded regularly by the U.S. Department of Labor and then uses its pumped-up influence to lobby for budget-busting social programs." Under the Older Americans Act, the Council received $35 million in 1982 to run a program providing jobs for the elderly. It was also vocal on various entitlement issues, such as subsidized housing for the elderly and subsidized heating.

Aside from the money question, how might the whole labor-Senior Citizens effort be evaluated? Specifically, how did the King-Anderson rallies go in other cities? Simulcasts of the Kennedy speech, sponsored by labor and the Senior Citizens organization, were beamed to thirty-one major cities. Many were a bust. The *Charleston Mail* (West Virginia) ran a story on the rally in that union stronghold with a photograph showing the lead attraction, Nelson H. Cruikshank, at the podium with only forty-six people scattered throughout the 3500-seat Civic Auditorium.[21] John Noonan's thesis gives this account of the day in Boston:

> In Boston, the President's hometown, the Donnelly Theater had been turned over to the local committee for a big rally. The theater seats about 3400 persons, but no more than 300 of those seats were filled on that bright Sunday afternoon. A Navy band was engaged to play a few selections to start the festivities, but as things turned out the rally turned into an afternoon band concert. The spectators were repeatedly asked to applaud the band vigorously to encourage the rendering of more selections.
>
> A Boston labor official assured the small group that the hall would be packed in a few minutes. It never happened. The President's personal representative, Secretary of Commerce Luther H. Hodges, spent a few uncomfortable hours on stage looking for the crowd that never showed. The people who were expected to storm the doors of all rallies did not.[22]

Despite the rebuffs, and in search of an issue, if not a legislative success, for the campaign in the congressional elections later in the year, the administration pressed for a vote on King-Anderson. It came that summer when the Senate took up consideration of a bill already passed in the House. The Medicare legislation—the King-Anderson bill—was attached as a rider, or amendment, to this bill by Senator Anderson, and the vote came on a motion to table; that is, to separate and not act upon the Medicare rider.

For the preceding three weeks, David Baldwin had stayed close to a room in the Statler-Hilton in Washington, assigned to writing speeches for senators who opposed King-Anderson. In the Senate, the opposition was orchestrated by Senator Kerr. Baldwin recalls,

> The great day came on July 17, and I don't suppose I'll see anything like it again. Every single member of the Senate was present. Senator Chavez, near death, was brought in sitting in a wheelchair. Vice President Johnson presided. The nose count we had made was so

close that we couldn't call it. The vote started with the first man on the roll call, Senator Carl Hayden of Arizona. We had his vote, but only on the condition that it was not needed to insure passage of the amendment. Hayden said, "Pass." A big surprise came when Jennings Randolph of West Virginia voted to table. We learned later he needed a big favor from Senator Kerr. In the end when Hayden was called again to vote he went with us. But that was because we'd won; the final count was 52-48.

We'd all been up in the Senate gallery while this was going on, counting the votes. Bert Howard was on hand; he was the head of the staff task force on King-Anderson. Afterward there was a mood of wild jubilation among all of us.

Not for two more years would King-Anderson come up for a vote again. And not for three more years would it pass both houses. While the propaganda war between the AMA and the labor-Senior Citizens-liberal Democrat coalition continued, the key to the legislation remained in the hands of the Chairman of the Ways and Means Committee of the House, Wilbur Mills. Supported by the votes of all the Republicans on the committee and a few Southern Democrats, he refused to report the bill out of committee. For one thing, he was not sure it would pass, and he abhorred defeats. For another, he was highly protective of the Social Security program, and he did not want to risk its solvency by using it to finance the health care of elderly people or anyone else.

It was his stubborn resistance that blocked the King-Anderson bill from the time of its introduction in 1961 until early 1965. President Kennedy could not budge him from his position, and, unwilling to start a head-on battle with Mills, the frustrated administration turned its wrath on the AMA, making the physicians, not Wilbur Mills, the villain of its political scenario.

In the months that followed the defeat of King-Anderson in the Senate, the AMA felt a growing confidence in its cause. Those with finely tuned antennae could even detect a loss of interest on the part of the President; at least his efforts to goad Congress into action slackened. Addressing the House of Delegates in December 1963, Ed Annis, who had by now become the AMA president, said, "…the tide of events has swung so dramatically in our favor…"

But the AMA tempo of activity did not slacken. To ease the burden of medical expenses on the elderly, the AMA suggested various tax forgiveness measures, including the use of tax credits (rather than deductions) on a sliding scale, which would most benefit people over sixty-five with the lowest taxable incomes.[23] The AMA suggested changes to make Kerr-Mills work more smoothly and pressured the state medical societies to expand local Medical Assistance to the Aged programs as rapidly as possible. At the same time, March 1963, the AMA launched Operation Hometown, a more formal drive to equip the local societies with materials and programs that would help them keep up the pressure on Congress.

To the public at this time the AMA presented a picture of strength, unity, and intransigence. Congressmen, HEW officials, the press, and others who saw the AMA at closer range noted the same qualities. But they were also struck and usually antagonized by the vehemence with which the AMA advanced its views.

Among those whose curiosity was aroused by the depth of animosity displayed by physicians in their opposition to the King-Anderson bill was Wilbur J. Cohen, the man the AMA considered its archenemy during the 1940s, 1950s, and 1960s. Some fifteen years after the Medicare fight was over, Cohen was asked, without warning, if he had any explanation for the intensity of the feeling. Cohen had a surprisingly full answer to offer, suggesting that the question had occurred to him before. He said,

> I can't say that I understand it completely, but I can give you three hypotheses. First, I think the most single, long-range factor was Dr. Fishbein's famous 1932 editorial, the one where he called the Committee on the Costs of Medical Care report inciting to revolution and to socialism and communism. His use of that incendiary language set the tone of the discussion for years to come. Then there was the note developed by people like Marjorie Shearon* in the 1950s and 1960s that national health insurance was some kind of socialist or communist plot. She got out a newsletter in Washington called *Challenge to Socialism*. I'd go on to what I call the devil theory of history. Doctors, of course, were not particularly sympathetic to national health insurance, and they could not explain to themselves or anybody else why all these other people were in favor of it. They really couldn't understand why other people wanted national health insurance, and they preferred to believe in this conspiratorial and devil theory, that somebody was trying to do something to them that was unjustified...They couldn't imagine anyone being for national health insurance the way I was, simply because I thought it was the right thing to do.[24]

*See Chapter 13.

Interesting as Cohen's hypotheses are, the intensity of the AMA's feelings at this time can also be explained by the attacks from the other side. They were incendiary too. During the King-Anderson rallies around the country in May 1962, for instance, speakers referred to opponents of the legislation as "liars," "blackmailers," "selfish interests," and "witch doctors."[25]

While the AMA may have presented a stone facade to the public, the physicians were not altogether of one mind. Many wished that the association's stand was not so uncompromisingly negative. Individual members, some county societies, and a few state associations informally submitted to the AMA hundreds of alternatives to King-Anderson. Although these ideas varied, they reflected a common conviction that the AMA needed to counter the public's criticism that physicians had no positive program to offer instead of the King-Anderson proposal that they found so repugnant. Frank C. Coleman, M.D., who was chairman of the Council on Legislative Activities through the end of 1964, remembers that at the direction of the board his council held a series of meetings, actually hearings, where anybody in the association could come in and express views on how the AMA ought to address the issue. "We had several such meetings," Coleman recalls, "most of them in Chicago, but some regional meetings too. The leadership of the whole federation came and spoke before our council."

Russell B. Roth, M.D., vice chairman of the Council on Medical Service in the early 1960s, was one of those sharply critical of the AMA's negative position. He thought the association was in a "profound state of auto-hypnosis." In a letter written at the end of 1962 to Joe Stetler, secretary to the Council on Legislative Activities, he said, "By virtue of the togetherness that develops at AMA official sessions, wherein we hear our own lobbyists reporting on their work, listen to the Senators and Representatives we want to hear, and engender in ourselves a collective sense of self-satisfaction and boldness, our top leadership has somehow convinced itself that the AMA is doing just fine. My view is that it is lamentably not doing very well at all."

In Roth's opinion, Kerr-Mills was a totally inadequate alternative to the sort of proposal represented by the King-Anderson bill. "When the AMA selected Kerr-Mills as the vehicle of its deliverance," he wrote in his letter to Stetler, "it picked a woefully creaky, sputtery and undependable glory-wagon." Roth and the Council on Medical Service were working on ideas and principles that could serve as a foundation for an AMA health insurance proposal. But Roth felt that even these preliminary moves were blocked by the Council on Legislative Activities and the Board of Trustees. When Stetler invited Roth to a January 1963 meeting of the Council on Legislative Activities to present his ideas, Roth offered his criticism of the leadership of the AMA and declined an invitation to what he called a "turkey shoot."

Max H. Parrott, M.D., a delegate at the time and a member of the Council on Legislative Activities, a target of Roth's, describes the mood of the House of Delegates in 1963-64. "There were two schools of thought on the matter of whether the AMA ought to have its own bill or not. No, let me amend that. There were three schools of thought: there was a left-wing element that thought we ought to go along with the administration; we had conservatives who didn't think we should have any bill; and there were liberals who thought we should have a bill to offset what was being considered in Congress. Bing Blasingame and the Board of Trustees, the establishment at that time, were in the conservative camp."[26] And for a long time, until 1964, the conservatives held the edge over the more liberal-minded physicians in the house. Bernard Harrison, who followed Stetler as secretary to the Council on Legislative Activities, recalls, "The only movement toward a positive approach then was coming from the Council on Medical Service and a small group in the house. They were pretty lonesome voices."[27]

The momentum that had appeared to be flowing in the AMA's favor from late 1962 through most of 1963 abruptly changed course that autumn when an assassin's bullet felled President Kennedy on November 22. The mood of the country turned somber, the gloom overlaid with an apparent feeling of guilt because his beautifully articulated social visions had not been translated into realities. In his successor, Lyndon B. Johnson, the country inherited a President whose political awareness began with the New Deal and culminated with his dreams of a Great Society. He believed in Medicare more ardently than Kennedy did. In addition, as majority leader of the Senate during the 1950s, he had become a master at working the levers of power on Capitol Hill. Better than any other man, Lyndon Johnson knew how to get what he wanted out of Congress. And he wanted Medicare.

Though he did not achieve his objective in 1964, the tide turned in President Johnson's favor that year. Some of the southern Democrats on the Ways and Means Committee began having second thoughts about their opposition to Medicare, and in the Senate there was enough movement that the King-Anderson, again attached as a rider to a piece of House-approved legislation, passed 49-44. When that bill went to a Senate-House conference committee to resolve the differences between the two bodies, Wilbur Mills stalled the measure once more. But in order to do so, he agreed that the legislation would be at the top of the agenda when the new Congress convened.

After the congressional adjournment that October, the AMA began an aggressive educational campaign against the King-Anderson legislation. In 1964, the AMA's expenditures for purchased advertising space and time totaled $1,813,000. The ads argued that King-Anderson was not needed, that the existing Kerr-Mills program could meet the health requirements of the elderly.

Whatever doubts may have lingered over the future of the legislation were dispelled by the election of November 1964. Not only did Lyndon Johnson trounce Barry Goldwater, who was attacked then as more of a Viet Nam hardliner than the President,* the Democrats took control of the Congress with better than 2-1 margins in both houses. According to its chairman, AMPAC was "outgunned." In comparison with the $402,050 spent by AMPAC (and about $125,000 by other medical organizations), the AFL-CIO's COPE disbursed $988,810 to support its candidates, with over $1 million from other labor-affiliated political action committees and $44,788 from an organization called Senior Citizens for Johnson and Humphrey. Democratic candidates for federal offices declared $5,735,555 in campaign expenses for 1964, Republican candidates, $3,368,568.

Whether it was money, a liberal mandate, an act of contrition over Kennedy, a rejection of Goldwater's conservatism and perceived hawkishness, or all four, liberal Democratic congressmen were now present in such numbers as to make AMPAC's strategy unworkable. There was no way that a conservative majority coalition of southern Democrats and northern Republicans could be formed. Wilbur Mills, in a speech that December to the Little Rock Lions Club, said,

---

*A Johnson campaign commercial showed a small girl plucking the petals from a daisy while a background voice intoned a solemn countdown, at the end of which the viewer saw the mushrooming of an atomic cloud. The implication was that Goldwater would start a nuclear war.

"I can support a payroll tax for health benefits just as I have supported a payroll tax for cash benefits."[28] A staff member of the Republican Congressional Campaign Committee, unruffled by his switch, observed, "Wilbur Mills can count, too."[29]

Going into the legislative session that began that January, Congress had before it two elements of a health care program for the elderly. One was the already enacted Kerr-Mills legislation, which promised comprehensive care; that is, hospital *and* physician services, for those over sixty-five who could establish variously defined conditions of neediness. Then there was the King-Anderson proposal, which promised, basically, sixty days of federally paid hospital or nursing home care, but virtually no physician services, to everyone over sixty-five regardless of neediness. A number of people, including Chairman Mills and the officers of the AMA, feared that if King-Anderson were enacted, an angry reaction would follow.[30] Because so many people thought the program covered more expenses than it actually did, the AMA called it a "cruel hoax."[31] AMA estimates indicated that it might cover only about 25 percent of the expenses of a more or less typical, serious illness. The AMA had criticized it for some time because it did not provide for physician services.

Up to the time in late 1964 when Mills began to change his position, the AMA had assumed that no health care legislation would reach the floor of the House of Representatives. All proposals, including King-Anderson, would be buried in the Ways and Means Committee, the AMA believed. But now the game was different. The historic process that creates legislation was about to begin— the bargaining, the compromising, the merging of ideas taken from competing legislative proposals. In the AMA House of Delegates, those who had felt for so long that the AMA should put forward its own legislative answer to the nation's health needs started to gain ascendancy.

The first signs of a shift in the AMA's viewpoint appeared at the November-December 1964 meeting of the house in Miami. Two resolutions that called for federal programs to assist the elderly were voted down. But a California resolution, which underwent considerable amending before it was adopted, reasserted the AMA's conviction that *no* person needing care should go without it because of an inability to pay. The resolution further urged the "fullest possible implementation of existing mechanisms...to the end that everyone in need, regardless of age, is assured that necessary health care will be available."[32] Among the existing mechanisms, of course, was the program authorized under Kerr-Mills, which permitted the state-administered programs to purchase private health insurance to assist those in need.

In that resolution the three key words were "regardless of age." What was so special about the health needs of the elderly indigent, the AMA was asking. Couldn't the Kerr-Mills program be extended to cover the health care needs of all people unable to provide them for themselves? What was being advocated here was what we know today as Medicaid, though the AMA did not get to the point of putting its idea into a formal legislative proposal.*

What did proceed to the point of formal proposal a few weeks later was a program that the AMA called Eldercare. Designed as an alternative to King-Anderson, Eldercare was put together in a sequence of meetings that extended throughout most of December 1964. One of them, on December 29, included representatives of Blue Cross, Blue Shield, the American Hospital Association, the American Dental Association, and the health insurance industry. The Eldercare proposal was a plan of comprehensive health care for the elderly needy. A simple declaration of income (not assets) determined eligibility. Federal matching grants and state funds underwrote advances, which varied with income, for the elderly needy to purchase private health insurance. Those least in need received little or nothing toward the purchase of a private health insurance policy; those with the lowest incomes, in effect, received a paid-up policy. The federal outlays were to come from general revenues, not social security, and would be used to match state funding. The states would administer the program. On January 27, 1965, two members of the Ways and Means Committee, Thomas B. Curtis (R.-Missouri) and A. Sidney Herlong (D.-Florida), introduced legislation that embodied the Eldercare concept. The AMA quickly backed Eldercare with an advertising campaign, the messages emphasizing that Eldercare would cost less than Medicare (because it would not cover the elderly who could afford private health insurance themselves), but would provide more generous benefits than Medicare

---

*On December 15, 1964, Blasingame met with Mills in Washington. The board minutes of December 20 give a summary of that meeting, which was related specifically to actions of the house at the recent Miami meeting in repeating its opposition to King-Anderson and "extension of Kerr-Mills legislation for those unable to pay for medical care..." One can speculate that Mills was also thinking in terms broader than the health needs of the elderly.

to the elderly who could not. The educational campaign for Eldercare cost the AMA $1,669,000 in 1965.

Like the AMA, the Republicans in Congress were moving too.
Stung by the defeats suffered in the fall elections, it shifted leadership in the House of Representatives from Charles Halleck to Gerald
Ford and backed a proposal of its own to provide comprehensive
health care for the aged. The bill was submitted by Congressman
Thomas W. Byrnes of Wisconsin. Like Eldercare, it called for coverage of hospital *and* physician services for the aged through the
purchase of private insurance. Administration, however, was to be
federal. Financing was to come two-thirds from general revenues
and one third from deductions on the individual pension checks of
those who voluntarily chose to participate in the program.

To ratify the board action creating Eldercare, the AMA speaker
summoned a special meeting of the House of Delegates in Chicago
for February 6 and 7. During the opening session on the morning of
the sixth, occupied heavily with official addresses and procedural
matters, there was some sniping at the board over the handling of
the Eldercare proposal. When the house reassembled after lunch to
take up the real business before it, James H. Sammons, M.D., a
delegate from Texas serving his first term, was recognized at one of
the floor microphones. Feeling that the board deserved praise for
responsible action rather than the muttered carping that could be
heard that morning, he proposed a standing ovation to convey the
supportive feelings of the house.[33] Not only did he accurately gauge
the overall sentiment of the house, but also when the delegates
arose to applaud, adoption of the Eldercare program was assured.
It was a shrewd political manuever as well as a reflection of genuine feelings.

Besides giving its endorsement to Eldercare during this special
session, the house re-emphasized the idea, first expressed at the
November-December meeting, that Kerr-Mills should be expanded.
Accordingly, it adopted a resolution asking the board to "proceed at
once, as indicated, with study of the desirability and feasibility of
extending the principle of federal and state aid to persons under the
age of 65 who need help..."[34]

Later that month the Ways and Means Committee concluded hearings and stepped up its executive sessions to consider all of
the health bills submitted: King-Anderson, Byrnes, and Eldercare.

Catching almost everyone by surprise, Mills proposed not a choice among the proposals but an amalgamation.

"In order to get a broad base of support in the House of Representatives," writes Robert J. Myers, then the chief actuary of the Social Security Administration and a frequent administration witness at the Ways and Means hearings, "he [Mills] proposed that the new bill incorporate the essential features of all three of the major proposals—the King-Anderson bill, the Byrnes bill and the Eldercare bill."[35] In the less formal wording used by Mills, what emerged was "a three-layer cake"—H.R. 6675.

Layer one, Medicare Part A, was very close to King-Anderson. It included hospital care for Social Security retirees, financed and administered by Social Security. Layer two, Medicare Part B, came out of the Byrnes bill—a supplemental, voluntary insurance plan covering physician services. It called for financing by uniform premiums from those beneficiaries who elected to participate and a matching contribution from general revenues.

Layer three, Medicaid, grew out of the Eldercare bill, Kerr-Mills, and the AMA's concern for the non-elderly needy as expressed at the November-December 1964 meeting of the house and at the special session in February 1965. Medicaid liberalized the eligibility requirements of Kerr-Mills and widened it to cover indigent people under sixty-five. It relied on matching federal-state funds and state administration, and permitted the use of private insurance carriers. Though it was regarded as something of an afterthought at the time, Medicaid proved to be almost as large and almost as expensive a program as Medicare.

In Congressional testimony before the Senate Finance Committee on May 11, the AMA stated its qualified opposition to the three-tiered measure. "While we recognize that there are parts of H.R. 6675 which commend themselves to Congress and the nation," President Donovan F. Ward, M.D., said, "Medicine is opposed to this measure as a total package."[36] He recommended Eldercare instead of Parts A and B of Medicare, even though Part B embraced many concepts that the AMA supported in principle: voluntary participation, the use of private insurance, financing from general revenues, and contributions by the beneficiaries. What the AMA objected to was the federal administration and management.

Ward told the committee that the AMA favored the adoption of Medicaid.

In expressing its overall opposition, the AMA offered several warnings, at least one of which was borne out by events. "There is no totally effective method or methods which will keep the costs of the program under control," Ward testified. Estimated at $6.8 billion a year,[37] the program cost more than double that in 1970, more than four times that in 1975, and nearly ten times the estimate in 1980. The overrun is attributable to many causes: general inflation, reimbursement procedures that had no cost-containment incentives, increasingly expensive technology. But the major factor was simple economic law: the legislation fueled an enormous and immediate demand for medical services, but no offsetting increase in their supply.*

Since the Senate had expressed itself favorably on King-Anderson the previous summer and had become even more liberal after the November elections, the test for Wilbur Mills' three-layer cake came in the House. There, bills reported by the Ways and Means Committee are considered under a "closed rule," which permits a vote only on the bill itself or a motion to recommit, with recommendation that a substitute bill be considered.

In late March, staff members of the AMA field service division and from AMPAC checked into the Congressional Hotel, which stands on the southern slope of Capitol Hill, and fixed a sharp eye on the proceedings in the House of Representatives. William R. Ramsey, assistant director of the AMA field service, headed that group; Joe Miller, along with David Baldwin, supervised the AMPAC staffers. As the debate and maneuverings began in the House, the two groups met daily to compare their vote counts. Baldwin recalls:

> It soon became clear that if it came to a straight up or down vote, those opposed would have been a very, very small minority. That would demonstrate that AMPAC, offered to doctors as a way for them to become politically effective, was unable to withstand the electoral landslide. So there was a little strategy discussed. We [himself and Joe Miller] decided to encourage a motion to recommit,

*Another expense that Medicare and Medicaid absorbed was that of the free care that most physicians gave to many of the needy. A state-by-state survey conducted by the magazine *New Medical Materia* and published in May 1961 indicated that physicians in private practice were providing $658 million annually in free medical services.

with the Byrnes bill as a substitute. A motion to recommit sort of fuzzes things up. We thought we could do better on it, and we were right. At one time our count even showed a majority who would vote to recommit, which would have meant the end of the bill.

But Wilbur Mills and Lyndon Johnson were alert to what was going on. William Ramsey of the AMA field staff remembers pressing Jim Foristel, a long-time AMA lobbyist, about the vote of a congressman named Everett from Union City, Tennessee. "If we don't have Fats Everett," Foristel growled, "we don't have anybody, and I'm not checking." When the motion to recommit came up and Everett voted against it, Foristel exploded. It emerged later that Mills had gone to Congressman Murphy, who represented the district adjoining Everett's. Murphy, like Mills, was a committee chairman, a member of an elite, powerful, and clubby group within the House. Mills asked him as a favor to put pressure on Everett. Mills, in fact, had done that to all the committee chairmen.

Baldwin recalls that soon after the talk of a motion to recommit began, "Lyndon's myrmidons came to with alarm and recognized that Mills' bill might be beaten. Whereupon they turned up the heat." On April 8, 1965, the motion to recommit lost 236-191. After that, the congressmen were no longer held by party discipline or other commitments, and they voted 313-115 for Mills' three-layer cake. In statutory terms these became amendments to the Social Security Act, Title 18 for Medicare and Title 19 for Medicaid. After final action by both the House and the Senate (on July 27 and 28), President Johnson flew to Independence, Missouri, to sign the bill in the presence of Harry S. Truman. It was a political gesture to please the liberal-labor constituency and an act of homage to the first President to commit himself to national health insurance.

Though the Medicare and Medicaid legislation had been written, the regulations had not. In many ways the regulations that are created to implement a new law are as crucial as the law itself, for the regulations define how the program will operate. Poor regulations can cripple a good law; good regulations can salvage benefits from a bad one. Thus, to a considerable degree, the ultimate success of the two new programs depended on the Department of Health, Education, and Welfare (HEW) drawing up sensible, workable regulations. That was a challenge of major dimensions, for the legislation, the most sweeping health measure ever to be enacted in the nation's history, would soon affect the financing of medical care for more than one American in five.

At the meeting of the AMA that June, when Medicare was already part way through Congress, the mood of the delegates was defiant. But beneath the pugnacious rhetoric, some voices of political realism could also be heard. From the floor, Russell B. Roth suggested that if the Medicare bill passed, which seemed likely, the board or the Council on Medical Service should be authorized to work out the regulations with HEW. Nothing quite that clear was done. But one resolution that was adopted urged "branches of government interested in the formulation, the enactment and the implementation of laws that deal with the provisions of professional medical services to the public to seek and utilize the advice and assistance of the physicians who will render such services."[38] The word "implementation" was construed to mean that the board could supply advice, guidance, and suggestions when and if the regulation-writing process started. Another part of the same resolution would also play a part in the events of the next few months. It read, "Resolved, That this House of Delegates restate its offer to meet with the President of the United States through our Legislative Task Force to discuss proposed medical care legislation with a view to safeguarding the continued provision of the highest quality and availability of medical care to the people of the United States..."

Soon after the meeting of the house ended on June 24, the requested letter was written and sent to the White House. Upon arrival, it was routed to Undersecretary Wilbur J. Cohen at HEW for comment. Emphasizing in a memo to the White House that the new legislation would require "the full cooperation of the physicians of this country to make the program work successfully," Cohen suggested a meeting between the President and the AMA's legislative task force on the day following final congressional approval of the bill, still about two weeks away. The suggestion was accepted and, as the date for the meeting approached, Cohen drew up a ten-point briefing memo outlining the tack he thought the President ought to take with the physician delegation. Sensing the need to make peace between the previously warring factions, he again stressed the need for cooperation, adding that the input of physicians would be welcome. He primed the President to remind the doctors that the legislation itself called for consultation with the medical profession on the selection of advisors.[39]

When the meeting got underway at the White House on July 29, the participants who ringed the table in the Cabinet room included not only the President and the physicians but also outgoing Secretary of HEW Anthony Celebrezze, incoming Secretary John W. Gardner, Undersecretary Wilbur Cohen,* and Social Security Commissioner Robert M. Ball. Roth, at the time Chairman of the Council on Medical Service, was in the AMA delegation and remembers Lyndon Johnson telling doctor stories and "making us feel welcome." The President asked for the AMA's help in developing the regulations and, dramatizing Cohen's straightforward memo, sternly told Cohen to listen closely to the recommendations the doctors had to offer. "It was a famous meeting." Cohen says. "The doctors all got a big kick out of the President telling me what to do. But I was really only telling myself." The President had simply added some Texas flamboyance to what Cohen himself had written.

Out of this "exploratory conversation," as the AMA called it, came the AMA's understanding that HEW would seek advice and guidance from the AMA before any Medicare and Medicaid regulations were made final.[40] To carry on further discussions the Board of Trustees appointed a seven-man advisory committee, its first session with Secretary Gardner scheduled for Monday, August 30. The preceding day, as the AMA advisory committee gathered in a suite in the Washington Hilton to plan the next day's agenda, members from the AMA Washington staff appeared with upsetting news. Another bill, this one calling for a program of regional referral centers to deal with heart disease, cancer, and stroke, seemed to be headed for quick approval in a House committee despite strenuous objections made by AMA witnesses. "It was a bad bill," Roth (who had been appointed to the advisory committee) remembers. "It established so-called centers of excellence with referral patterns that seriously departed from the standard patterns."

The advisory committee decided it would have to shift gears and go to the HEW Secretary and say, as Roth phrased it, "Before we start discussing ways and means by which we can help on the Medicare regulations, we have got to tell you that this heart disease, cancer and stroke thing is a disaster from our viewpoint. If it goes through as is, we're going to be facing an emergency meeting of the house, at which there could be action to stop anyone from trying to come down here to try to make bad laws into good programs."

The next morning, when the advisory committee members said as much to Gardner and Cohen, they struck a nerve. A meeting was

*Cohen succeeded Gardner as Secretary of HEW in April 1968.

hastily scheduled with the President that afternoon. Cohen drafted a memo for the President itemizing the physicians' objections. Some members of the advisory council had to catch their planes. But at five that afternoon, Charles L. Hudson, M.D., Raymond M. McKeown, M.D., Roth and two staff members, Ernest B. Howard, M.D., and Bernard Harrison, were ushered into the Fish Room for the meeting with President Johnson. Roth recalls, "We sat around the big table and once again we heard Lyndon Johnson's funny stories about doctors and how he'd never do anything to disadvantage doctors because he loved them so dearly."

Cohen had given his memo to Johnson, listing the things the AMA felt it could not live with and asserting that HEW could go along with some changes the advisory committee had thought necessary. The President, dominating the meeting, got tough. He said he was strongly for the bill and would oppose amendments that would gut it. The AMA was making little progress. In the midst of this, an aide interrupted. Former President Eisenhower had arrived for an appointment to discuss with Johnson—it turned out later—how to handle the news of his (Johnson's) upcoming gallbladder surgery.

At least one of the AMA group was concerned that nothing had really been settled. As Johnson went around shaking hands goodbye, Roth said to him, "Mr. President, I have the unhappy feeling that we have not communicated to you our real reason for being here. If the heart disease, stroke, and cancer bill comes out the way it looks like it is going to come out, we will be forced to withdraw any participation in the writing of the regulations for the implementation of Medicare."

With that Johnson turned to Secretary Gardner and Wilbur Cohen. "Stay here with these fellows," he said. "We can't stop the bill. But make it acceptable to them." Within a day the AMA advisory committee and Bernard Harrison, who was helping to staff it, worked out some twenty changes in the legislation with Cohen. Cohen then persuaded the House committee chairman to accept them, and they became part of the final wording of what became the Regional Medical Program.[41]

The two presidential meetings and the events of the following months established a new relationship between organized medicine and the federal government. Instead of glowering at each other across a political battlefield, hurling slogans and accusations, the two sides now addressed each other in civilized tones around a conference table. As the AMA President (and member of the advisory committee) James Z. Appel, M.D., told the House of Delegates that fall, "The health care of the people is no longer a personal matter between the patient and the physician." Unless the AMA wished to repudiate all its statements about working for the best possible care for the people, it had little choice but to work with government and make the new programs as productive of quality care as possible.

In the Medicare legislation, one of the sections called for a Health Insurance Benefits Advisory Council designed to insure physician input into the program. Samuel R. Sherman, M.D., chairman of the Council on Legislative Activities, initially represented the AMA on this sixteen-member council, and nearly 25 percent of the 200 people serving on the six committees under the council were AMA choices. The government had invited the medical profession's participation, and the AMA had accepted. The AMA board committed the association to a policy of constructive advice and guidance.

Wilbur Cohen, among others, looks back on this period as something of a turning point. "It didn't mean the AMA had to agree with the government," he says. "But it did mean that it was desirable to have discussions and constructive suggestions for change growing out of that kind of dialogue. The meetings with the President helped to break the strong feeling against governmental action. Now it was possible for the medical profession to feel that at least it could discuss its views and its attitudes and its opposition and its constructive suggestions with government."

But the AMA rank and file—a large number of delegates, anyway—was marching to a different drummer. At the meeting the previous June the threat of nonparticipation dominated the business of the house. But no action was taken, the delegates deciding to wait and review "in a special session if necessary" the effect of the law. In mid-September, as they may do under the constitution and bylaws, enough delegates from enough state medical associations petitioned for a special meeting. It was held on Saturday and Sunday, October 2-3, at the Palmer House in Chicago.

As well as any others, the words of E.S. Rifner, M.D., of Indiana convey the anger that surged through the House of Delegates at that moment. He said,

We...feel let down, bewildered, shocked and dismayed as we attempt to assess the probable damage of the collusion between the ruthless power of Federal Government and organized medicine; we are torn by the forces of apathy, incredibility, submissiveness, ignorance and anger...

We have learned that the AMA leadership is negotiating with the federal employees who for 30 years have been trying to impose socialized medicine on physicians of the country, and we hear such words as collaboration, cooperation, and deals, which leave us ever more confused and ever more bewildered.[42]

He might as well have accused the AMA leadership of treason, and he sat down to applause.

But in the end, the house did not go along with Rifner or those who felt as he did. For one thing, he was followed by A. Leslie Hodson, the AMA's outside legal advisor, who told the house that individual physicians had the right to do as they pleased about participating in Medicare. But if the house passed a resolution recommending that physicians refuse to see Medicare patients, it would be a violation of the antitrust law.

What carried the day (the delegates sat for seven and a half hours as a reference committee) was something said to the house at the very beginning by President Appel, who, like Cohen, acted as a peace-maker. Even were it perfectly legal to endorse a non-participation motion, he said, it would still be "unwise." A boycott, he told the house bluntly, would be "a foolish and petulant action." Having lost the battle over Medicare, he said, "We are now expected by the public, the press and the Congress to act as reasonable and mature men and women."[43] It was not what the delegates, conditioned by the fighting rhetoric of Ed Annis, wanted to hear right then.

The immediate reception of the president's speech was as quiet and as chilling as anyone could remember. But the following day, when it came time to settle the issue by a vote, the delegates accepted Appel's leadership. Nothing more was said about the boycott, and they endorsed a policy of working with HEW to translate the Medicare law into a beneficial program.

Although both programs attracted critics, mainly because of their seemingly uncontrollable costs, Medicare and Medicaid achieved the broad objective of lowering, if not removing, economic barriers to medical care for the elderly and the indigent. Persons in the lowest income brackets started seeing physicians with more frequency than those in other income classifications. And among people over sixty-five, hospital admission rates rose almost 25 percent after the passage of Medicare; the rate of surgical procedures climbed 40 percent; and the number of hospital days per person over sixty-five jumped 50 percent.[44] Rapidly and dramatically, medical and hospital care for the two groups became more accessible. Since that was the intended result of Wilbur Mills' legislative recipe, his three-layer cake was a culinary triumph.

Medicare and Medicaid did not close all the gaps in the American medical care system, but they did cover the major hardship areas, and, in the case of Medicare, sizeable non-hardship areas as well. One way or another, between government programs and private health insurance, an estimated 85-95 percent of Americans now get at least some assistance with their medical bills. Enactment of Medicare and Medicaid was a watershed decision, for after 1965 the politics of medicine began to shift, focusing less on the accessibility of care and more on its cost.

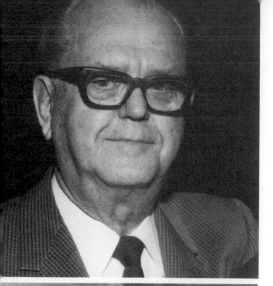

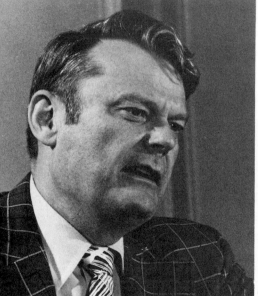

A CHANGE IN LEADERSHIP led to the dismissal of F. J. L. Blasingame (below), the executive vice president from 1958 to 1968. A strong-willed administrator, Blasingame ran into a board that thought he failed to consult them sufficiently, especially on financial matters. He also found himself philosophically out of step with new and politically pragmatic trustees such as (left, top to bottom) Burtis E. Montgomery, Max H. Parrott, and John R. Kernodle, who served successively as chairmen of the Board of Trustees beginning in June 1968.

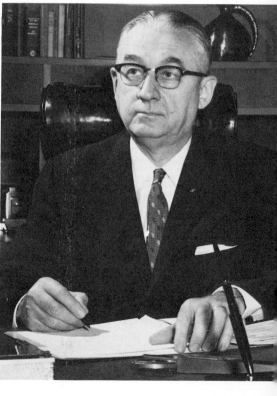

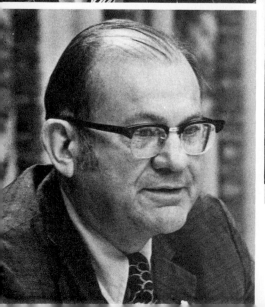

Chapter Sixteen

The Pragmatists
Come to Power

No organization can undergo what the AMA underwent and remain the same. It had battled a generally hostile press, two Presidents of the United States and three Congresses—and lost. It had taken an uncompromising stand upon a major health issue, laid its principles on the line and committed its resources—only to fail. People were weary of physicians calling programs they did not like "socialism" and looked unsympathetically on the AMA's inability to develop an alternative plan for the care of the elderly needy until it was too late. The size of the final vote on Medicare, almost three to one in the House of Representatives, underscored a disjunction that had opened between the AMA and society.

Outwardly, the association appeared unscathed. No one was calling for resignations; no one was looking for a scapegoat. Nevertheless, feelings of disenchantment and unrest were running through the House of Delegates. With the enactment of Medicare and Medicaid, medical policy-making—a lot of it, anyway—moved to Washington, and the AMA needed ways to deal with the new center of power. A better ongoing relationship with the federal government would have to be established in order to respond to the regulatory requirements of the new health care programs. It was to be expected, also, that the forces that had backed Medicare would soon seek to broaden the government's role in medicine. That raised further questions. If another bruising political struggle was in the cards, was the present leadership, both elected officers and staff, adequate to the challenge? Did the AMA organizational structure need an overhaul? New committees with different responsibilities, for example? Or new staff departments with different assignments?

Even before the Medicare legislation was passed in Congress, the House of Delegates began to raise such questions. At the June 1965 meeting the North Carolina delegation introduced a resolution calling for a permanent advisory committee on policy and planning. Noting that medicine was caught in the forces of political and social change, the resolution advocated that a committee be appointed to analyze the trends of the day and "advise" the house and board as to "projected policies and programs." At the special meeting in October, John H. Budd, M.D., (later a trustee, and president in 1977) made a more specific suggestion. Calling attention to the well-established staffs of government agencies and national non-government organizations (i.e., labor) that were "continually engaged in developing future legislative proposals," his resolution proposed an AMA committee to perform a similar function and a staff to support it. At the November-December 1965 meeting, two Michigan resolutions went farther. One, observing that "certain other well organized craft and professional groups...have been amazingly effective" and that, until unified, "medicine will be repeatedly reminded of its ineffectiveness," demanded a study committee to develop an improved organizational structure. The other suggested that the AMA establish an independent, "objective" think-tank, an institute, to develop socioeconomic data and act in an advisory capacity in the formation of policy.[1]

Though they did not do so directly, the resolutions raised questions about the AMA's leadership. The subjects they covered—data gathering, trend analysis, future planning, legislative development, political strategy—were responsibilities already assigned to the Board of Trustees, the Council on Legislative Activities, and the Council on Medical Service. If those bodies had been operating effectively and providing the association with the leadership it needed, there would have been no problem, or so the thinking seemed to go. But as it was, the reference committees that considered the resolutions had to ask, what was the use of another committee? Unable to see any benefit in appointing one, they referred the resolutions to the board. The board did appoint a Study Committee on Planning and Development in late 1965, but it concentrated on planning techniques and procedures; it could not have changed the leadership of the organization even had it wanted to. Such a change, which was what most of the resolution-writers wanted, would have to be accomplished by other means—in the board itself, in the house, and at various other pressure points throughout the association.

From the late 1950s until well past the mid-1960s, the man whose personality, convictions, and intellect dominated the AMA was its executive vice president, F. J. L. Blasingame, M.D. A southerner, a political conservative (though no extremist), a man of administrative strength and unfailing courtesy, Blasingame's basic sympathies lay with the "purists" within the AMA, those who stressed its scientific and educational traditions. Although he backed AMPAC originally and certainly understood the legislative process in Washington, Blasingame took great pride in the AMA's array of councils and committees that concentrated on scientific questions. He was deeply interested in the scholarly pre-eminence of the AMA's journals, the AMA's Biomedical Institute, founded in 1963, and the size of the AMA's medical meetings, which at that time were attracting as many as 25,000 physicians, more than any other medical meetings in the world.

But as events drew the AMA deeper and deeper into socioeconomic matters and politics, he seemed to grow uneasy. He did not particularly like what he saw happening in the choice of the AMA's elected leaders. Up until the time of the Medicare battle, the usual route to high office in the AMA lay through one of the scientific or educational councils of the AMA. With occasional exceptions, people rose within the organization through interest and accomplishment in those fields. "What you had now," says Blasingame, referring to the early 1960s, "were people interested in political action, people who liked that kind of life." He regarded the election of Edward R. Annis as president-elect in 1962 as a profound change in direction. "The Council on Legislative Activities pushed him and AMPAC pushed him," says Blasingame. "He was speaking more and more. Here you had a man with a golden tongue, and pretty soon you had a groundswell of support for him in the House of Delegates...Annis represented a shift in the life of the AMA from what I usually label the scientific-educational to the socioeconomic-political."[2]

Nor was the Board of Trustees, which listened closely to Blasingame, especially responsive to the mounting legislative, political, and governmental relations needs of the AMA. Few on the board at that time had any experience in political activities or even took much interest in the workings of government. Russell B. Roth, M.D., recalled that one of the trustees at the meeting with President Johnson and the top officials of HEW at the White House in July 1965 had to be told who Robert M. Ball was, even though Ball was the commissioner of the Social Security Administration and a major figure in the development of social legislation. Ted Lewis, Jr., who quit the *Wall Street Journal* in 1959 to cover medical news in Washington for *AMNews*, found the AMA leaders naive about politics. "Going from Washington to an AMA meeting in the 1960s," he recalled, "you felt you were back in 1949. They were not looking at reality."[3] A number of physicians, some in the House of Delegates, more who had come to prominence in their state political action committees or through AMPAC, were beginning to feel the same way about the incumbents on the board.

At the first board elections to be held after Medicare passed, those in June 1966, two such physicians won election as trustees. Burtis E. Montgomery, M.D., who had been on the politically sophisticated Council on Medical Service, had little trouble winning the seat of Percy E. Hopkins, M.D., a fellow Illinois physician who had served as the chairman since November 1962 and now chose not to run. Max H. Parrott, M.D., of Portland, Oregon, had a tougher time. Easily identifiable as what Blasingame would regard as "political," Parrott's ultimately successful campaign for a board position was headed by a fellow Oregon delegate, Blair Henningsgaard, M.D., who was rising rapidly in AMPAC.

At his first board meeting Parrott got a surprise. He had always thought that the chairman ran the board, and he did. The surprise was Blasingame's influence over the chairman. "I didn't realize," Parrott says, "that Dr. Blasingame had that kind of a hold on the board. He was the father figure, although things came down to the board laundered through the chairman. Whoever was aligned with Blasingame sat at the head of the table, and that's where control of policy lay."[4]

Parrott, from his seat far down at the board table, noticed something else. "Any neophyte coming on the board then who knew anything at all about politics could see that there were six or seven men there who weren't doing anything. They weren't given any jobs to do. If you did not do what the head of the table wanted you to do, you didn't get any assignments, and that meant that you didn't move up."

At some point during that first year, the other new trustee, Montgomery, a man several years older than Parrott, sat down next to him and said, "Now, look. We're not getting anywhere with these guys. So why don't we reorganize the board? We can probably get the votes to do it." The two went to work. The following June, right after the house adjourned its meeting, the board retired as usual to elect officers and form its executive committee for the year ahead.

At the meeting Parrott and Montgomery had eight votes, enough for control. They decided not to unseat the chairman, Wesley W. Hall, M.D., because they thought it would be embarrassing. "That turned out to be a mistake," Parrott decided later. "But we outvoted the head of the table, electing Burt Montgomery to the executive committee. That caused quite a bit of consternation on Dr. Blasingame's part."

The next year (June 1968) there were even more significant changes. Two trustees of the Blasingame head-of-the-table group were defeated for re-election. At the same time, two physicians closely identified with AMPAC were elected, John R. Kernodle, M.D., and John M. Chenault, M.D. Elected a trustee at the same time was Raymond T. Holden, M.D., of Washington, D.C., also considered to be politically sophisticated. To make the insurgents' ascendancy unmistakably visible, Montgomery was chosen to be chairman. Thus in the three years following Medicare, there was a new character to the board, a new alignment. Blasingame's influence within the board was sharply trimmed, and the AMA's leadership now included a majority of men with a different perception of the AMA's role in government relations, public affairs, and politics.

The turnover also frustrated Blasingame's most strongly held ambitions. As the first person to occupy the position, he thought the function of executive vice president went beyond making recommendations and administering the staff operation. According to Ernest B. Howard, M.D., who served as his deputy for ten years, "Bing Blasingame wanted to revert to the Morris Fishbein sort of administration. He wanted to be the permanent president of the AMA and have the board act as an advisory committee to him. That was Bing's primary motivation. He and I absolutely disagreed about that, and that was the basic reason he was terminated...Bing was constantly irritated by the board, sometimes by its slowness of action, sometimes by its differences of opinion, sometimes by its failure to grasp a point. His whole attitude was: 'I am the leader. I have the experience and the knowledge.' He wanted to be to medicine what George Meany was to labor: a full-time president who clearly set the policies."[5]

Simultaneously with the shift of power within the board, the initiative and dynamism within organized medicine seemed to shift from the AMA to AMPAC. William R. Ramsey, the assistant director of the AMA field service division under Aubrey Gates, remembers a palpable let-down after the Medicare bill passed. "There was a lack of clarity as to where we should go. People were looking for things to do. Hell, I was trying to find out how to keep twelve field men busy." He remembers a time in late 1965 or early 1966 when an outside consultant addressed a staff meeting. To illustrate the AMA's changed circumstances, the consultant drew a large circle on the pad of his flip chart and put a dot in the middle, which he labeled, "leadership." Then he redrew the picture to show how Medicare had changed things. The dot remained more or less in the same place, but the circle, representing the universe of medicine, was shifted, leaving the leadership dot not at the center, where it had been, but well off to one side. "We went through a hell of a lot of soul-searching," remembers Ramsey, who resigned to become the executive director of the American Society of Internal Medicine in early 1968. "We were trying to find something to coalesce around."[6]

No such problem existed at AMPAC. The political lessons of Medicare were easy to read, and they were not lost on physicians. They could readily connect labor's power in Congress with its power at the polls, and many physicians who had not previously grasped AMPAC's importance to their future did so now. Medicine, demoralized over the loss on the Medicare issue, now seemed to coalesce (in Ramsey's term) around AMPAC. "The 1965-68 period was one of disappointment and unhappiness," Joe D. Miller remembers, "but those feelings were offset by the success we were having in developing the AMPAC organization, building the state organizations and membership. Let me underscore something. The explosive growth AMPAC was experiencing was not a foreseen or planned event. It just *happened*. And it would have happened without me or without the original AMPAC board. It was an idea whose time had come."[7]

AMPAC was new and glamorous and dynamic. It was suffusing organized medicine with new life, new energies, new initiatives. It was bringing forth a younger generation of medical leadership. For a number of reasons, including the threat to his own power, Blasingame did not like it. "It was a tougher crowd," he remembers. "More aggressive."

First underestimating the appeal that AMPAC would have and then refusing AMPAC the sort of support that might have strengthened his own position, Blasingame finally tried to curb its growing power. A rankling conflict broke out, which centered around the two field staffs. Both the AMA and AMPAC employed eight to twelve field men who had the same basic function: maintaining liaison between the state and county organizations and the head-quarters in Chicago. The AMA field service division, whose operations also included the Washington legislative staff, had the job of keeping the AMA headquarters and the local medical associations up to date on legislative and regulatory developments in Washington. It was the field men's job to determine the reactions of the local organizations to pending legislation and, when appropriate, to bring grassroots pressures to bear in Congress. The AMA-state relationships were cordial and effective in a large number of cases, cool in some, and almost hostile in a few. The AMA field men worked on membership recruitment; they listened to complaints; they interpreted AMA policy to the local societies and tried to iron out differences when they arose. They had a lot of the same duties as a sales force. But their primary function was legislative.

The AMPAC field staff focused on political programs—conducting educational workshops, organizing local political action committees, helping candidate support committees get going, showing local physicians and the auxiliaries what to do, propagating the AMPAC faith. Unlike their AMA counterparts, who lived in Chicago and commuted to their territories, the AMPAC field men stayed in their assigned areas, sometimes with offices in the houses where they lived. Though their duties were technically different, both groups of field men saw a lot of the same people: the state and county society staff executives and the state and county medical leaders.

This is where frictions and jealousies arose. Out in the field, among the members and the constituent medical societies that make up the AMA, physicians wondered which was the dominant leadership organization, AMPAC or the AMA? Which one was going to accomplish what the physicians wanted? Aubrey Gates, the director of the AMA field service, had not liked the idea of an AMPAC field staff from the beginning. Blasingame was originally reluctant for the AMA board to grant AMPAC enough funds to start a field service.

As time went on, disputes broke out over a variety of issues; interference with each others' assignments, for example. The charges and counter-charges mounted in frequency and intensity. Though the arguments focused technically on the field staffs, they went deeper than that; they were really manifestations of the struggle going on in the board room between the conservative medical "purist" group, personified by Blasingame, and the "pragmatists," clustered around Montgomery, Parrott, and the leaders of AMPAC. As time went on the suspicion and distrust grew. Blair Hennings-gaard, M.D., chairman of the AMPAC Board of Directors, who was doing a lot of traveling and speaking to local medical societies to encourage local political action committees in the summer of 1968, frequently found himself, as he put it, "attended" by AMA field men. "I believe they suspected that my trips were being used to organize political activity within the House of Delegates. By following me, I suppose, they expected to uncover an attempt to create an AMPAC coalition in the house."[8] Joe Miller says he met with Gates and Blasingame several times, "suggesting on more than one occasion a compromise to ease the situation. Finally," says Miller, "it got to the point where we'd have to give up the AMPAC field staff altogether if we were going to coexist with Bing."

Blasingame was vulnerable on other counts. His main flaw—the fatal one, as it turned out—was his desire to exercise more authority than the board, especially the new board, was willing to grant him. The AMA bylaws are not very specific on this point; they say only that the executive vice president shall be the chief executive officer and shall administer and manage the activities of the association. They do make clear, however, that in a showdown between the administrator and the board, the board has all the votes. There was also the matter of Blasingame's management style. He was a taskmaster, a perfectionist. There was a rigidity about him, a perceived aloofness when it came to dealing with elected officers.

The course that Blasingame had chosen in handling the field staff problem led him into a collision with a group of his critics in the summer of 1968. Of those who opposed him, the adversary with the most immediate complaint was the AMPAC field staff. In trying to restrict and control the AMPAC field men, Blasingame did not seek the support of his own board. Nor was the AMA board aware that the AMA field staff was apparently keeping an eye on the moves of AMPAC officers, such as Henningsgaard, when they accepted invitations to speak to local groups interested in political action activities. In mid-August Miller, who was the AMPAC executive director, and Frank C. Coleman, M.D., a soft-spoken member of the AMPAC board, went to see Blasingame to try to smooth over the difficulties by offering some compromise guidelines on the relationships and management of the two field staffs. Miller says that they reported back to the AMPAC board that Blasingame was not receptive. "In fact," recalls Miller, "he was pretty arrogant."

The AMPAC directors, unhappy, invited Blasingame to attend a meeting scheduled at one of the hotels near O'Hare Field. Blasingame agreed to go. For some reason, when the meeting started, no one suggested an executive session, which would have excluded the staff people. "We sat there," says Miller, "and witnessed one of the damnedest conversations I've ever heard. Every member of the AMPAC board had a bone to pick with Bing, and, for the most part, this was not done politely. Bing's posture was tough, even arrogant at times. That meeting did more than anything else to assure Bing's termination, because the AMPAC board, representative of a young, emerging leadership, had a lot of influence with the AMA board. Bing made a bad mistake, for he caused the AMPAC board to dedicate itself to his demise."

The issue was resolved three weeks later when, by coincidence, both the AMPAC Board of Directors and the AMA Board of Trustees had meetings scheduled in Chicago, September 5-8. Both boards were also staying at the Drake Hotel on Chicago's lakefront.

Before the AMA board began its first sessions, the Montgomery-Parrott group had already decided to introduce a motion calling for Blasingame's resignation, and they had enough votes on the board for that. But Montgomery, recognizing how controversial the step would be, insisted that it be backed by a unanimous vote of the board, and his count for this fell short.

As the arguing surged back and forth in executive session, the crucial issue centered on a charge that Blasingame had not kept the board fully informed on financial matters. The trustees were uneasy about the way a number of things had been handled, and, though there was no suspicion of Blasingame's personal conduct, the financial management of the association had become a sensitive point. In its efforts to assert its independence from Blasingame, the new trustees had recently formed a finance committee of the board for the first time in several decades. The trustees were taking their fiduciary responsibilities a great deal more seriously than their immediate predecessors. Blasingame, on the other hand, considered all but the major financial decisions were his to make, a part of his regular administrative duties. When Blasingame withheld the auditor's annual management letter from the board, the trustees were affronted. The report was not a particularly important document or especially confidential. All it really contained was a financial critique and some suggestions for new procedures. But withholding it threw down a challenge and raised a larger question. Who was responsible for running the American Medical Association, its executive vice president or its Board of Trustees? Those who had started out non-committal on the motion to seek Blasingame's resignation started to change their minds.

The Montgomery-Parrott group finally got a unanimous vote,* and the chairman, Montgomery, and the president, Dwight L. Wilbur, M.D., left for Blasingame's office to offer him the opportunity to resign. But he refused. "Never let it be said that Blasingame was easy," Miller said years later. "He acted as a professional. He refused to accept their offer and almost derailed the whole effort. As a matter of fact, if he had offered just one simple compromise, he might still be in the job; the opposition to him was about to fold. But he was unyielding."

The refusal to resign forced the board into an even tougher decision: to fire the executive vice president. When the board finally adjourned that Saturday afternoon, no unanimous decision to fire Blasingame had been reached, and a number of the members of the opposition had started to lose their appetite for the ouster proceedings. Joe Miller was with a group in the Drake that night which included most of the anti-Blasingame leaders. Four of the AMA trustees were there: Montgomery, Parrott, Kernodle, and Long. The AMPAC board was represented by Henningsgaard, Sammons, Gardner, Wood, and Coleman. Two former presidents were present, Ed Annis and Milford Rouse. The latter, being the immediate past president with a vote on the board, was routed out of bed by his fellow Texan, James H. Sammons, M.D., to join the group near the end of the evening. From the staff there were, in addition to Miller, the deputy director of AMPAC, David Powers, and the AMA assistant executive vice president, Ernest B. Howard, M.D.

Even within this hard-core anti-Blasingame group a certain indecisiveness had taken over. Blasingame, after all, had proved himself to be a generally able executive, and not so long before the board had raised his salary by $25,000 a year and extended his contract. There was a lot of talk that maybe the idea of ousting Blasingame should be abandoned. This grated on the AMPAC chairman, Henningsgaard. Uncharacteristically for him, he remained rather quiet throughout the evening. Finally, about midnight, his exasperation with his friends overwhelmed him. Setting down his drink and rising to his feet, he repeated his earlier objections to having Blasin-

*The unanimity was not exactly 100 percent. Gerald D. Dorman, M.D., president the following year, abstained, and Wesley W. Hall, M.D., ducked out of the room at the crucial moment.

game continue in office. Then he announced in loud, assertive tones, "I am going to pack my bag," he said, "and leave Chickens-ville." The word left a deep mark on his friends, Burt Montgomery and Max Parrott especially. "After he had gone," remembers Miller, "they regrouped. He'd put a little starch in some backbones."

The next morning the board voted to give Blasingame until the close of business the next day to resign (which he did not do) or be dismissed, and designated Howard as the acting executive vice president.

"Dr. Blasingame always maintained that it was AMPAC that dumped him," Max Parrott claims. "Some of the movement did of course start with John Kernodle when he was on AMPAC, with Blair [Henningsgaard], Jim Sammons and Joe Miller. The PAC certainly had a piece of that action. But that was not the only factor, and many of the trustees who voted against Blasingame had nothing to do with AMPAC."[9]

A more thorough evaluation of Blasingame and the board's reasons for dismissing him are to be found in a letter of explanation that Montgomery wrote on November 1 to O. M. McCallum, M.D., the chairman of the Tennessee Medical Association, who had asked about the reasons for dismissal. "Massive new demands on the profession," Montgomery wrote, "have created many new challenges requiring imaginative and active functioning. It was clear that the requirements had grown but the capabilities of the executive vice president in meeting them remained attuned to past procedure...Our explorations showed a tighter and tighter rein on all information, suggestions and planning done by staff and many of the bodies of the AMA. Many matters of considerable importance did not come to the attention of the board so it could consider and act on them."

As for Blasingame, he took his dismissal without any public expression of rancor. The board settled his contract by continuing him at two-thirds salary until February 1, 1972, and similarly extending his fringe benefits. Invited to address the house at the December meeting, he said, "No ill will is harbored by me toward the AMA." He did, however, admit to feelings of "amazement, regret and sadness." He told the delegates, as might be expected, that there were internal difficulties at the AMA. He also voiced a thought that had bothered him for many years. "How can a dichotomy be avoided in matters of medical service and research on the one hand and legislative and political [matters] on the other?" He hoped that the concerns, frustrations, and motivations that led to his dismissal would be the cause of a review "not only of management but of the entire structure of the AMA." Later in his address he said it might be time to convene "a sort of constitutional convention" to revamp the AMA, though he did not mention an idea which he sometimes spoke about: a bicameral House of Delegates, one chamber to deliberate on medical and scientific matters, the other to concern itself with socioeconomic and political issues.

With the departure of Blasingame and the appointment of Howard,* the shift in leadership that began in 1966 with the election of Montgomery and Parrott to the board was complete. The new executive vice president differed from Blasingame in several important respects, not the least of them being his understanding of his authority. Howard was by no stretch of the imagination a subservient person; he was not a soldier. But, at fifty-nine, neither was he so ambition-driven that he wanted to dominate the board, as Fishbein and Blasingame had done. In his perception of what the AMA had to do to improve its performance in the area of public policy he was closely in tune with the new leadership of the board.

His background was urban Boston, Harvard, the Boston University School of Medicine, a masters degree in public health at Harvard, then the Massachusetts Public Health Service, the Army Medical Corps and, for a brief period, the Department of State, under whose sponsorship Howard developed a post-World War II medical program in Peru. As a consequence, he could look on the AMA as an outside observer might. He brought a detachment to the job, a perspective, that his predecessor, who had moved through the chairs of organized medicine, did not have. Howard knew how to roll with a punch; he was good with the press, coming across to interviewers as a moderate, candid, articulate, urbane executive. He had been through all the AMA's political battles and seen the victories and mistakes. Where Blasingame tended to be unyielding, Howard could be flexible, fully appreciating the uses of compromise and negotiation. Like the majority of the men on the board who had just made him the AMA's chief executive officer, Howard was a pragmatist, not a crusader.

---

*A search committee was formed and interviewed other candidates. But the board confirmed its confidence in Howard by removing the "acting" from his title in March 1969.

Immediately after his appointment, Howard tackled the problem that the house had thrust on the board during the November 1966 meeting. What the house, in essence, had then said was, "If agencies of the federal government and labor unions can be successful in developing legislative programs and getting them passed by Congress, why can't the AMA? What is wrong with us that we cannot do what they can do? Do we need new people? Structural changes? A new planning committee? What?"

The answer that Howard proposed called for the creation of a new, important administrative unit within the AMA. Maybe it would not take care of all the problems that the house had identified, but it would take care of some of them, and many of the most immediate. Among other things, his plan would head off any future rift over the AMPAC and AMA field staffs, the sore that had afflicted both organizations for the last two or three years.

He approached Joe Miller about returning to the AMA to head the new unit. Beginning in the pre-AMPAC days when Howard had asked Miller to do an informal study of political pressure organizations, the two had become close, developing a good working relationship, a respect for each other's administrative abilities, and a mutual personal liking. What emerged from their discussions now was the design of a new entity within the AMA to be called the Division of Public Affairs. It would be responsible for the AMA's relations with the federal government, and it would serve as the link between the AMA and the state-county organizations. Structurally, it would include the existing field service division, which had been created by Blasingame in his 1958 reorganization of the AMA and had been headed since that time by Aubrey Gates.

Because of his ties to Blasingame as well as his opposition to the AMPAC field staff, Gates could not now expect a major operational assignment. Besides, he was nearing retirement age. His position, already diminished, was not helped when the board received a letter from his friend, Wilbur Mills, asking for assurances that Gates' retirement benefits were not in jeopardy (they were honored, Gates remaining on the staff in an advisory capacity until he reached retirement age in the spring of 1969).

In addition to the field service, the new public affairs division was also given the AMPAC field staff operation, together with many of the educational and research activities that AMPAC had been conducting. AMPAC would continue its political activities, and it would have the new, combined field staff at its disposal during election years. Unspecified "broader responsibilities" for the new division were mentioned, alluding to changes in the Washington office, the organizational placement of the Department of Legislation and the staffing of the Council on Legislative Activities. On the Sunday following the Sunday when the trustees dismissed Blasingame, the executive committee members of the board returned to Chicago to approve this revision in the AMA's structure. During a telephone conference call the day after that, the entire board endorsed the Division of Public Affairs and confirmed the appointment of Joe D. Miller as its director.[10]

Though the delegates had been the ones to call for change and new direction, the house, as it gathered for its December 1968 meeting in Miami, was not ready to accept the recent actions of the board without comment. The moves that had been made were too sudden, dramatic, and extensive. Always protective of its role as the premier policy-making body, the house resented the board's failure to consult. An invitation to Blasingame to speak his mind at this meeting was an attempt to embarass, as was the introduction and recognition of Gates on the floor of the house. But two resolutions aimed at hamstringing the new public affairs division were argued down, one after a speech from the floor by Sammons, a delegate and the AMPAC vice chairman. The board had acted within its authority, and the opposition could not muster enough votes to make a serious challenge.[11]

Howard spent the first months of 1969 on further organizational changes. As with the establishment of the Division of Public Affairs, these were aimed at strengthening the non-scientific side of the AMA's operations. With the advice of Philip Lesly, an outside public relations counselor, the communications division was reorganized.* Assisted by Cresap, McCormick and Paget, the management consultants selected by the board in the fall to do an overall study of the AMA, the Washington office was restructured. For the first time since it was opened in 1944, it was headed by a seasoned public affairs executive rather than a physician. The new director, Harry R. Hinton, made his mark first as an AMA field man and then as a lobbyist. He also carried the title of deputy director of the Division of Public Affairs, reporting to Miller.

---

*Among the changes, the weekly newspaper became the *American Medical News* rather than the *American Medical Association News*. The new title reflected an emphasis on broader coverage and the articulation of policy on the editorial page rather than in the news columns.

In the summer of 1969 Howard appointed two assistant executive vice presidents. One was Hugh H. Hussey, M.D., to whom the directors of the scientifically oriented divisions were to report. The other was a newcomer to the AMA staff, Richard S. Wilbur, M.D., a grandson of an AMA president, Ray Lyman Wilbur, M.D.; the nephew of the immediate past president, Dwight L. Wilbur, M.D.; and an attractive, politically active physician who had risen to be chairman of the California Medical Association. The directors of the non-scientific divisions, including Miller, reported to Wilbur, and Howard referred to him as "my principal deputy." Although he had no authority to designate his successor, Howard let few occasions go by without saying, or giving the impression, that Wilbur was his heir apparent. A few years later, this was to create a problem of major dimensions.

While the AMA was buffeted by the process of internal change during the late 1960s, the nation was rocked by repeated outbursts against the Viet Nam war and shrill demands for the righting of perceived social wrongs. Students seized control of universities; blacks burned and looted urban ghettos; flower children stuffed daisies down the rifle barrels of soldiers lined up to protect the Pentagon; an estimated 250,000 protesting the war in Viet Nam converged on Washington in November 1969. It was a period of widespread tension and anger, and every traditional institution seemed to be a target for the young.

Certainly the AMA was. At the June 1968 meeting in San Francisco members of the Medical Committee for Human Rights and a group called the Poor People's March took over the platform microphones at the opening ceremonies and harangued the assembled delegates. A year later, in New York, demonstrators again burst in upon the ceremonies, seizing control. This was the occasion when an American Murder Association placard appeared and a young physician climbed to the podium and burned what he said was his membership card. In contrast to a reasonably restrained reaction at San Francisco, the delegates shouted obscenities back at the protesters this time. A few delegates had to be restrained from physical violence; someone hurled an ashtray. At the June 1970 meeting in Chicago, demonstrators again appeared, but, shunted into a hearing room where they could vent their feelings, they "confronted"—a favorite word—AMA leaders without disrupting the meeting.

Like other organizations of young people, the Student American Medical Association had some things to say to its elders. They, however, said them with comparative restraint, establishing a legitimate medical "left" and paving the way for increasing participation in the affairs of the AMA in the 1970s. It is interesting to note, in the following excerpts from speeches by various presidents of the student association to the AMA house year by year, the mounting tempo of their societal concerns.

1965. It has been a year of sweeping social change...SAMA's House of Delegates has expressed growing concern over the student's lack of exposure to family practice...SAMA has established formal liaison with AMPAC...officers met with the AMA Board of Trustees for the first time in an official capacity...

1966. What is the medical student of today really like? He is dedicated to his profession...He realizes that medicine involves not only the practice of an art and a science but also continuing involvement in the social and political interactions that have shaped our past and will shape our future.

1967. We established a committee to stimulate local SAMA chapter involvement in urban and rural community health projects to help educate our members in the development and the delivery of health facilities to the medically indigent...We supported liberalization of abortion laws.

1968. We have a high infant mortality rate; we find severe shortages of physicians and allied health professionals in many areas; and we find that the health statistics of the urban and rural poor often resemble the health statistics of an underdeveloped country.

1969. The controversy, the hostility and the violence seem to be increasing even in a society where our prosperity and technological advances continue undiminished...How do you explain away children who are dying of lead poisoning in the ghettos and hungry children in Appalachia?[12]

Such was the societal climate in which the new AMA leadership came to power. It was not an easy time. But there seemed to be a new "give" to the AMA, a new responsiveness to events, a new recognition, at least, of identified needs.

Early in 1970, invited to deliver one of the Lowell lectures at Boston University, the new executive vice president, Howard, felt so confident that the AMA had made a break with past rigidities and orthodoxies that he spoke with disarming candor. After briefly describing the wide scope of AMA activities, he said, "It has the resources, human and material, to promote that art and science of medicine and the betterment of the public health as its founders intended. Has it done so or has it failed? The answer is not an unqualified yes, for it has failed in some respects." He said that the association had failed to anticipate the rising demand for services in the 1950s and was slow to recognize the need to expand the supply of physicians. It had failed to recognize the problem of escalating costs.

But he was hopeful that in June "the house will establish a planning mechanism that I am sure will focus on the gaps in our health care system...and permit effective, early action." He went on to catalog a full list of new AMA responses to societal needs, including efforts to develop the allied health professions, to get physician volunteers into ghetto areas, to work with the Office of Economic Opportunity on the establishment of neighborhood health centers, to focus attention on infant mortality problems, especially among blacks, and to liberalize the AMA's traditional and strongly conservative stand on abortion.

Acutely aware of the mounting social pressures pushing for actions that carried the label "reform," he summarized the agenda of the new AMA leadership as it looked ahead to the coming decade. "Today," he told his university audience, "the nation faces a crucial decision: Whether to change radically the entire system of health care as we know it or to identify the gaps and deficiencies that do exist and take responsible action to correct them."[13]

A GENERATION ANGERED by the Viet Nam war and other perceived injustices took aim at virtually all institutions in the late 1960s and early 1970s. The targets included organized medicine. At the 1969 annual meeting, some protesters picketed the AMA headquarters hotel in New York (right) while others broke into the opening session of the House of Delegates and took over the dais. In the photograph below, Russell B. Roth, the vice speaker, is visible top center, his face above and slightly to the right of the clenched fist. Walter C. Bornemeier, the speaker, can be seen to Roth's left. In the lower right foreground, a young physician burns what he claimed to be his membership card.

At the 1970 annual meeting in Chicago, (opposite page), the protesters were directed into a reserved room where they were given an opportunity to "confront" such AMA leaders as Malcolm C. Todd (center, holding his glasses) who became the AMA president in 1974.

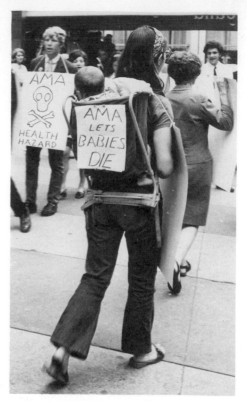

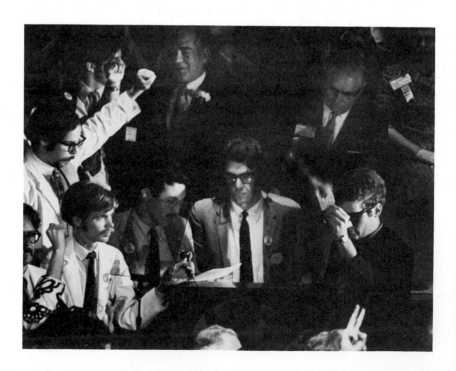

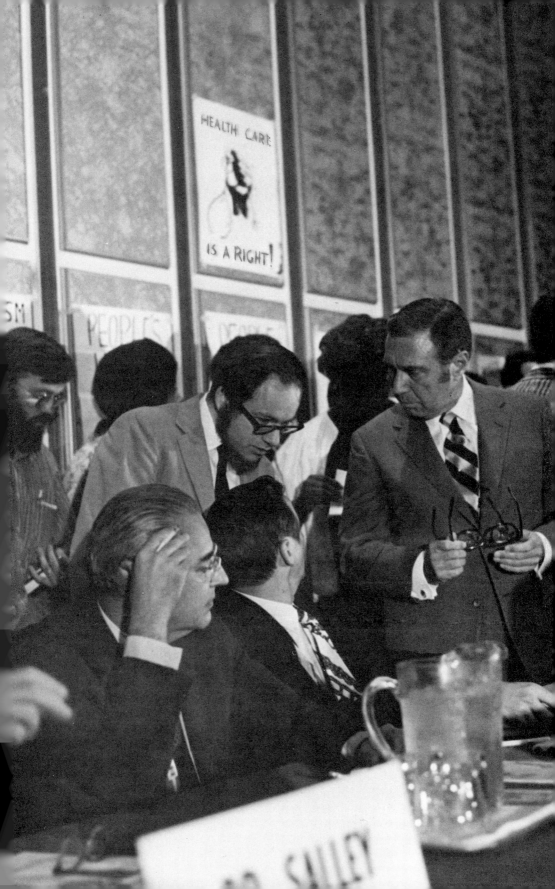

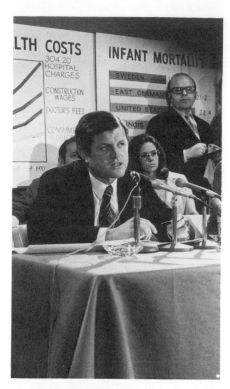

PRINCIPAL PLAYERS in the legislative drama of the early 1970s backed competing health insurance bills. At left, Senator Edward M. Kennedy, assisted by the staff of a Senate subcommittee on health (which he chaired), is shown during a five-week, nationwide roadshow in 1971 to generate support for his Health Security Act. At the same time, the AMA concentrated on developing support in Congress for its Medicredit bill. Seated (below) in shirtsleeves in a Washington hotel room, Russell B. Roth (left) and Max H. Parrott (right) get ready for Congressional testimony the next day. Harry R. Hinton (left), then head of the AMA Washington Office, is briefing them on the sort of questions to expect.

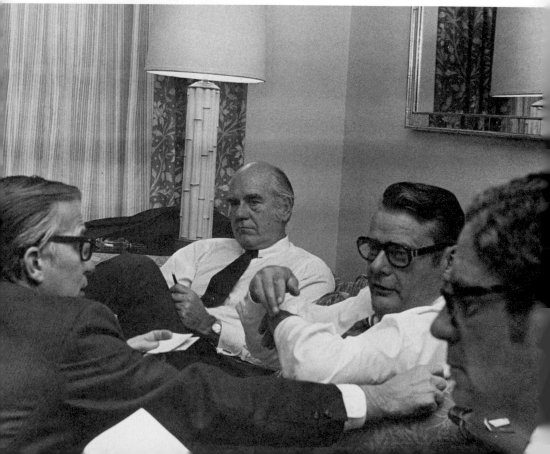

Chapter Seventeen

National Health Insurance: The High-Water Mark

The delegates who saw Medicare as only the prelude to a larger, all-inclusive national health insurance program had all their fears and forewarnings validated in November 1968. Speaking first to the annual meeting of the American Public Health Association in Detroit and later at a press conference, the President of the United Auto Workers, Walter P. Reuther, declared the nation's health care system to be in a state of "crisis" and announced the formation of a group, with himself as its chairman, to promote the urgently needed remedy: a federally financed, federally administered program of "universal" national health insurance.[1]

To those who remembered the contest over the Wagner-Murray-Dingell bills in President Truman's time, Reuther's announcement evoked a sense of *déjà vu*. Here was the familiar labor-liberal Democratic coalition again. Here once more was the Committee for the Nation's Health, now reconstituted as the Committee of One Hundred for National Health Insurance. Like its predecessor, this committee was preparing to develop sales materials, generate publicity, mount a nationwide campaign, and lobby the Congress to change the way medical care was financed and delivered in the United States. Here again, this time as technical consultant, was Isidore S. Falk, the veteran of the Federal Security Agency who had helped write the original Wagner-Murray-Dingell bills. Here again, this time as vice chairman of the new committee, was Mary D. Lasker, who had done so much to bankroll the campaign for national health insurance in the 1940s.*

---

*The other vice chairmen were Michael DeBakey, M.D., the famous cardiac surgeon, and Whitney Young, Executive Director of the National Urban League.

But familiar as the scenario first appeared to be, it could not play on the old track. Too much had changed. Back in 1945-50 national health insurance was advocated as a way to remove the financial barriers to medical care—to make physician and hospital services universally accessible by making them "free," except for the taxes necessary to finance the system. But since then the spread of private health insurance and the institution of Medicare and Medicaid had diminished the problem of access that national health insurance was originally designed to solve. In the same period, the medical system itself had also changed. The specialties had expanded. Treatments and procedures had grown more complex. Great new medical centers emphasizing tertiary care had sprung up across the nation. And with the purchasing power supplied by government programs and private insurance, the rate at which people made use of the system had accelerated.

Under the impact of a sharply increased demand for medical services, and little response in terms of increased productivity, costs had spiraled upward. A growing uneasiness had developed, and a deep concern with costs had come to overshadow virtually all health care policy decisions. In the case of national health insurance, the changed socioeconomic environment imposed a new frame of reference on the decisions. The central focus was no longer a matter of sociology, which it had been, but one of economics.

Something else had changed too: the AMA, the traditional opponent of national health insurance. Its new leadership was inclined to take a more worldly view of policy questions now. There was certainly a more sophisticated understanding of the legislative and political process. This time the AMA was not, as it had been, locked into an all-or-nothing position. Where before it had relied on the confining tactics of frontal assault to defeat legislation it opposed, now it was preparing for a war of maneuver.

The policy that the AMA pursued in respect to national health insurance from 1968 to 1978 began to evolve as early as 1961. At that time the AMA supported the Kerr-Mills bill, which provided for limited assistance to the elderly. But the association opposed the King-Anderson bill, and for a long time was convinced that Wilbur Mills and the Ways and Means Committee of the House would stop all health legislation, including the King-Anderson bill, before proposals could emerge onto the floor for a vote. Except in the very last moments of the Medicare fight, the AMA maintained that Kerr-Mills was enough to meet the needs of the elderly.

"We were always saying no," recalls Bernard P. Harrison, who was secretary to the Council on Legislative Activities before Medicare. "It was never 'No, but' or 'No, here's a better approach.'"[2] Despite the AMA's obstinate position, some physicians within the AMA disagreed with its generally negative stance, thinking— among other things—that it might be better tactically if the association had its own proposal for financing health care.

Three physicians who had come to that conclusion, Charles J. Ashworth, M.D., Willard A. Wright, M.D., and Russell B. Roth, M.D., were uniquely positioned to advance their decidedly minority view. Two of them, Ashworth and Wright, were delegates to the house, and all were members of the Council on Medical Service.* Since the council was a council of the house, members could make decisions independently of what was then a very conservative Board of Trustees. Besides being a member of the Council on Medical Service, Roth chaired a committee of that council, the Committee on Federal Medical Services, whose special responsibility was liaison with the various agencies of the federal government that conducted medical care programs, such as the armed forces, the Social Security Administration, the Veterans Administration, and the Division of Indian Health, a part of the Public Health Service.

More familiar than most of their colleagues with the workings of the federal government, Roth and others on the council were also more sophisticated than many of their fellows in their political thinking. "The three of us came to an agreement that the AMA was at a disadvantage if all it could do was sit on the sidelines and throw slings and arrows at the proposals other people made," Roth says. "We ought to be able and willing to come up with some kind of program to which physicians could subscribe. Agreed that there was a role for the federal government and for the federal dollar in the financing of health care, we thought we should say how that should be done."[3]

Working through Roth's Committee on Federal Medical Services, the three physicians developed the general outlines of a legislative proposal for national health insurance. Once these had been reviewed and agreed upon, they went to the Council on Medical Service, which, after a struggle, gave approval for proceeding seriously with a detailed legislative proposal. "We had an outside consulting

*Roth became a delegate in 1964, vice speaker of the house in 1965, speaker in 1969, and president in 1973.

firm come in to help out with that," says Roth. "Their accountants did all sorts of studies, breaking down the various components of medical care, making cost analyses for each of the elements we put in the bill."

Pleased with the progress being made late in 1962, the Council on Medical Service decided to take the idea farther up the line, submitting a short report for consideration at the November 1962 meeting of the house. The statement said that "despite general lack of public awareness" the AMA did have a program for medical care for people of all ages and that this policy position is "capable of being expressed as a legislative program." The report urged that the house instruct the board, the Council on Legislative Activities, and the Council on Medical Service "to undertake promptly, with full, adequate consultation, to present a clear legislative expression of AMA policy to the members of the association and the public at large."[4]

Temperate as the suggestion was, it came at a bad time. Just over four months before, the King-Anderson bill had been beaten in the Senate. Now was the interim period when the AMA thought it had won its battle. Accordingly, the board saw little reason to develop or back a legislative alternative. Thus, when the proposal from the Council on Medical Service came up for consideration, the trustees opposed it and the reference committee brushed it off, stating that its ideas were "essentially covered" in two other reports, both from the Board of Trustees. When the reference committee report came before the house for a vote, the house supported the board, and the Council on Medical Service was, in effect, told to go back and sit down. The house would continue backing the board in its standpat position on Medicare.[5]

At this Roth, as he puts it, "took great umbrage." He felt that the board had used its power arbitrarily and unfairly to stifle consideration of a proposal that merited more discussion than it had received or was going to get. It was this sort of action that led him to observe that he thought the AMA was in a "profound state of auto-hypnosis."

But five years later, after the passage of Medicare, the ascendancy of the pragmatists, and the growing power of trustee Burtis E. Montgomery, M.D., himself a member of the Council on Medical Service from 1961-66, the prospects for a more positive approach looked better. The AMA legislative proposal was carefully reviewed and restudied over a sixteen-month period, worked over by outside consultants, discussed with representatives of other groups (including labor, business, and the insurance industry), and finally endorsed by the Board of Trustees.

In June 1968, it began its way through the House of Delegates. A report from the Council on Medical Service, after expressing the belief that "society is moving inexorably and rapidly in the direction of a system of financing health care for all persons," called for the development of financing programs that would meet the needs of everyone under age sixty-five. It also urged changes in existing AMA policy to accommodate several features in the contemplated legislation. A longer report from the board and its Committee on Health Care Financing offered a set of twelve carefully worded principles as the philosophical underpinning for a legislative proposal, which the report also outlined. The reference committee to which the reports were given noted "an enthusiastic response" to the council report, accepted it and the board-approved report from the Health Care Financing Committee, and sent both of them to the board. A resolution from the Florida delegation, affirming the principle of using graduated income tax credits for premiums for adequate health insurance, was adopted "as approved policy."[6]

At the December meeting that year, just a few days after Walter Reuther announced labor's intentions, the board resubmitted the report of the Committee on Health Care Financing—the one that contained the twelve principles and the outline of the bill—and the house adopted it.[7] Going a step farther, the house also adopted a resolution that asked the AMA to "vigorously promote the enactment of federal legislation which would translate the concept of income tax credits for health insurance premiums into law."

From this came the Comprehensive Health Care Insurance bill, or Medicredit as it was named. It called for the retention of Medicare, for voluntary participation, for reliance on the existing health care system. Basically, it was a program establishing the use of federal income tax dollars to subsidize private health insurance policies for everyone except the Medicare population—100 percent subsidization for the poor, and subsidization on a graduated scale and tax credit incentives for everyone else.[8] Early in 1969 Senator Paul J. Fannin (R.-Arizona) and Representative Richard Fulton (D.-Tennessee) introduced a prototype of the bill into Congress.

It is important to understand Medicredit for what it was and what it was not. No one in the AMA was so naive as to think that a Medicredit bill would pass. At no point were there enough votes for that, and, besides, the law-making process does not work that way. Yet Medicredit represented more than a diversionary ploy. It was a way of saying to Congress, *if* you decide that federal dollars shall be broadly used to finance health care, then here is the way we think it should be done.[9]

In approving the Medicredit proposal, the House of Delegates broke sharply with history. For many years the AMA had argued that those who earned their living in the private economic system were appropriately served through a private medical care system.* The exceptions—and the AMA sanctioned many of them over the years—applied to people with special claims on society, those wounded in military service, Indians, crippled children, the indigent, and others. The AMA's support for Kerr-Mills, its opposition to King-Anderson, and its sponsorship of Eldercare were all consistent with that policy.

But Medicredit represented a philosophical departure, for it relied on federal tax money to subsidize universal participation— for the affluent as well as the needy—in health insurance plans. It should be emphasized, however, that Medicredit worked on a sharply graduated scale; the benefits tapered off swiftly above the lower income levels.

Meanwhile, Reuther and the Committee of One Hundred were proceeding at a measured pace. They recruited Senator Edward M. Kennedy to their cause in January 1969, but it was not until the summer of 1970 that their legislative proposal, the Health Security Act—or the Kennedy-Griffiths bill as it became known—was introduced to Congress.

As originally conceived, this bill established the federal government as a fiscal agent to provide the nation's health care. Through a combination of social security taxes and general tax revenues, the federal government was to authorize a pool of money each year to be allocated by HEW to its 100 regional offices, which, in turn,

---

*It should be noted that beginning about 1912 American physicians started developing an enthusiasm for compulsory health insurance programs modeled after those in Europe, particularly in England and Germany. (See Ronald K. Numbers, *Almost Persuaded* [Baltimore: Johns Hopkins University Press, 1978]: 33-36, 102-105.) These plans were, however, state rather than national in scope and were referred to as "state medicine." They relied on financing through contributions by the employee, the employer, and the individual states; they were designed to protect workmen earning less than a certain amount. Initially supportive, the AMA lost interest when the United States entered World War I and finally voted its opposition at the annual meeting in 1920.

would contract with hospitals, clinics, physician groups, or individual practitioners to provide health care for everyone. A person in need of medical attention would simply present himself to a participating institution, group, or physician. There would be no fees, deductibles, or co-insurance payments; care would be "free." The system was compulsory in the sense that all those with taxable income would have to finance it. But patients could choose their physicians from among those in a group, consult an individual participating doctor, or select a non-participating physician and deal with him or her on a privately paid fee basis.

With moderate enthusiasm, the Nixon administration also submitted a bill that relied on a combination of public and private financing mechanisms. The Comprehensive Health Care Insurance Program, or CHIP, called for mandated employer-employee insurance, state-assisted plans for low-income and high-risk populations, and improvements in Medicare for the elderly. Senators Russell Long (D.-Louisiana) and Abraham Ribicoff (D.-Connecticut) introduced another bill, a catastrophic insurance bill providing benefits for the victims of exceptionally long and expensive medical episodes.[10]

Early in the 1970s a whole range of proposals, ten to fifteen separate bills in all, lay before Congress. The major constituencies had been heard from—the Republicans and the Democrats, the liberals and the conservatives, the insurance industry and labor, the hospitals and the doctors—and the press was moving the issue forward on the nation's political agenda. Once again national health insurance was to be tested in the court of public opinion and then subjected to the legislative decision of Congress.

A term that everyone likes to use but means different things to different people, public opinion plays a major role in the process by which public decisions are made. But what is it? In part it consists of what the press has to say: the print media, including some 1,700 daily newspapers, syndicated columnists, news magazines, and journals of opinion; and the broadcast media, with its emphasis on a more narrow range of network newscasts, commentators, talk shows, and documentaries. Besides participating in or even leading the debate on an issue, the press performs two other functions in the formation of public opinion. First, it sets the agenda by determining which issues have sufficient relevance to be discussed at all. And then it provides the vehicle for much of the dialogue.

A far less visible but nevertheless important part of public opinion is the consensus of a group of "thought leaders:" university professors, corporate officers, executives of big banks, influential people in think-tanks and foundations, and leaders in law, labor, government, politics, religion, and ethnic and racial communities. Their information is usually good, their insights and experience are valued, and their viewpoint is therefore respected. At the same time, public opinion also finds partial expression through the trends in society: the placards on the picket lines, the shouts of the demonstrators, the slogans of the marchers. These demand attention not because they show where we are but because they may indicate where we are headed.

Finally, public opinion includes the great majority of the population that is usually quiet and is slow to respond to doctrinaire issues. Most of the time this part of the public seems indifferent to, or at least inarticulate about, all but the simple and immediate issues of jobs, taxes, prices, and street crime. This is variously referred to as Main Street, the silent majority, or Peoria, where political scenarios may or may not play. Though mainstream opinion commands only a small amount of attention, few major policy changes are made without at least the tacit consent of Middle America.

Anyone examining public opinion in the late 1960s or the early 1970s has to be struck with the strong element of anti-institutional bias that was present. Almost no part of the establishment escaped a persistent and angry antagonism. This was the time of the "me" generation, whose members demanded to know why their interests were not being better served by the traditional institutions of society. Youthful idealists—the sort of persons who joined the Peace Corps in the Kennedy administration—now rallied under Ralph Nader's consumerist, environmentalist, anti-establishment banner. It was a difficult time for institutions. The Harris Survey, which started measuring public confidence in institutions in 1966, reported in 1971 that public respect for the leadership of most institutions had "fallen drastically." The number of people expressing "a great deal of confidence" in major business corporations dropped by 50 percent; in the Supreme Court, 55 percent; in education, 39 percent. Medicine fared comparatively well, experiencing only a 12 percent drop to remain the one institution out of the sixteen studied in which a majority of Americans expressed high confidence.

For medicine, the temper of the times was reflected in the demand for health care as a "right." Though the term can be found in

AMA discussions at least as far back as the state medicine proposals before World War I, it emerged in the 1960s with a new truculence, often conveyed in the tones used earlier to demand the extension of civil rights. The term caused medicine no end of trouble, because there was no agreed upon definition of what the right to health care included. Physicians acknowledged both their ethical duty to respond to requests for assistance in an emergency and the ethical and legal strictures against the abandonment of a patient. In this sense, they agreed that there was a right to care.

But at the same time they were protective of their own right to choose the patients (non-emergency patients, that is) whom they would serve. They worried whether the "right" to health care implied an endorsement of a national health service like England's to fulfill that right. And they asked about the individual's responsibility for his own health—a responsibility to adopt a sensible life-style and to seek professional care when warning signs appeared.

The right to care grew into a touchy issue, its prickliness nowhere more evident than at the June 1967 meeting of the AMA House of Delegates. During his inaugural address that year, President Milford O. Rouse, M.D., noting the changes that had taken place in medicine, said, "We are faced with the concept of health care as a right rather than a privilege."[12] Not overly mindful of the context of Rouse's words, some of the reporters covering the meeting pounced on the new president and on the AMA for suggesting that health care had ever been other than a right. An angry flare-up followed, causing the house to develop and adopt a resolution in 1969 saying that it was the basic right of every citizen to have adequate health care available to him and that the medical profession should endeavor to make good medical care available to every person.

The question, "Do you believe in health care as a right?" took on added currency as a way to bait AMA policy spokesmen. If the AMA officer replied positively, he found himself in a tangle from which it was hard to emerge without endorsing a nationalized health program to assure citizens that the health care to which they had a right would be provided. If, on the other hand, he responded negatively, then he risked being branded as a political troglodyte. The question, "Do you believe in health care as a right?" was rarely useful for purposes of elucidation.

As for the press, it was staffed by younger people and sensitized to change (which is itself a definition of news). Journalism took on much of the anti-establishment coloration that was so widespread.

At many papers and television stations the restrained who-what-why-where-when-how reporting traditions gave way to advocacy journalism, wherein the "personal statement" of the reporter, that is, his or her feelings, assumed equal importance with the facts of the story being reported. Objective news coverage began to yield to subjective comment. The respected Harvard sociologist, Daniel Bell, recognizing the presence of what Lionel Trilling called an adversary culture, thought that its protagonists "substantially influence if not dominate the cultural establishments today: the publishing houses, museums and galleries; the major news, picture and cultural weeklies and monthlies; the theater, the cinema and the universities."[13]

Given the reform-minded climate and the advocacy mindset of the press, it is hard to imagine an easier task of presentation than Senator Kennedy faced in launching his health proposal. Placing it officially before the Senate on August 27, 1970, and borrowing much of his rationale from Walter Reuther's early words, he declared a "crisis in the availability and delivery of essential health service."

The American medical system, he went on, was the "fastest growing failing business in the nation." Health services were on the point of "collapse." As evidence of the failures of the health care system he cited international statistical comparisons, asserting that the United States trailed twelve nations in infant mortality rates and six nations in the percentage of mothers who die in childbirth, "shameful evidence of the ineffective prenatal and postnatal care our minority groups receive." Pointing out that the United States was the "only industrial nation that does not have a national health service or a program of national health insurance," he urged the adoption of his proposal as a way out of a "crisis of disorganization and spiraling costs."[14] It was an argument tailor-made to appeal to the prevailing anti-institutional mindset.

For a time in the early 1970s, comparisons of the international infant mortality statistics made surefire headlines. The data, published in the *Demographic Yearbook* of the United Nations, was used to measure the quality of medical care in the United States against the quality of that in other nations. This argument held that because the infant mortality statistics were better in Sweden (and other nations) than in the United States, it followed that the United States could improve things by remodeling its medical care system after Sweden's nationalized system of health care.

The argument ignored at least three relevant points. One, it is not valid to compare the demographic characteristics of a nation with a large, heterogeneous population (such as the United States) to those of a nation with a small homogeneous population (such as Sweden); the populations are not comparable. Two, it is not *just* medical care that determines infant mortality statistics; they are also significantly affected by a wide array of genetic, cultural, social, and economic factors. Three, inconsistencies exist in the definitions of terms used in different countries. There are some births for which it is difficult to decide whether the infant should be classified as having been born dead or having been born alive and then dying a short time later. The Kennedy bill backers and parts of the press continued using the unqualified infant mortality figures to suggest that the American system of medical care was behind the times.

The press gave the Reuther-Kennedy arguments a generous measure of attention and, at times, echoed them. *Fortune* magazine, for example, opened a single subject issue on health by stating, "American medicine, the pride of the nation for many years, stands now on the brink of chaos...the time has come for radical change."[15] CBS-TV aired a documentary on health in two one-hour segments. One of its Washington correspondents, Daniel Schorr,* used the material afterward for a book called *Don't Get Sick in America*. NBC-TV televised an hour-long documentary also, with heavy emphasis on "horror" stories of people purportedly needing care and being denied it for lack of insurance—or postponing it for fear of catastrophic financial consequences.

The NBC-TV show, "What Price Health?," featured the plight of an appealing four-year-old girl needing a blue baby operation. There was a chance, the program suggested, that her father, employed as an assembler at a Cleveland manufacturing plant, might not be able to afford the life-saving operation. Here the theme music of the program swelled. "If you can't afford to live," went the show's ballad, "you die."

However, the episode cost the program its credibility later when investigation by the Ohio State Medical Association and the AMA discovered that the girl had been successfully operated upon five weeks *before* the air date and that the father's employer-employee insurance covered the bulk of the expenses. If it had not, the operation would have been taken care of under the Ohio State-Social Security crippled children's program.[16] The *New York Times* televi-

---

*Schorr was married to Lisbeth Bamberger Schorr, the AFL-CIO staffer who worked with Nelson Cruikshank on Medicare. See Chapter 15.

sion critic (with no time to verify the facts on the program) did not hesitate to hail it as "unblinking confrontation...precisely what TV news (sic) might be all about." But in fact, instead of being a victim of the current health care system, the AMA wrote to NBC, the young girl was an obvious beneficiary.

Labor maintained its unwavering support for the Kennedy program despite Walter Reuther's death in a plane crash in May 1970, just as the campaign for the Kennedy bill was getting underway. Leonard Woodcock, who succeeded Reuther as president of the United Auto Workers, picked up the standard, and George Meany of the AFL-CIO never flagged in giving his all-out support to universal health insurance.

Because the auto workers and most other big unions already had good health insurance programs, won over the years through bargaining at contract time, one might be curious as to why the unions took to the cause of national health insurance with such enthusiasm. Weren't their members already covered?

The matter was one of elementary economics—a pork-chop issue. In testimony before the Senate Committee on Labor and Public Welfare, Woodcock made it clear that if a national health insurance program like Kennedy's went into effect, what the employers had been spending on health insurance for their employees could be converted into a pay increase. "We are now spending, with the three big automobile companies," he said, "30 cents an hour on what could otherwise be wages for the purchase of our existing sickness insurance."[17] Labor was thus as interested in a pay raise for its members as it was in national health insurance for everybody. Passage of the Kennedy bill could be translated into more dollars in the pay envelope.

As the legislative and public relations contest developed, the AMA's Medicredit bill put the association in a strong position, certainly a more aggressive one than it had been able to take in previous considerations of national health insurance. Defending a totally negative position presents difficulties because it forces you to refute the deficiencies cited by the opposition in support of the legislation it wants to see passed. Denying such deficiencies can be difficult. But having a positive proposal of your own allows you to undercut your opponent by maintaining that any deficiencies that truly exist can be corrected by other means.

Legislatively, the Medicredit bill had the advantage of giving the AMA's congressional allies a place to go. They too could answer the

Kennedy proposals for "reform" with something more substantial than a hardline "No." To voters who might be critical of their rejection of the Kennedy bill, congressmen could respond, "I have a better solution to the problem." It is frequently better politics to offer alternatives than to say "Nay," because backing an alternative may create fewer enemies. It is that reasoning which underlies the historic political dictum: You can't beat something with nothing.

There is an even stronger argument for having your own bill introduced when the real possibility of new legislation exists: Those with a program to offer get a seat at the bargaining table, a part in the negotiations that precede the writing of what may be a final bill. Those who have simply said, "No," are left out, for the simple reason that they have contributed no ideas.

In contrast to Kennedy's sweeping legislative proposal, the AMA counseled moderation. At the hearings in 1971 before Kennedy's Subcommittee on Health in the Senate and the Ways and Means Committee in the House, Max H. Parrott, M.D., the chairman of the AMA board, positioned the organization on middle ground. "Let me begin," he told the Senate Subcommittee, "by saying we are not here to testify that the American medical and health system is perfect. It is not. Nor are we here to testify that the American medical system should be scrapped. It has problems, and we are here to advocate some positive approaches to solve these urgent problems, to suggest how improvements can be made."

He rebutted the argument that Kennedy had advanced to prove the "failure" of the United States medical system, America's surprisingly poor showing in the international health comparisons. After stressing how health and medical factors both affect vital statistics, Parrott told the Ways and Means Committee "...it is idle to argue whether it is the quality of medical care or the quality of a child's environment that is the more important factor in infant mortality. These cannot really be separated. No matter how good the medical care system is, mortality rates cannot be lowered below a certain point unless improvements are made in the social environment. Nevertheless," he continued, "you might consider the U.S. record on infant mortality. In 1940 there were 47 deaths per thousand live births; in 1950, 29.2; in 1960, 26; and in June 1971, 19.2. That is better than a 25 percent drop just in the last decade. We might look at longevity too," he said. Between 1940 and 1970, life expectancy at birth in the United States had risen from 62.9 to 70.8 years. "We *are* making progress," he said.

Challenging Kennedy's claim that his health bill would halt rising costs, Parrott reminded the Ways and Means Committee of the three basic dynamics of a health care system: the desire for universal access; the desire to restrain costs; and the desire for high quality. Balanced properly, he said, the three forces can function as "a magic troika." But, he said when you couple unregulated access with the promise of high quality, which the Kennedy bill did, the combination has to exert an upward pressure on costs. To support his argument, Parrott cited the 614 percent increase in health expenditures from 1950 to 1966 when Sweden instituted its national health plan, and the 213 percent increase in Canadian hospital expenditures between 1950 and 1967 when a compulsory hospital insurance program went into effect there. In the same period American costs rose more slowly, 174 percent and 148 percent, during comparable time periods.

Testifying alongside of Parrott on both occasions was Russell B. Roth, M.D., who, as its principal author, presented the AMA's case for the Medicredit proposal. Medicredit, he told the Kennedy committee, "builds on the very real accomplishments of American medicine. It stresses that the major contribution be made by the private sectors of the economy. It takes advantage of the achievements of private institutions and industries. It attempts to hold to a minimum its demands on government, both for tax dollars and for the inevitable controls that go with them. It is a program for now …which seems certain to enlist the support of the practicing medical profession, which endows it with a far greater chance of success than would a program for which doctors have small appetite."[18]

To increase the stature of the Medicredit bill, the AMA lobbyists intensified their campaign to win congressional co-sponsors for the legislation. When a member of Congress puts his name on a bill, it does not commit him to vote for it. All co-sponsorship does is signify a philosophical agreement with a piece of legislation. As the AMA lobbyists canvassed the House and Senate,* they found themselves beneficiaries of the preceding nine years of work done by AMPAC. Mindful of medicine's support back home at election time, many congressmen and their staff assistants lent the AMA an attentive ear. During the rounds of office calls and on the continuous Washington reception circuit, the AMA lobbyists explained the philosophy and provisions of the Medicredit bill. Special attention

---

*The AMA spent $114,800 on lobbying in 1971, a crucial year.

focused on members of the four committees with jurisdiction over health legislation: Finance, and Labor and Public Welfare in the Senate; Ways and Means, and Energy and Commerce in the House. In rounding up co-sponsors, the lobbyists did a praiseworthy job. By 1971 they had more than 150; eventually they enlisted 175 supporters. Those backing the Kennedy bill, the AFL-CIO lobbyists especially, pursued the same strategy but not as successfully, for they came out second in the sponsorship numbers game. Though it finally amounted to almost a third of the Congress, the total of AMA sponsors did not foreshadow passage of the Medicredit bill, nor was it supposed to. What it did accomplish, though, was to announce the presence of a viable alternative to the Kennedy and the administration bills, and a sizeable measure of philosophical support for the Medicredit financing approach to national health insurance.

Appealing for public support as well, the AMA, as it had in the past, undertook an advertising campaign in 1971-72, spending $1.7 million over the two years. This time, however, the shrill warnings of "socialized medicine" were absent. Instead, the messages stressed organized medicine's role in public health measures, health education of the public, its interest and concern for a healthy nation. Only at the very end did the legislative proposals get attention, and then in restrained, low-key language. Other public relations efforts stressed the Medicredit bill, with a special effort to encourage editorial writers, columnists, television commentators, and reporters specializing in medical news to treat Medicredit as one of the three major pieces of health insurance legislation that were up for consideration. As the list of Congressional sponsors grew, that task became easier. The AMA communications division was busy preparing responses to unfair press coverage, "advocacy" outbursts like the NBC-TV show, for example. It encouraged a better understanding of the international health statistics and their dubious value as a measurement of national medical care systems.

Unlike the Kennedy adherents, the AMA took the view that the statistical comparisons meant little. For one thing, even their source, the *Demographic Yearbook* of the United Nations, warned that the medical definitions (of a live birth, for example) varied country by country.[19] For another, as the AMA emphasized, factors other than medical care (genetic and cultural differences, for example) had a significant influence on a nation's medical statistics. Despite all the arguments to prove "failure" or "crisis" in the American health care system, the public opinion polls continued to show high satisfaction by the public with the care it received. Though people expressed concern over the rising costs of medical care, they did not rank national health insurance as an urgent societal issue. When Louis Harris and Associates did a study for Congress in 1973 to identify what the public saw as the nation's most serious problems, inflation took top priority; health care delivery was way down on the list, rated fifteenth out of the sixteen issues listed.[20] Reflecting a few years later on all the negative publicity medicine had received, HEW Assistant Secretary for Health Theodore Cooper, M.D., remarked, "Never has anything sounded so bad that has actually been so good."[21]

For all the energy expended on the issue, the Congress made only one serious try at a national health insurance bill during the whole decade of the 1970s. It came in August 1974 immediately after President Nixon resigned, an event that opened up time on the congressional calendar that had been unofficially earmarked for the expected impeachment proceedings. In his inaugural address on Monday evening, August 12, the new President, Gerald Ford, suggested that Congress "sit down and sweat out a sound compromise ...Why don't we write a good health bill on the statute books before this Congress adjourns?" he asked.

At the time he made his suggestion, the capital was abuzz with speculation that some of the major sponsors of national health insurance legislation were in a mood to compromise. The day before, NBC's *Meet the Press* had telecast a one-hour special on health legislation with an unusually star-packed cast. It included: Casper Weinberger, Ford's HEW Secretary (representing the administration's CHIP program), Congresswoman Martha Griffiths of Michigan (representing the Kennedy-Griffiths-labor bill), the immediate past president of the AMA, Russell B. Roth, M.D. (Medicredit), Chairman of the Senate Finance Committee Russell Long (the catastrophic health insurance bill), Chairman of the Ways and Means Committee Wilbur Mills, and former HEW Secretary Wilbur J. Cohen.

For the most part it was a show and tell session, each of the proponents plugging his or her bill. But at the end, Lawrence Spivak, the regular host of the show, asked each of the participants what he or she thought was going to happen. Roth said, "I don't think we are ready for national health insurance." But the others gave answers stirring speculation that some sort of compromise bill might be possible. Wilbur Mills, people thought, just might be able to construct another multi-layer health insurance cake to suit everyone's taste, as he had done in 1965.

The day after Ford's address to Congress, the Ways and Means Committee assembled in its 400-seat committee room in the Longworth House Office Building. Overhead, recessed into the ceiling and reflecting a soft, indirect light over the room, glowed a galaxy of silvery, five-pointed federal stars painted against a light blue sky. Listening to the committee members, who occupied a graceful arc of twenty-five seats behind a curving table, the spectators were puzzled. The business being discussed by the committee seemed hardly relevant to the President's call the evening before. The more savvy observers suspected that the liberal bloc on the committee was staging a small filibuster in response to a word from labor headquarters to stave off action on health insurance for the year. Walking across the street to the Capitol after the morning session, Chairman Mills told a friend that he saw through the stratagem and said he would offer a compromise bill, force a vote on it, and thereby end the delaying tactics.

When Mills gaveled the committee to order Wednesday morning, the first witness was HEW Secretary Casper Weinberger. Mills said he was thinking of a bill that would include mandated employer-employee-financed health insurance (the CHIP proposal supported by the administration), catastrophic insurance (supported by Russell Long) and a federalized Medicaid system. Carefully choosing his words, Weinberger indicated that Republican support for such a proposal might be forthcoming if the financing role of Social Security was confined to just the catastrophic part of the program. Mills said, "I do not disagree." By giving in on that point, Mills struck a compromise with the Republicans. During the exchanges, however, the committee members looked on silently, showing few signs of enthusiasm. At lunch time Mills briefed Senator Kennedy on developments. Having broken with labor in this instance, Kennedy was working with Mills on the compromise bill. The AMA Washington office was, in fact, referring to it as the Kennedy-Mills-Weinberger bill.

For the remainder of the week, Mills labored over various financial aspects of the bill, such as whether it would include deductible and co-insurance payments by the insureds, and what size premiums employers might be expected to pay. Mills also reported on a meeting he had had with a delegation from the AMA that included

Chairman Richard E. Palmer, M.D., President Malcom C. Todd, M.D., former President Roth, Trustee Raymond T. Holden, M.D., and Executive Vice President James H. Sammons, M.D., who had been chosen to succeed Ernest B. Howard, M.D., just five months earlier. The physicians had told Mills that they objected strenuously to any Social Security role in health insurance financing because of the "tremendous problems" they had experienced with Social Security in the Medicare program. Their opposition on this point was adamant.

On Monday of the next week, August 19, the Mills compromise seemed headed for clear sailing. Mills had drawn up a twelve-page description of the plan to guide the drafting of the legislative language. Frank Carlucci, Weinberger's deputy at HEW, gave the developing bill the administration's blessing again.

But on Tuesday, August 20, when Mills called the committee together to go through the bill in detail, he walked into a minefield. Wayne W. Bradley, then director of congressional relations for the AMA, remembers being in the handsome committee room that morning. "It was a mark-up session," he recalls, "but for some reason it was open. There was an air of excitement, almost a feeling of destiny. After all, it was the first time that a major health insurance bill had come to a vote in committee since Medicare. The place was packed."[22]

On the agenda was a series of votes on the basic concepts in the compromise bill. As a staff member started to read the sections of the Mills proposal to the committee, Representative Joel Broyhill (R.-Virginia), one of the leading sponsors of Medicredit, said he thought the committee should have the opportunity to vote on alternative methods of financing for the proposed program, including consideration of the use of tax credits as envisioned in the Medicredit bill. Mills stalled him for a while, but just after the section on the financing of the employer-employee part of the plan had been read, Broyhill insisted on a vote on his amendment calling for tax credit financing rather than Social Security financing of the catastrophic part of the bill. The vote ended in a 12-12 tie, which meant it lost. But the narrowness of his victory disheartened Mills. Among the Medicredit sponsors who voted with Broyhill against the chairman were five Democrats. Next came a vote on another suggestion for alternative financing methods. This one lost narrowly too, 13-12. The compromise effort was in trouble.

At this point a friend of Bradley's on the staff of the Ways and Means Committee approached him at the back of the committee room, asking, "What can we put together?" Bradley said, "Nothing."

The AMA had been locking up every vote it could against the use of the payroll tax to finance health insurance. In any case, Bradley had no authority to make a deal. That requires a decision by elected AMA officers. At the afternoon session Mills lost another round when the committee voted 11-7 to make a part of the plan voluntary rather than compulsory. Mills angrily adjourned the session. The next morning, scarcely half an hour into the agenda, he threw up his hands. "I've never tried harder on anything in my life than to bring about a consensus on this bill," he announced. "But we don't have it. I'm not going to go before the House with a national health insurance bill approved by any 13-12 vote."[23]

This was as far as national health insurance progressed in the 1970s. Though it lingered on—the AMA kept introducing the Medicredit proposal through 1978—it seemed to many to have received the last rites at this moment. During the two middle weeks of August 1974 the time for national health insurance had suddenly come and gone.

No one factor accounts for the rejection. The medical profession, in wide agreement with the AMA position, was overwhelmingly opposed to national health insurance. Avoiding the mistakes of earlier campaigns, the AMA this time made good use of a skillfully developed political base, an effective legislative strategy, and believable public relations. In Congress, nothing close to a consensus formed. Members with ties to labor refused to compromise, insisting on an all-out, sweeping approach such as the first Kennedy bill embodied. Others in Congress either wanted no legislation at all or legislation that would minimize federal involvement, such as the Medicredit bill. Wilbur Cohen believed that Congress was afraid of a big health bill that would suddenly "transfer $40 billion or $60, $70, or $80 billion from the private to the public sector." Something that size was too much. Only an incremental approach might have worked, Cohen believed.[24] After Ford's inaugural speech, the White House never threw its full weight into a legislative push.

As for the public, it never exhibited anything that could be interpreted as enthusiasm. In poll after poll, people expressed high levels of satisfaction with the care they were receiving. They showed widespread interest in the concept of national health insurance but little appetite for the additional taxes that such a program would require. Unmoved by the demagogy and the cries of "crisis," people did not think of national health insurance as something that was urgently needed.[25]

In putting forward its Medicredit proposal, the AMA was sometimes accused of acting hypocritically. The charge is not a fair one. To be sure, the AMA did not advocate national health insurance, and, in this sense, it did not push hard for the passage of Medicredit. But if the time had come when Congress felt compelled to pass a national health insurance bill, financing everyone's health care with federal funds, then the AMA would have supported Medicredit fully as the best way of accomplishing that objective. Many members of Congress shared that view, and they regarded Medicredit not as an act of deviousness but an acknowledgment of political realities.

Chapter Eighteen

The Politics of Rising Costs

Not long after Medicare and Medicaid were in place, the American health care system began to exhibit worsening symptoms of the inflationary disease that was beginning to sweep through the whole economy. Seemingly immune to control, annual health expenditures mounted so relentlessly that the legislative initiative, so recently focused on the expansion of programs and the extension of services, started to shift direction. The spirit of largesse that suffused the Kennedy and Johnson administrations began to give way to a search for economies. The spreading alarm over rising costs not only helped slow the drive for national health insurance; it came to dominate nearly all the major health initiatives of the 1970s.

Inflationary pressures actually began to build early in the 1960s. Even at that time, increases in the medical care total of the Consumer Price Index were moving ahead of all other items. But the annual increments remained slight, a bit over 2 percent. In the 1967-71 period, however, they jumped sharply upward. While the Viet Nam war drove the whole Consumer Price Index higher, increases in the medical care total outstripped the general rise.[1]

It is an over-simplification to blame it all on Medicare and Medicaid. The fact is that the private health insurance industry was also fueling the demand for services by putting spendable health care dollars into millions and millions of new consumer pockets. Between 1960 and 1970 the number of persons privately covered for hospitalization, for example, grew from 130 million (72.3 percent of the population) to 175.4 million (86.4 percent of the population).[2]

Yet there is no way to deny the sudden impact of the federal programs. The year that Medicare and Medicaid were enacted, the medical care total of the Consumer Price Index went up 2.1 percent; in 1966, when Medicare became operational (on July 1), it went up

2.9 percent; but in 1967, the first full year of the program, the inflation rate for medical care leapt to 6.5 percent.[3] By its very nature, Medicare placed a special demand on the health care system, for insuring the health of older people is costly. Those over sixty-five years of age represent about 10 percent of the population but account for about 30 percent of total medical expenditures because they need more medical care than younger people.[4] Referring to the launching of Medicare and Medicaid, Walter J. McNerney, former president of Blue Cross-Blue Shield, describes the effect as "a demand added on top of a demand that was already accelerating." McNerney, an authority on hospital and medical economics, adds, "Very subtly, the major concern in health care began to shift from a supply problem to a demand problem."[5]

As general inflation grew politically troublesome in 1971, President Nixon, in an isolated and ultimately unsuccessful action, imposed price and, for a while, wage controls on broad sectors of the economy. His measures included ceilings on physician fees and hospital charges. His short-lived Economic Stabilization Program drew wide criticism—from the AMA, among others—partly because price controls without wage controls caused disruptive imbalances, partly because the controls tended to do more harm in the long run than they accomplished in the short term.

As expected, the controls did work temporarily, holding price increases in medical care to 4.7 percent in 1972 and 3.1 percent in 1973.[6] But in 1975, after the controls in the health care field were lifted (they remained in place longer than the others), the medical care total of the Consumer Price Index promptly spurted ahead at a 12.5 percent annual clip.

In the late 1960s, zeroing in on one specific problem stemming from rising medical costs, the administration and Congress reacted with dismay to what they saw happening to the estimates for Medicare and Medicaid. Medicare Part A for example, the hospital insurance part of the program, was going to cost $5.8 billion in 1970, not the $3.1 billion that Congress had "conservatively" estimated it would cost five years previously. Taking a long range view and foreseeing a $131 billion deficit in Medicare Part A alone over the next twenty-five years, President Nixon requested an increase in taxes. Faced with that, both the executive and legislative branches sought ways to escape the difficulties brought on by rising medical care costs.

In February 1970 a report prepared by its staff put the problem bluntly to the Senate Finance Committee. "The Medicare and Medicaid programs are in serious financial trouble," the report announced.[7] The control mechanisms in the original legislation were not working. These included review by committees of hospital physicians of the utilization of hospital services (Did the patient need hospitalization in the first place? Was his stay too long?). The procedures also called for claims review by the insurance intermediaries for the programs (Is the stated charge for the appendectomy correct?). The various states established review procedures for their Medicaid programs. To improve on the sort of supervision then in effect, the staff report recommended a more active involvement of organized medicine in the monitoring of care and its cost.

In the House of Representatives, Wilbur Mills was voicing a parallel concern. In March 1970 he invited AMA representatives to join his Ways and Means Committee in executive session to discuss ways to control costs and end abuses. As a result of those discussions, the AMA developed a formal peer review program,[8] put it into legislative language, and added it to the Medicredit bill, introduced as a bill formally sponsored by the AMA that July.* The Peer Review Organizations in Medicredit called for the Secretary of HEW to contract with state medical societies or organizations they might designate to conduct review programs. At that time most state and many county medical societies maintained grievance committees to hear patient complaints, review physician charges for services, and evaluate the quality of services provided by physicians.

What the AMA sought to do was extend this sort of on-going, workable review process into a legislative format. If peer review were established for the Medicare and Medicaid programs, physicians could go over the work of other physicians, checking on the appropriateness and quality of the care provided. Although these review organizatons would identify "problem" physicians—those, for example, who were following outdated or inappropriate procedures—the objectives were educational rather than punitive.

Actually, for well over fifty years, the peer review concept had been an established part of the medical education process. Even the hospital tissue committees, which compared pre-operative diag-

*Congressman Richard L. Fulton (D.-Tennessee), borrowing heavily from the Medicredit concept, introduced what was considered the first Medicredit bill on April 2, 1969. This bill did not contain any review mechanism such as the Peer Review Organizations envisioned in later Medicredit legislation.

noses with the pathology reports on the excised tissue, conducted their programs not to penalize a surgeon who missed a diagnosis but to improve his diagnostic skills.

But Congress, with money on its mind, pushed in a different direction. Its desire to act took on new impetus when a study initiated by Senator Wallace Bennett (R.-Utah), a member of the finance committee, revealed that only 40 percent of hospitals had functioning utilization review programs in place, even though they were mandated by the law. Guided by Bennett, Congress established what it called Professional Standards Review Organizations (PSROs). This concept drew heavily from developments in the private sector—the AMA's proposed peer review organizations, and a computerized review system being used by the San Joaquin Medical Foundation, an offshoot of the county medical society in Stockton, California. But the purposes of a PSRO differed from those of a peer review organization, one stressing cost surveillance, the other emphasizing quality of care factors.[9] The AMA looked to peer review as a teaching method; Congress saw it as a system of internal audit. Thus, a basic disagreement over priorities arose.

As the legislation developed in 1971 and 1972, the AMA contested many provisions in the evolving bill, frequently with success. But in the end, the AMA registered its opposition. The stress on "norms" of treatment and "profiles" bothered many physicians. Would alarm bells go off when the "limits" of accepted practice were violated? Was this going to bring on "cookbook medicine?"

Doctors sensed an erosion in an agreement written into the Medicare and Medicaid legislation that medical decisions in the two programs would be left to physicians. Now they worried that some of the authority was being surrendered to a medical review system sponsored, financed, and directed by the federal government. Fears about the musclebound ways of the federal bureaucracy surfaced. But what really solidified medicine's opposition was the priority placed on cost over quality. Physicians looked at the final wording— "to promote effective, efficient and economical delivery of health services of proper quality"—and had to conclude that in a contest between the considerations of cost and those of quality, the desire to save money would take precedence. That bothered them.

After the enactment of the PSRO legislation, known as the Bennett amendment, on October 30, 1972, the AMA had the same policy dilemma it faced after the passage of Medicare. As it had before, the AMA leadership recommended a constructive course

designed to develop regulations that would get an acceptable program underway. That was its initial reaction at the November 1972
meeting, and the house authorized an Advisory Committee on
PSROs to provide input from the medical profession. Headed by
Robert B. Hunter, M.D., a trustee, the advisory committee created
eight task forces, eventually involving sixty-three physicians, to explore such aspects of PSROs as the definition of norms, the training
of personnel, and the development of a uniform data support system. HEW, meanwhile, commissioned Arthur D. Little, Inc., to analyze the PSRO legislation and develop working models of PSROs.
Establishing a network of peer review organizations for the two big
federal health care programs was not going to be easy.

Then why help? asked a number of physicians as 1973 wore on.
Annoyed originally when the AMA could not stop the Bennett
amendment from passing, they were now angered because the
AMA was helping translate the law into a program. The most vehe-
ment in their denunciation of the AMA leadership clustered around
two rigidly conservative medical organizations, the Association of
American Physicians and Surgeons and the Council of Medical
Staffs, both of which seemed to enjoy carping at AMA policy decisions. Recognizing the resentment caused by the PSRO legislation,
they kept stirring it afresh and accusing the AMA of a "sellout."

Jose L. Garcia Oller, M.D., a New Orleans neurosurgeon who
headed the Council of Medical Staffs (later the Private Doctors of
America), stumped the circuit of medical society meetings with
demagogic assaults on the AMA. He charged Russell B. Roth, M.D.,
with writing a book "to tell us how to implement PSROs," though
all Roth had done was to agree to sit on an advisory panel for the
Arthur D. Little study as a devil's advocate. Garcia Oller also accused Bernard Harrison, director of the AMA legislative department, of writing the AMA's peer review program and getting it
introduced into Congress before anyone in authority at the AMA
had a chance to go over it carefully. To those familiar with the way
the AMA operates, the accusation brought smiles.

Denying both charges at a state medical society meeting that
Garcia Oller had addressed the preceding day, the board chairman,
James H. Sammons, M.D., said, "I consider the tactics being used by
the Council of Medical Staffs and its leader as among the most
divisive in American medicine."[10] Emotions were running high on
the PSRO issue, and AMA leaders like Sammons and Hunter, who
thought the wisest policy was to work constructively on the regula-

tions, took growing amounts of heat. Sammons occasionally shook his head over what he characterized as the "give-me-liberty-or-give-me-death" mentality of the die-hard PSRO opponents.

As physicians crowded into Anaheim, California, for the December 1973 meeting of the House of Delegates, they showed minimal interest in the offerings of Disneyland next door. Instead, they seethed over the PSRO issue, now crackling with ideological voltage. On Saturday, the day before the meeting officially opened, six to seven hundred doctors jammed a conference on PSROs especially scheduled by the Board of Trustees. One purpose was to improve everyone's informational background; another was to provide an opportunity for blowing off steam. Both exercises, the board hoped, would lead to a more reasoned consideration of the PSRO issue when the house met.

The session offered a debate, the affirmative side led by Claude E. Welch, M.D., a delegate from Massachusetts, one of the nation's top abdominal surgeons and, of all the delegates in the house, probably the man most respected as a physician. Welch expressed misgivings over the PSRO law but said, "It would be a tragedy if medicine turned its back on PSROs." Taking the other side of the question, J.W. Johnson, M.D., whose views had recently won him the presidency of the San Diego County Medical Society, called for repeal of the law. "It takes a sophomoric outlook to believe that this law will either improve the quality of care or lower costs," he said. Serving as an informational panel for the meeting were: Henry E. Simmons, M.D., Deputy Assistant Secretary for Health of HEW, in charge of the PSRO program, Ernest W. Saward, M.D., head of the government's PSRO physician council, and Robert B. Hunter, M.D., the AMA trustee who headed the advisory committee on PSROs and also served as the AMA representative on Saward's council.

At the end of several hours of discussion, AMA President-elect Malcolm C. Todd, M.D., tried to summarize the sense of the meeting. "PSRO poses a greater threat to the private practice of medicine than anything ever developed by the Congress of the United States," he said. "Repeal may ultimately be required. But now is not the time for such action—it would be unrealistic, politically naive and unattainable. The wisest choice is to continue to work within the program in hopes of having a significant impact on the implementation."[11]

Though Todd's summary was reasonable, it did not settle anything. Even the Sunday session of the convention, usually ceremonial, proceeded under ideological storm clouds. AMA President
Roth devoted his address to a historical survey of peer review.
Charles C. Edwards, M.D., the assistant secretary for health at HEW
and a former AMA executive, spoke in conciliatory tones about the
need for a joint approach to peer review. But all the palliative efforts
were offset when the speaker gave permission to a Georgia physician, John P. Heard, M.D. (who was not a delegate but nevertheless
emerged as the leader of the anti-PSRO militants at the meeting), to
read a letter addressed to the house and signed by thirty-four congressmen opposed to the PSRO legislation. It is a bad law, the letter
said; it should be repealed. "Unfortunately," it continued, "although
many of us want to work for the repeal of PSRO, we have been
handicapped by the AMA's failure to continue its active opposition
to the law."[12] If the anti-PSRO fires had been cooling, that accusation
rekindled the flames.

On Monday Reference Committee A received a major load of
PSRO business—no fewer than sixteen resolutions and two reports,
one a joint report of the board and the Council on Medical Service.
Over 500 physicians attended the four-hour hearing on this one
subject. "No speaker's time was limited," the committee report
stated, "except by fatigue. The discussion was often heated and
emotional." Tuesday brought a day of relief, but on Wednesday
morning the reference committee report came before the house. To
free the discussion from parliamentary restrictions, the rules were
relaxed to permit "informal consideration" of the reference committee report. But after fifty minutes at least nine amendments or
substitute amendments cluttered the agenda.

At this point, the speaker, Tom E. Nesbitt, M.D., called a fifteen-
minute recess. During the break the contending factions agreed to
some compromise wording for insertion in the joint report from the
Board of Trustees and the Council on Medical Service, which the
reference committee was recommending for adoption. When the
house returned to business, the amended report was adopted. It
called for the AMA to develop appropriate regulations and to support constructive amendments. But at the same time it said that
repeal of the law would be in the best interests of everyone. It was a
thoroughly contradictory resolution of the controversy.

Heard, who had argued long and hard for repeal of the PSRO
legislation, calling it "immoral to support a law we believe to be a

bad law," was not yet through. Emphasizing words in the final action that instructed the AMA "to inform the public and legislators as to the potential deleterious effects of this law on the quality, confidentiality and cost of medical care," he issued a threat. "We've given the officers and staff instructions on what we want done," he said. "We'll be keeping book on them, and when we meet again next June, we'll hold them accountable."

The militants had a final card to play. Midway through the Wednesday morning session, Philip M. Crane appeared in their midst, an Illinois congressman of ultra-conservative leanings and one of those who had signed the letter Heard had read to the house on Sunday. Crane had come, most people thought, at Heard's invitation. Recessing for the second time that morning, the house interrupted its business session, agreeing to hear what the congressman had to say.

The AMA was taking a self-defeating stance on the PSRO law, Crane began. "The doctrine of inevitability is the most pernicious doctrine ever put forward by Karl Marx," he declared. "To accept that doctrine is to be removed from the battle...If you, the people who will be most affected [by PSRO], won't stand in the vanguard of this battle, then we may very well go down the tubes. They'll take us salami style, a slice today, another slice tomorrow." The house was through with the issue, however, and Crane's oratory changed nothing. James H. Sammons, M.D., recently elected chairman of the Board of Trustees, pointed out that thirty-five to forty congressmen were not very many and said that his best information from Washington indicated "no political viability whatsoever" in an effort at repeal. But the multidirectional action of the house—calling simultaneously for the amendment, repeal, and implementation of PSRO law—remained in place. The issue had not been settled.[13]

Over the next seven months, the need for decisive action grew increasingly urgent. When the June 1974 meeting convened, no fewer than twenty-five resolutions on the PSRO law occupied the agenda. A substantial percentage of the medical profession probably was resigned to the legislation, having taken what AMA President Roth called a *Porgy and Bess* attitude. This he described in a bit of doggerel that he sang to the tune of "It Ain't Necessarily So" before a meeting of the Utah State Medical Association:

There's nothing but misery and woe,
To expect from a PSRO;

But thanks to the amendment,
And Senator Bennett,
There's no other way we can go-o-o-o.

Nevertheless, there were those physicians who were stoutly opposed, not just to the law, but to the AMA's leadership position of assisting in its implementation. For a time, it looked like the anger of the Anaheim meeting would erupt again.

A reference committee spent all of Monday in hearings on just the PSRO question, the most divisive, observers agreed, since Medicare in the early 1960s. The committee remained in session, it reported, "until 5:30 p.m. arrived and no speakers remained standing." The committee, in its report to the house, estimated that sixty-four physicians had spoken, some "ardent for a policy of repeal," others "ardent" against. When submitted to the house, the report of the reference committee faced down the militants, calling for the AMA to help develop constructive amendments and regulations.

On the floor, the delegates braced themselves for another grueling session. As the various advocates were clearing their throats, William B. Hildebrand, M.D., a delegate from Wisconsin, gained recognition at one of the floor microphones. Bluntly he told the house, "This is the fourth time in two years we have dealt with this issue, and I, for one, have heard nothing new in this year's discussions. Therefore, Mr. Speaker, I move the question." The delegates seemed to gasp in surprise; but then, apparently recognizing how much time would be wasted in debate, they voted four to one in favor of Hildebrand's motion to end discussion, in effect, before it began.

Then they voted 185-57 for the policy recommended in the reference committee report: that the AMA seek constructive amendments and sound regulations. By implication, the quest for repeal of the PSRO law was dead for the time being, and with a sense of catharsis, the house broke into applause. However, one delegate, John R. Schenken, M.D., of Nebraska, asked to have his negative vote recorded. "I did not vote for tyranny," he said.[14]

No one welcomed the AMA's now clearcut position more warmly than Robert B. Hunter, M.D., the trustee who had been put in charge of the PSRO advisory committee in late 1972. Though he was acting at the board's direction and though the board was carrying out policy adopted by the house, Hunter had nevertheless been treading on thin ice. For eighteen months he had had to commit himself to a program to which the AMA itself was not unreservedly committed. He had invested a sizeable amount of his own time in the difficult work of negotiating sound, sensible PSRO regulations, and he had laid his own future in the AMA's elective hierarchy on the line.

Part of his job was to defend the AMA's implementation policy, making him, in the eyes of some of the die-hard militants within the AMA, a Quisling. A bigger part of the assignment was missionary work, convincing doctors that they should participate in the program once it was underway. A talk he gave to a regional medical conference in Atlanta in early 1974 typifies the appeal he was making to the profession. He began by saying that in his capacity as head of the PSRO advisory committee, he had flown some 250,000 airline miles and that he had ridden more comfortably "knowing that the pilot and the co-pilot were required to undergo periodic fitness examinations." Warming to his subject, he continued, "No individual, group or profession can hold itself aloof from inquiry, which, in many respects, is healthy. We welcome the visit of bank examiners to those institutions which have custody of our funds. Why, then, should our profession draw back in alarm at the possibility that our judgments and our actions should be subject to review?"

A voice of reason, Hunter's explanatory efforts helped prepare physicians to accept the PSRO program. Eventually, it would fail. But the failure was not brought on by a physician boycott. It is remarkable, in fact, that the PSRO program so vigorously attacked when initiated, received the support it did. In 1981, in what might be regarded as a post mortem, Helen L. Smits, M.D., director of the national PSRO program for the Carter administration, observed, "With the total PSRO membership now comprising over 50% of all physicians in areas with active PSROs, there seems little question that doctors have been willing to take on the responsibility of reviewing cases."[15]

While the AMA struggled to clarify its position in early 1974, the federal government began to establish the PSROs. As a first step, HEW designated 203 PSRO areas. In some cases, the areas conformed to state boundaries; in others, they followed county lines; in still others the designations fell in between—western Virginia, for example, was a PSRO area. The local medical societies were, of course, forbidden to become the PSRO in a designated area, even though most of them had been performing review functions on a voluntary basis.

What would happen, in most cases, was that physicians with interest and experience in existing review activities would form a corporate "shell" and apply for appointment by HEW as the recognized PSRO for the designated area. Before that could happen, however, a poll of physicians in the area would have to show approval for those heading the PSRO. An element of threat was also involved: if physicians did not come forth and start a PSRO, HEW could name an "alternative" PSRO, designating an insurance carrier, for example, or an existing medical group to do the review work.*

As the new groups began to function, they concentrated on utilization review, that is, the use of hospital facilities. This is where the most expensive forms of medical treatment are given. The review of hospital use was, of course, written into the original Medicare law, and many state Medicaid programs also monitored hospital use. In the case of Medicare, the review of utilization originally was "retrospective," taking place after the patient's discharge. Upon findings of improper use, the insurance carrier for the Medicare program would deny payment, setting off squabbles among the hospital, the admitting physician, and the patient as to who was responsible for the bill. When the existing utilization review processes were absorbed into the PSROs, one of the major changes made was a shift to "concurrent" review, which took place while the patient was still receiving hospital treatment.

Norms of care were established, which might indicate, for example, the normal number of hospital days for a particular illness or surgical procedure. If a patient was running substantially over the norm of hospital days for the procedure, a notice went to someone connected with the PSRO. Physicians' profiles were kept too, indicating, for example, how long Dr. Smith usually hospitalized his patients. If Dr. Smith's profile showed he was customarily hospitalizing patients 30 percent longer than his colleagues for treatment of the same conditions, the PSRO would call him in for a talk. Concurrent review also had the advantage, simply because it was current, of eliminating the post-hospitalization denials of payment.

It was the apppropriateness of hospital admissions and length of stay that PSROs concentrated on; in only a few instances were they

*In some cases, in Louisiana for example, "alternative" PSROs were imposed when the local physicians did not form them. In Nebraska, however, whose senior delegate asked that his negative vote be recorded (against "tyranny"), no PSRO of any sort was established. The utilization review program set up by the original Medicare legislation did, however, remain operative.

able to develop ways to review long-term (nursing home) care or ambulatory care (office visits).

Early in 1975, again looking for ways to curb the cost of its programs, HEW issued regulations intended to advance the utilization review process even further. The objective this time was to get a review of the medical necessity of a hospital admission within twenty-four hours. What HEW now sought also proposed the use of non-medical personnel in the review process. The profession balked. Wasn't this encroachment on the doctor's authority? The original Medicare legislation said that there would be no interference with a physician's medical judgments and specified retrospective review. And the law had not been changed. The AMA challenged the regulations, seeking an injunction to stop HEW from carrying them out. A federal district court issued a restraining order, upheld upon appeal, which found Secretary Weinberger had exceeded his statutory authority.[16]

As the rise in Medicare costs persisted, HEW decided in early 1977 to strike out on a different front by releasing the names of physicians receiving over $100,000 in federal payments in preceding years. Although it maintained it had to make the names public because of the Freedom of Information Act, physicians saw HEW as acting on its own initiative out of a desire to embarrass and intimidate them. Whatever the case, it quickly became evident that HEW had sprung its own trap. The list of physician recipients—presumed guilty in the predictable headlines about "medical rip-offs"—was astonishingly inaccurate. Of the first 112 physicians to be checked by the AMA and state medical society staffs, only thirty-two said the HEW information was completely correct. One physician, listed as practicing in Illinois and receiving $233,871 from Medicare in 1975, was located in Arizona where he had retired twelve years earlier. Another, listed as receiving $258,139 in 1975, had actually died in 1974.[17] The story in the press turned quickly around; less attention focused on the so-called "Medicare fatcats" (who were not individual recipients, by and large, but usually heads of physician groups receiving payments for services rendered by a whole group) and more on the errors spewed out by the HEW computer. HEW beat a retreat, and an injunction sought by the Florida Medical Association and the AMA prevented the release of all names of physicians and the amounts of income they allegedly generated from Medicare in 1978.

Right from the beginning, and for all involved, the PSRO program launched a parade of frustrations. Not only did the doctors raise initial objections; the states erected obstacles to protect the review procedures in their own Medicaid programs, and some of the insurance carriers, also with review mechanisms, grew defensive. Even within HEW there was a problem for a long time. Where should the direction of the new program be placed administratively? Medicare was part of the Social Security Administration. Medicaid was part of the Social and Rehabilitation Service. To avoid hurt bureaucratic feelings, the administration of the PSRO program was given to the Public Health Service. Not until 1977, when Medicare, Medicaid, and PSROs were all gathered under a new administrative unit, the Health Care Financing Administration, did a unified effort become possible.

As time went on, the bureaucratic ways of the federal government turned physicians off. When their suggestions were sat upon and local needs and conditions were ignored, doctors began to lose patience with the PSRO program.

The way the federal government tried to bring PSRO to Texas illustrates the sort of insensitivity to local preferences that can cause rigidly drawn and rigidly enforced federal programs to founder.

At the start, Texas was split into nine PSRO areas, a policy decision not entirely consistent with what HEW was doing elsewhere. Texas physicians, having formed the Texas Institute for Medical Assessment with the strong backing of the Texas Medical Association, fought for a single, statewide PSRO. HEW fought back, and the dispute went to court, to be resolved in the doctors' favor. The U.S. District Court for western Texas found that the designation of nine PSROs in the state was "unlawful and invalid." But HEW's insistence on having things done its way eventually resulted in the absence of any PSRO in the state until September 1980, by which time the Texas physicians, who once were more than willing to get a program started, were now opposed to it.

Confidentiality—the protection of physician and patient privacy—was also a worry to physicians. Congress did not pass the kind of law desired by physicians to exempt PSROs from the Freedom of Information Act. When the Nader-associated Health Research Group used the act to obtain PSRO data identifying individual practitioners and institutions, a federal district court ruled that PSROs were indeed not exempt and were, as the physicians long feared, to be considered agencies of the federal government insofar as the

Freedom of Information Act was concerned. An appeals court reversed that decision, but it was not until late in 1981 that there was
a clear ruling. Until that time, some doctors remained uncertain
about their participation in a PSRO because the data it generated
were subject to Freedom of Information requests.

Efforts at improving the PSRO program, instead of being welcomed, were occasionally pigeonholed without explanation. This
alienated physicians even further. For example, through contracts
with the federal government, the AMA developed criteria to assist
local PSROs in their review process. The documents were not to
establish standards of care; they were simply tools to help a local
PSRO formulate review criteria. It was an appropriate use of private
sector resources to assist the program. However, the submitted documents simply gathered dust in Washington and were of no use to
the local PSROs, for which they were drafted.

At its December 1980 meeting the House of Delegates finally
decided to give up on federally mandated peer review, voting narrowly, 104-100, to seek repeal of the PSRO law. In testimony on
March 23, 1981, before the Health Subcommittee of the Senate
Finance Committee, Joseph F. Boyle, M.D., then a trustee, later chairman and president of the AMA, spoke for the clinicians who had
first objected to the program, then tried to make it work.

The AMA reversal of position, he said, "is a natural, eventual
result based on the growing dissatisfaction that developed from the
often fruitless and frustrating efforts to work with the federal bureaucracy and improve the PSRO program...I emphasize strongly
this should not be considered a withdrawal of our support for
professional peer review of medical services to ensure quality care.
What the AMA is rejecting is a federally directed review program
where the federal direction is no longer interested in patient care or
quality service, but has become devoted to the single-minded purpose of restricting health expenditures." In adopting a set of voluntary peer review principles at this December 1981 meeting, the
AMA took note of the pluralistic nature of the review systems in
place across the nation as well as the increasing demand for review
services by state and local governments, businesses, and insurers.

After nearly ten years, the PSRO program was judged a failure.
At the operating level, physicians consistently thought the program's
priorities were wrong. At the administrative end, Carter administration PSRO Director Helen L. Smits, M.D., saw as one major problem "the federal bureaucracy's predictable discomfort in managing

a program based on local professional decisions." She thought the program should be judged on its professional competence and local effectiveness.[18] Congress, taking a third view, looked for ways to measure the financial benefits of the program against its costs. It did not completely accept one well-publicized interpretation of data indicating that for every dollar spent on review there was only a ninety-cent savings to the federal government. But when the Congressional Budget Office, the Health Care Financing Adminstration, and the General Accounting Office could not "prove" that the PSRO program generated sizeable net economies, Congress started to phase out the program.

As Congress began developing its PSRO legislation in the early 1970s, the Nixon administration rolled out another engine to fight the inflationary fires: the health maintenance organization, or HMO. Billed (many thought overbilled) as a new concept in medical care delivery, the HMO offered a different anti-inflationary strategy— the encouragement of market competition rather than the imposition of regulations.

Credited to Paul M. Ellwood, Jr., M.D., a Minneapolis physician who concentrated on the study of alternative delivery systems rather than clinical practice, the term HMO initially puzzled many people. What was so different about HMOs? Were they not the same as existing prepaid medical groups, such as Kaiser-Permanente on the West coast, the Group Health Association in Washington or the Health Insurance Plan of Greater New York (HIP)? Yes, they were like that, said spokesmen in the Nixon HEW. But there was a difference.

In the HMO the physicians would concentrate on "wellness" rather than sickness, on maintaining the health of enrollees, on the prevention of illness rather than its treatment, on health education programs and screening programs to detect problems early. In the prevailing fee-for-service system, so the rationale went, costs were high because physicians had an economic interest in the illnesses of their patients; they had incentives to treat, even to overtreat, and run up the bills. Conventional health insurance insulated both patients and physicians from concerns over costs.

In an HMO, by contrast, the economic incentives theoretically worked the other way. Since the HMO enrollee paid a fixed amount per year regardless of how much medical attention he or she required (the basic contractual arrangement of an HMO) and since the physician depended on an income geared to the financial performance of the HMO, the physician had an economic incentive to keep the patient well. Should the patient become ill, then the physician had an incentive to limit treatment to the essentials—no frills. Whenever possible, the patient would be taken care of on an ambulatory basis; HMOs gave physicians a strong incentive to hold down on hospital admissions. On paper at least, the HMO concept had a strong allure for those concerned with the cost of medical care.[19]

The AMA reacted with skepticism. Beyond such procedures as immunizations, Pap smears, periodic checkups, and prenatal and well-baby care, what were physicians to do in the way of health "maintenance" that they were not already doing? Was the orthopedist to set broken bones for so many hours and then teach little league baseball players the techniques of the hook slide? The public already seemed well provided with educational materials on smoking, diet, exercise and so forth. What could the physician add to those efforts that might bring down the incidence of such expensive illnesses as heart disease, cancer, and stroke? A great many physicians thought the HMO spiel on "wellness care" belonged on Madison Avenue. Traditional fee-for-service doctors also resented the charge that they were running up bills for economic reasons. "If some doctors are so unscrupulous as to overtreat patients for economic gain," John H. Budd, M.D., then a trustee, occasionally asked, "why won't there be physicians unscrupulous enough to undertreat patients for economic gain in an HMO?"

Careful to avoid a break with the Nixon administration despite policy differences, the AMA showed restraint in voicing its reservations. These echoed the old objections to contract practice. Didn't an HMO set itself up in such a way as to skew the participating physician's loyalty from the medical needs of the patient toward the financial, corporate interests of the HMO? Wasn't that basically the sort of thing that the lumber and mining companies did back in 1905? Nevertheless, the House of Delegates did not adopt a policy of objection; the AMA fell back instead on the pluralistic policy it adopted in 1959—that a physician should be free to practice under any system of care he or she preferred and that patients should have free access to whatever system of health care delivery suited them. However, the house did object to HMOs if they were to be "the exclusive or major means of providing health care delivery."

Introduced first in March 1970 by HEW Undersecretary for Health John Veneman as an alternative for Medicare Parts A and B,

federally supported HMOs got their start without any formal legislation being passed; existing loan, grant, and research funds financed the first programs. By early 1972, 110 planning and development grants had been made, and President Nixon in his health
message proclaimed that HMOs "ought to be everywhere available
so that families will have a choice." HEW Secretary Elliot L. Rich-
ardson was shooting for 1,210 HMOs by 1980, enough to be available to 90 percent of the United States population. His cost estimates: $1.1 billion, plus another $2.8 billion in loans. Never one
to be upstaged in matters of health, Senator Edward M. Kennedy
plumped for a five-year HMO program to cost $8 billion. Congress,
raising sharp questions about the authority of federal agencies to
proceed, was getting ready to develop legislation.

When its turn came to testify at the hearings, the AMA urged
caution. "There is much to be cautious about," AMA Vice Chairman
John R. Kernodle, M.D., told the Subcommittee on Public Health and
Environment of the House Interstate and Foreign Commerce Committee, April 13, 1972. Kernodle cited the failures of many HMO-
like plans in the past for lack of consumer support. Not everyone
liked HMO medicine. "Conceivably the HMO could solve some of
our problems. But that is not yet proven...we should first gain
experience with test models and see if they fly before we order a
whole fleet." Believing that the government should not favor one
form of medical care delivery over another, the AMA urged Congress to restrict federal financing to pilot programs.

In 1973, when President Nixon signed the Health Maintenance
Act, it called for spending $375 million over the next five years, far
less than the figure Senator Kennedy had in mind, less than early
adherents in the Nixon administration sought. Paul G. Rogers, the
Democratic chairman of the health subcommittee of the House
Interstate and Foreign Commerce Committee and an important
figure in health legislation in the 1970s, echoed the AMA's Kernodle.
"We want to see if [the HMO concept] works before making a
wholesale federal commitment to the idea," he said. As passed, the
bill also contained provisions pre-empting the laws designed to prohibit the corporate practice of medicine that existed in twenty-two
states. This was regarded as a setback for the AMA, even though the
AMA had long since changed its policy and the contract practice
laws had already been invalidated by the courts or otherwise rendered ineffective. The bill also required employers of twenty-five or
more people who provided employee health insurance benefits to

offer HMOs as an additional health insurance option if a federally qualified HMO were available. The new, federally underwritten HMOs were free to promote themselves and advertise their services, a use of tax dollars to which many physicians strongly objected.

Backed by the federal grants and backed even more strongly by the private sector, predominantly Blue Cross-Blue Shield and the commercial health insurance companies, HMOs slowly established themselves. A number of them—12 percent of the federally backed plans—failed. A number of others required federal bail-outs. But enough succeeded that the AMA could pursue a question implicit in its 1972 congressional testimony: How well did the HMO "test models" fly?

In October 1975 the AMA established a National Commission on the Cost of Medical Care. It was a group of twenty-seven people drawn from a variety of backgrounds—industry, labor, insurance, hospital services, HMOs, government, medicine—who met frequently over the better part of two years seeking answers to the problem of growing costs. One of its conclusions was that HMOs had a potential for strengthening cost consciousness among patients, physicians, and hospitals.

When the cost commission's recommendations reached the House of Delegates at its June 1978 meeting, the house agreed, at the same time recommending that a "neutral" public policy be pursued and that fair market competition should prevail among the varying systems by which health care is delivered—HMOs, fee-for-service, and others. The house also asked the board to initiate "an objective assessment of HMO...and other group arrangements with respect to their impact on access, quality and cost of health care."

That turned out to be a large order. It led first to an exhaustive study by the Council on Medical Service, which extended over almost two years and finally resulted in a 183-page report.[20] Together, the council members and the AMA staff developed a study in two parts, the first a review of fifteen HMOs based on information from detailed questionnaires and site visits, the second a comprehensive review of the literature published over the last twenty years. As the work progressed, there were ten meetings of the council and the staff working with it. Many of the sessions were tense, the council members aware that they had been handed a hot political potato, the staff intent on gathering objective data. One thing that bothered the council was the *soi disant* character of so much of the information, the main source for data on HMOs being the HMOs themselves. Though it continued to take a skeptical view of the data submitted to it, the council wrote a report contradicting many of its initial preconceptions.

When it was submitted to the house in July 1980, the report confirmed many physicians' opinions that health maintenance organizations did not "maintain" patient health appreciably better than fee-for-service systems. Actually, the talk about "wellness" care had died down considerably. In the view of at least one independent HMO authority, that was all political rhetoric anyway, invented to rally support for a federal program to widen the distribution of what were, basically, prepaid medical groups.[21]

These had been in business for a long time, controversial in the eyes of some physicians as contract medicine, but of satisfactory service to some populations, and, since the famous 1932 cost committee report, thought to provide quality medicine at costs lower than conventional fee-for-service medicine. In summarizing its long report for the house, the Council on Medical Service reaffirmed the AMA's belief in fair market competition, restated its objections to favoring one form of health care delivery over another, and recommended that "the HMO approach to health care delivery be recognized as one which may result in care for enrollees at a lower total cost than for comparable groups in other health care delivery systems..."[22] The HMOs, the council believed, achieved savings primarily through lower hospital admission rates.

While generally supportive of the council's report, the house extracted the recommendation on costs and referred it to the board for further examination. The house was afraid that the statement might be interpreted as a conclusive AMA judgment on the absolute cost-effectiveness of HMOs. The Council on Medical Service findings stopped short of that, and the house did not want to go quite as far as the council.

Researchers who attempt cost comparisons of HMOs with insured fee-for-service medicine find one major difficulty in doing so. There is inherent logic in the HMO rationale that the economic incentives work against costs. The preponderance of the evidence and the majority of opinion point sharply toward HMO cost-effectiveness. This is what the Council on Medical Service found.

But a great deal of the evidence offers only apple and orange comparisons. The populations enrolled in HMOs tend to be employed populations that include few retirees and few welfare recipients. For that reason alone HMO cost figures could be superior. Getting precisely comparable populations for study is not easy. In addition, HMOs show varying cost performance in the same way that different parts of the United States show different utilization rates. For example, the length of an average stay in a non-government, non-profit hospital in New England in 1980 was 8.1 days; it was 6.4 days in the Pacific region; 8.7 days in Minnesota; and 6.8 days in Texas.

The problem may be further complicated by attitudinal differences. HMOs emphasize the austerities of medical care, stressing ambulatory rather than hospital treatment wherever possible. Does that sort of policy attract the Spartans among us? The Council on Medical Service suspected it might. One of the council's reports states, "There is...some evidence which suggests that people who choose HMO membership are less prone to seek medical care. Similarly, the possibility has been suggested that the physician joins an HMO if his style of practice complements that of the health maintenance organization."[23] In its final report relating to the 1980 study, the Council on Medical Service remained "convinced that...HMOs may be able to provide care at lower total costs." But it had to conclude with a warning, "It should be recognized that varying factors in different health care delivery systems do not permit an absolute direct cost comparison between HMOs and traditional practice settings."[24]

As Congress started to phase out the federal HMO grant program in the early 1980s, it turned the future of the HMOs over to the judgment of the medical marketplace. Prepaid medical groups—a classification that includes the 106 HMOs started with federal funds during the 1970-80 decade—altered the pattern of health care only to a modest extent. They grew from 26 plans to 236; the number of people enrolled climbed from 2.9 million (about 1.4 percent of the population) to 9.1 million (about 4 percent of the population).[25] One must remember, however, that of the total, more than half are registered in the five largest plans, all started before 1970, with more than a third of total enrollees served by just one HMO, Kaiser-Permanente. Though far from universally popular, HMOs are clearly attractive to many people and to many physicians as a way to practice. And they have a role to play in the economics of medical care, the competition they offer probably exerting downward pressures on the price of traditional systems of care.

With passage of the National Planning and Resources Development Act in the last days of 1974, Congress tried to get a grip on rising medical costs by federalizing the planning process of the nation's health care system. Heretofore, this was predominantly a local responsibility, performed on a volunteer basis and often accomplished with commendable cooperation between local government agencies and the local medical organizations. Starting in 1964, twenty-three states had enacted certificate-of-need legislation aimed at controlling the duplication or over-expansion of facilities and services. A degree of federal intervention was present in the local planning process through Hill-Burton, the Regional Medical Programs, and the Comprehensive Health Planning Act of 1966. Largely ineffective, the state planning agencies set up under the planning act took on new power in 1972 when Medicare/Medicaid started paying less than full reimbursement to hospitals that expanded facilities without approval. Compared with what was to come, however, this extension of federal power was minimal.

The planning act of 1974 created a broad new authority for the Secretary of HEW, placing him atop a complex, multi-layered hierarchy—a national advisory council, state planning agencies, state coordinating councils, and, at the base of the extensive pyramid, 204 local planning groups, to be established by the secretary after consultation with the appropriate governors.

In defining the composition of these local Health Systems Agencies, their jurisdictions generally aimed at population clusters of 500,000 to 3 million people, Congress added an unusual—and, as it turned out, fatal—gimmick to an otherwise undistinguished piece of regulatory legislation. Its eye on a trendy new desideratum in politics, "participation," Congress specified that the local planning groups were to consist of a majority of "consumer" members. There would be a minimum of one third providers (who could be doctors, hospital administrators, pharmacists, paramedics, etc.) and a maximum of one third public officials.

The composition of the agencies thus provided for a small number of those expected to bring some expertise to the task (the providers) and for a large number of people with unspecified, undefined, or non-existent qualifications (consumers and "officials"). That generalization may be unfair in cases where knowledgeable consumer members made solid contributions. But overall, a lack of people in the Health Systems Agencies who were trained, qualified, and experienced in health care planning assured the failure of the program.

The 204 local agencies had the job of establishing health goals for the community, developing plans for future needs, and, through the administration of certificate-of-need laws now required of all states by the new planning act, passing judgment on plans to expand or construct facilities or to broaden services. Their work was not helped in 1978 when guidelines from Washington were issued specifying the number of permissible hospital beds per 1,000 population per health service area. This was interpreted to require the closing of some hospitals and the sealing off of wings or floors of others. It was regarded as a stupefying act of bureaucratic effrontery, and the outcry put the health officials in Washington to flight. The guidelines were withdrawn.

As originally contemplated, the 1974 planning act had an even broader scope than the final version of the bill. What especially alarmed the AMA in the early concept of the bill was a proposed public utility approach to the regulation of the health care system. In March 1974 when Russell B. Roth, M.D., the president of the AMA, testified before Senator Kennedy's Subcommittee on Health of the Senate Labor and Public Welfare Committee, he stressed the "radical thrust" of the legislation as then written. One idea it originally expressed was that each state should create a health commission, designated by the HEW secretary, with authority to review and set health care rates. The commissions would, for example, set hospital and nursing home rates just as various public service commissions set rates for electricity and telephone service. Given that authority, said Roth, and "accompanied by their licensing and certification authority, the health commissions would, in effect, become public utility commissions. Even more ominous," he continued, "is the heavy hand of the Secretary of HEW in the regulatory process." The legislation as proposed would make him a health care "czar." Would there be others, Roth asked, to exercise public-utility type controls over equally essential sectors of the economy such as food, clothing and shelter?[26] In Washington at the time, it should be noted, there were those who looked upon the powers in the planning bill as a necessary prelude to the sort of national health insurance plan that Kennedy was then pushing for.

In the end, the public utility aspects of the bill were considerably toned down. Surviving, however, was authority in the final version for grants to demonstrate the effectiveness of rate regulation to not more than six states that already had rate regulations (for hospitals, mainly) or were intending to put them into effect in the near future. The AMA objected to that as well as several other features in the bill: the lopsided emphasis on consumer, or non-expert, representation on the Health Systems Agencies; the requirement of certificate-of-need laws in all states, the expansion of the HEW secretary's powers and, in fact, the whole idea of transferring so much authority from the local to the federal level.

"Without reiterating the many provisions in the legislation which authorize federal intervention into matters of health traditionally vested in local and state jurisdictions," Roth told the Kennedy committee, "I want to emphasize that there is no justification for this usurpation by the federal government of these state functions."

At the end of the year, within a week after President Ford signed the law (despite an AMA plea that he veto it) the AMA announced it intended to challenge its constitutionality. The AMA had opposed the bill in the legislative process, successfully stripping it of several features odious to medicine. But it was still a bill the AMA opposed.

A question remained as to the federal government's right to determine for states what aspects of the health care field should be regulated. The situation in North Carolina looked particularly promising for the constitutional challenge. There the state's supreme court had previously found that the state's certificate-of-need law violated the state constitution. Could the federal government, under such circumstances, insist on new certificate-of need legislation? Evidently it could. A federal district court and the United States Supreme Court found against the AMA and the State of North Carolina, the principal plaintiffs.[27]

By the time the Reagan administration announced its determination to reverse recent history by transferring many federal powers and programs back to the jurisdiction of the states, the planning program could offer little reason for its continued existence. Billed in *Medical Economics* as "the most damning report to date," a report by the General Accounting Office leveled devastating charges against the program. The Health Systems Agencies set goals that were sometimes too vague, the report said, sometimes too ambitious, sometimes too numerous. The American Health Planning Association, representing the local agencies, made invalid claims about the amount of money the program was saving.

Among the examples cited in the report was one involving an application for a nursing home. The first time the proposal came up before a local planning agency, plans for a $1.4 million building were rejected. A few months later, modified plans for a $1.42 million structure were turned down. But finally, on the third application, the agency gave the green light to plans for the $1.42 million nursing home. All very well. But the planning association added the sums of money involved in the two turndowns, a total of $2.82 million, and counted that in its tabulation of the money the Health Systems Agency was trimming from the nation's health care budget![28]

Inevitably, the horse-trading and log-rolling that characterize municipal government (and all government) came to dominate many of the local planning agencies. In a review of the local Health Systems Agency, Karen Garloch of the *Cincinnati Enquirer* reported:

> Its 30-member board hardly ever says no to requests for new hospital beds or new equipment. Moreover, it frequently rejects the labored recommendations of its own paid staff and its own adopted health systems plan when faced with a particularly political or emotional issue...A hospital administrator commented, "We are as insidious in our politics as anybody else." Hospital administrators lobby consumer members by taking them on tours and pointing out the needs of their facilities. Administrators then vote for each other's projects or quietly abstain. It's all accepted practice.[29]

Few mourned when Congress authorized a phase-out of funding for the planning program in 1981. Virtually everyone agreed that planning through a federal structure had failed. For two years the program limped along at a greatly reduced level of activity. In August 1983 it appeared that the Reagan administration had backed away from calling for immediate repeal, envisioning instead a two-year phase-out of the program. The responsibility for planning shifted back to where it had traditionally been, and the AMA, developing a set of voluntary health planning principles, strongly urged the involvement of its members and local societies in community planning efforts.

Independent of congressional and administration efforts to bring medical costs down, the Federal Trade Commission issued a complaint against the AMA in December 1975, charging it with anti-competitive practices. Because the AMA was restricting trade, the FTC alleged, physician fees were higher than they otherwise would be. Specifically, the complaint sought to end the AMA's supposed ban on all physician advertising and its alleged intervention in the contractual arrangements between a physician and a hospital, medical group, or HMO. Were a more free-wheeling medical marketplace to prevail, the complaint implied, competition would reduce physician fees and group practice prices.

The AMA asked for the dismissal of the complaint. Because the Federal Trade Commission had conducted no investigation beforehand, the AMA suspected that it was unaware of the association's current position on advertising and HMOs; some of the commission's assumptions might be based on outdated practices and policies. When dismissal was denied, the AMA challenged the allegations through the commission's quasi-legal machinery.

These proceedings hardly offer the impartiality of regular law courts. In fact, there is an *Alice in Wonderland* quality about them: the prosecutor, the administrative law judge (who also acts as the jury), and the appeals panel are all employees or officials of the Federal Trade Commission. What emerged first from the commission's action was the opinion of the administrative law judge that organized medicine should play no role *at all* for a period of two years in setting guidelines for ethical promotional practices. Advertising by physicians, the opinion said, should be regulated exclusively by the federal government. Medicine could speak on the subject only if it first obtained the permission and approval of the commission.

The AMA's outside legal counsel, Newton N. Minow, who had served as President Kennedy's Chairman of the Federal Communications Commission, was particularly affronted by that opinion. As a lawyer he objected to some of the legal conclusions. To establish the commission's jurisdiction in the case—the Federal Trade Commission has clear authority only over persons, partnerships, and for-profit corporations—the administrative law judge found the AMA to be in existence for the profit of its members because it offered them a retirement plan and opposed certain forms of national health insurance. Minow protested too, in a speech he gave to the House of Delegates in December 1978, that the AMA was being judged on statements made in the 1930s, 1940s, 1950s, and 1960s, "in a vastly different legal and social climate." He was also offended at what he saw as an assault on the professions, an erosion of their historic authority, role, and responsibilities.[30]

Appealing the administrative law judge's decision to the commissioners of the Federal Trade Commission, the AMA gained some satisfaction. They overruled the judge by saying, yes, the AMA did have a proper role to play in formulating and enforcing ethical guidelines with respect to false or deceptive advertising and to the personal solicitation of patients. But the AMA could not, ruled the commissioners, restrict truthful, informational advertising. Nor

could it interfere with the terms of a physician's contractual arrangement with any entity.

Contesting the trade commission's jurisdiction in the case—its
authority to regulate the professions and their non-profit associations—the AMA took its suit to the courts. But a 2-1 ruling by the
federal Court of Appeals, Second Circuit, went against the AMA,
and a final appeal to the Supreme Court ended in a 4-4 split decision, effectively upholding the findings of the appeals court.

While the appeal process was going on, the AMA joined others in
seeking a legislative remedy. Proposals to clarify the trade commission's jurisdiction were introduced in Congress; the original Federal
Trade Commission Act, while not mentioning regulatory authority
over non-profit or state-regulated bodies, still left openings by
which the commission could intervene in the affairs of the professions and non-profit associations. The AMA also encouraged proposals that would reform the procedures used by the commission in
hearing objections to a complaint. In testimony on behalf of the
bills, the AMA made it clear that it was not seeking the end of
all regulation. Should the trade commission's authority be limited,
medicine would still be subject to the antitrust laws as well as the
regulatory functions of the various states.

Though phrased in legalese and fraught with warnings and requirements of notification, the commission's final order, issued in
May 1982, accomplished little other than the beating of a long-dead
horse. The practices it attacked and forbade—medicine's alleged
attempt to interfere with a physician's participation in prepaid
group plans—were practices abandoned thirty or forty years earlier. The positions it called for with respect to advertising were
positions already adopted by the AMA.

Here, for example, is what the *Opinions and Reports of the Judicial Council* had to say as far back as 1962: "The Principles [of
Medical Ethics] do not proscribe advertising...The public is entitled
to know the names of physicians, the location of their offices, their
office hours, and other useful information that will enable people
to make a more informed choice of physician. The physician may
furnish this information through the accepted local media for advertising or communications..."[31]

The Federal Trade Commission's final order differed very little
from that. In fact, after studying it carefully, the AMA announced
that it would not have to change anything to be in compliance.

Looked at in retrospect, the commission launched a costly, seven-year, legal campaign merely to establish the *status quo ante bellum*.

And since what the commission ordered had been in effect all along, its intervention had no economic impact on the prices in the medical marketplace.

At the time the Federal Trade Commission was pursuing its complaint alleging anti-competitive practices, it tried to weaken and embarrass the AMA in other ways. In 1977 the commission appeared before the federal Office of Education seeking to end the AMA's role in the accreditation of medical schools. This function had been performed since 1942 by the Liaison Committee on Medical Education, a group composed principally of members from the AMA and the Association of American Medical Colleges. The trade commission argued that the liaison committee could not be counted upon for impartial decisions because of the presence of the AMA members. In taking its position, the commission struck at the traditional responsibility a profession has for the educational standards of its future members. If not through its largest professional association, how should the medical profession have a say in the quality of education being offered in medical schools? Who besides a physician can be counted upon to know whether such a complex subject as medicine is being competently taught? After a hearing and review, the Liaison Committee on Medical Education, with AMA members, was provisionally recertified as the officially recognized accrediting agency.

Undeterred, the commission then opened an investigation into the alleged efforts of the AMA to restrict the number of medical school graduates. This, of course, related to the old accusation that, through the AMA, doctors kept the number of physicians down in order to keep the fees up. Given the thrust of the commission's efforts at the time, evidenced by its complaint of anti-competitive practices against the AMA, it may be assumed that if such evidence existed the FTC would have pounced upon it with relish. However, no formal complaint or report was issued, and the commission's staff official in charge of health matters was quoted in the press as saying that the AMA may not have restricted entry into medical schools after all.[32]

As the government floundered in the tide of rising costs, what sort of lifeline did the private sector of medicine have to throw out? It had no quick and easy rescue to offer, but it was deeply concerned. In 1975, with medical care—and just about everything else—40 percent more expensive than it had been five years earlier, the AMA began a series of actions that responded in a variety of ways to the inflationary alarm.

The first step, and a major one, was the formation of a National Commission on the Cost of Medical Care, charged with developing during the next two years an overview of health care costs and ideas for stabilizing them. This was something the AMA had tried before, in 1960-64, an attempt that achieved little success because the base of representation was narrow.

This time, too, the medical establishment was generously represented. The twenty-seven-member commission included: the three most recent AMA presidents; the presidents of the American Hospital Association, Blue Cross, Blue Shield, the Health Insurance Association of America; a trustee from the American Dental Association, and two additional AMA appointees. But they were in the minority. The others on the commission represented a diversity of interests and disciplines: the director of employee benefits of General Motors; the chairman of the railway unions' health and welfare committee; two recognized economists, one the chief staff economist at the Rand Corporation; two leaders in the development of HMOs; a former vice chairman of the Reuther-Kennedy Committee of One Hundred for National Health Insurance; two legislators, one a federal congressman; and representatives from three of the most prestigious medical clinics in the country. An official from HEW attended and participated in the discussions but did not vote because HEW had already established its cost containment policies. It was as diverse and as able a group as anyone might have assembled for the task.

Moreover, it was independent. Though sponsored by the AMA and chaired by outgoing AMA President Max H. Parrott, M.D., and though staffed by AMA people, with Executive Vice President James H. Sammons, M.D., a vigorous but non-voting participant, the commission nonetheless had a charter to conduct its own analysis and draw its own conclusions. If, later, the AMA Board of Trustees or House of Delegates wanted to adopt and take action on its recommendations, well and good. If the AMA preferred to reject them *in toto*, the commission recommendations would nevertheless stand as a matter of record.

At the time the commission began work, the concern over medical care costs focused less on what was happening to federal expenditures—the major issue of the early 1980s—and more on the overall, growing percentage of the Gross National Product being spent on health care. People looked at the current rate, 8.4 percent in 1975, and asked if that was too much. Was it really necessary to spend that large a share of income just to stay healthy?

The commonly perceived villain was the health care system itself. Because so many patients were so protected by insurance, it was argued, there were few incentives for them to hold down costs. Hospitals demanded the biggest, the best, and the latest in buildings and equipment. Doctors developed ever more costly procedures. To many, the health care system was operating without response to other societal needs.

When the commission got down to business, its members agreed that the market forces of the health care system were working in such a way as to produce some results that were, from a societal standpoint, undesirable. A discussion at the initial meeting in March 1976 identified the factors that determined the cost of care. The members then grouped them into four categories: technology, supply, demand, and the marketplace. Organizing themselves along those lines, the commissioners divided into four task forces. As the work progressed, the task forces heard presentations at their meetings from outside experts, from selected commissioners, or from some of the staff members, drawn from the AMA Center for Health Services Research and Development. After the presentations there were free-wheeling discussions. At first the talk concentrated on informational or analytical topics; then it moved to the discussion of policy options.

As the commission's time limit approached, the task forces presented their conclusions and recommendations to the whole commission. The task force on technology reflected opinions then current that new technologies, such as CAT scanners, renal dialysis, open heart surgery, and radiotherapy, constituted a major source of health care cost inflation. Its recommendations took a more regulatory approach than those of the other task forces, stressing such measures as certificate-of-need laws, criteria by which state and local planning bodies could regulate the location of expensive facilities and equipment, review of the utilization of high-cost services, and cost evaluation of new technology.

The task force on supply, noting physician shortage areas and a trend toward over-specialization, nevertheless concluded that a further increase in the number of doctors would probably increase costs rather than generate a trickle-over effect that would cause substantially more physicians to locate in rural or inner city areas. It recommended stronger emphasis on family practice, more active recruitment of students from underserved areas, and fewer restrictions on allied health personnel. It did not think there should be new efforts to increase the number of medical school graduates until such time as necessity for change might be clearly evident.

The task force on demand, pointing out that health insurance covers much of the personal cost for care (68 percent), urged changes that would cause people to seek only needed care, and that in the least costly locations (i.e., non-hospital settings) whenever possible.

The task force on the marketplace identified four ways in which the health care system diverges from the textbook version of a classic economic market: (1) insurance takes a large cost burden off the consumer; (2) employees have little choice among employer-financed health insurance programs; (3) employers and employees both receive favorable tax treatment on health insurance—the employer gets a deduction for the cost of the premiums and the employee pays no income tax on the premiums paid on his behalf; and (4) the consumer is largely ignorant as to the cost, necessity, and efficacy of medical services. The remedy recommended by the task force: an emphasis on price consciousness.

After the entire commission had absorbed the findings of the task forces, it submitted a summary report to the AMA board, which in turn sent it to the house with its responses to the commission's forty-eight recommendations. A few of these involved regulatory action: certificate-of-need, for example. But the thrust of the report was contained in a statement that the house, upon the recommendation of the board, adopted: "The commission believes that the greatest hope for cost containment in the provision of health care lies in strengthening price consciousness in the health care marketplace."[33]

Lynn E. Jensen, Ph.D., director of the AMA Center for Health Resources and Development, summarized the report by saying that it "proceeds on the assumption that market forces do operate in medical care, that physicians and patients both respond to economic incentives. If you structure reimbursement appropriately, you can get solutions that meet your objectives."³⁴ In Jensen's opinion, the philosophical thread of the cost commission's report is contained in its first eight recommendations. These call for the strengthening of consumer and provider cost consciousness. Among many things encouraged or given incentives were: low-cost, tightly-run health insurance programs; consumer cost sharing of insured medical services; HMOs and fair market competition among rival health care delivery systems; informational directories, with price information, enabling consumers to select physicians and hospitals on a cost basis; and experiments with new methods of financing care through the use of hospital or physician groups that demonstrate an ability to deliver quality care at below-average cost. In coming down on the side of strengthening dollar consciousness, the commission did not reject altogether the idea of public utility regulation. The report said, "Some mechanisms must be put in place to assure that no group of consumers is denied quality care due to inability to pay." Regulation, it said, could avoid the needlesss duplication of facilities and expensive equipment.

Yet the overall thrust of the report was market-minded. The commission favored a health care system shaped, insofar as possible, by consumer decisions. If regulations were kept at a minimum, the national health care system, including its spending level, would be determined by the aggregate of individual consumer decisions. This is what the commission thought desirable, rather than a health care system whose scope might be decreed by fiat at, say, 9.8 percent of Gross National Product. But at the same time, if the system were to remain basically free of regulation, cost would have to be contained.

The best way to do this, the commission reasoned, was to infuse cost-reducing incentives into the system at various levels and in various ways. The first recommendation of the commission exemplified this approach. It suggested that employees be given a choice among employer-sponsored health insurance plans priced at varying levels. Though differently structured, the plans would have to meet approved minimums. To encourage as many employees as possible to choose the low-cost, low-benefit plans, an incentive would be offered: employees who selected the cheaper plans would be allowed to pocket the difference. To encourage employers to offer such a range of plans, a change in the corporate tax structure was recommended. Contributions to an employee health plan were to be tax deductible only up to a certain point—enough to finance a minimal program. Thus, there would be no tax subsidy for high-benefit, high-cost health insurance, only for what might be called economy programs.

Except for the development of directories—a suggestion that was referred to the board because of possible price-fixing implications—the House of Delegates reacted in a generally positive way to the recommendations for strengthening price consciousness.[35]

But changes in health insurance programs, a key in the establishment of price consciousness, would have to come from many sources. The benefit structures of health insurance policies are not designed by the AMA; they are determined to a great extent by employers and the unions that represent their employees in wage and benefit contract negotiations. Once management-union agreement is reached, the insurance carriers draw up the health insurance plans to embody principles the negotiators have worked out. Though the AMA and the commission might argue and persuade, action would have to wait upon a willingness to act on the part of a number of others—Congress, employers, unions, insurance companies, and so on.

That would be tough. Victor M. Zink, director of Employee Benefits and Services at General Motors, told his fellow commissioners in 1976 that his company would like to increase the employee's concern about the cost of the General Motors medical plan, but, he added, "We want peace with the unions."[36] Walter J. McNerney, president of the Blue Cross Association at the time and also a commissioner, stressed a different point at an earlier session of the entire commission. Wider cost sharing was emphasized as a way to make a beneficiary of a health insurance plan more aware that the ride was not entirely free. But, warned McNerney, "If deductibles and co-insurance are large enough to effectively impact utilization, they also tend to result in unjustified under-utilization and lack of salability in the marketplace." In other words, there is a danger. If cost sharing is so high as to discourage unnecessary use of the health care system, it may also be so high as to keep people who genuinely need medical care from seeking it.[37]

There is a further complexity to health insurance: the apparent desire by the insureds to benefit from their policies periodically. In this respect, health insurance differs from life insurance or fire insurance on a dwelling, both of which protect against a catastrophic event. Health insurance structured to protect someone against rare, highly expensive disaster has never been easy to sell; health insurance covering the more common, moderately expensive medical episodes has proved to be more marketable. Many people have therefore concluded that Americans have insured the wrong (i.e., low) end of medical expenses.

While the deliberations of the commission continued, so did the rise in costs, especially hospital costs. In 1977, the Carter administration proposed putting a cap on hospital prices. Congress showed scant enthusiasm for the legislation, recalling the futility of the wage and price controls imposed by President Nixon in 1971.

Just as Congress was about to adjourn for the year in late 1977, having failed to take action, Chairman of the House Ways and Means Committee Dan Rostenkowski, (D.-Illinois), suggested to the American Hospital Association, the Federation of American Hospitals (representing the for-profit hospitals), and the AMA that they "develop a meaningful program of cost containment."[38] Having lobbied hard against controls on hospital prices, the private organizations responded promptly and energetically with a program—named the Voluntary Effort—that gave initial promise of effectiveness, at least enough to remove the pressure on Congress to enact the controls that few really wanted. By 1982, however, it was becoming clear that the Voluntary Effort was failing to accomplish its objectives.

At that point, the hopes for a private solution to the problems of rising medical care costs seemed to rest with local, voluntary initiatives. In many areas, groups of businessmen, doctors, insurance executives, hospital administrators, union leaders, and consumers had sprung to life, united in their determination to solve some of the health care cost problems in their own community or section of the country.

In late 1981 the AMA, which had been supporting such coalitions since 1978, joined the American Hospital Association, Blue Cross-Blue Shield, the Business Roundtable, the Health Insurance Association of America and the AFL-CIO in a statement of endorsement. That made it easier for the county and state organizations to participate—the local medical societies, regional hospital groups, area-wide insurance plans. Having the AFL-CIO endorsement sent a similar signal to various union locals and district councils.

The major initiative, however, came from the business sector. Squeezed from several directions, employers were taking a careful look at both the scope and price of health benefits purchased for their employees. They were struck especially with the way surgical rates, physician/population ratios, and hospitalization rates could vary so much on a regional basis without any apparent difference in morbidity and mortality figures. Costs surely could come down without much difference in outcomes, they thought.

In 1976, just as the work of the commission was getting underway, AMA President Max H. Parrott, M.D., wrote an article for the policy forum section of the *National Journal*, a magazine based in Washington and concentrating on the discussion of major policy issues. At the end of his discussion of medical costs, Parrott outlined three broad options:

> The United States can have lower cost medical care and, at the same time, universal access to it, if it is willing to limit the quality of the care given.
>
> The United States can have lower cost medical care and the present high quality of care if it is willing to limit access by shifting more of the financial burden back on the individual.
>
> Or, the United States can provide universal access and the best medical care there is, if it is willing to accept the high cost.[39]

In the 1960s, when just about everyone, including the AMA, stressed access to health care as a right—meaning that all Americans should have unrestricted access to mainstream medicine regardless of ability to pay—the third option probably reflected public opinion accurately. Public opinion seemed to stay that way into the 1970s. But in the 1980s, as federal deficits caused increasing concern, a shift seemed to develop toward option two.

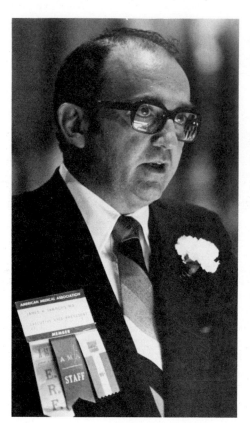

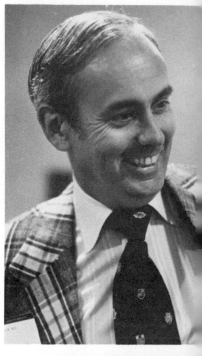

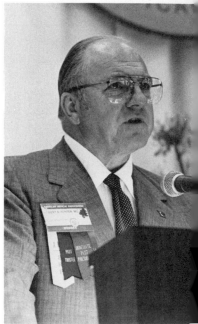

EMBATTLED LEADERS of the mid-1970s faced continuing controversy. The new executive vice president, James H. Sammons (above) had to deal with the AMA's worst financial crisis; Joseph T. Painter (above, right) headed a special committee to investigate it. Raymond T. Holden (top left, opposite page) was secretary-treasurer at the time, later board chairman. Tom E. Nesbitt (top right, opposite) presided over the stormiest session of the house that anyone could remember. In a less tense moment, Ernest B. Howard (wearing lei, lower right) shares a laugh with Presidents Todd and Palmer. Robert B. Hunter (lower right, this page) handled the sensitive PSRO issue and, like Nesbitt, went on to become President.

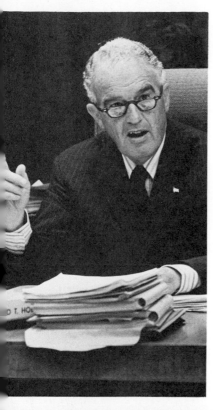

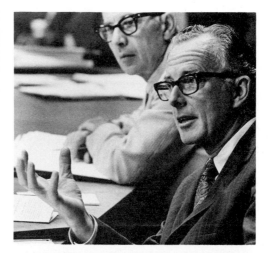

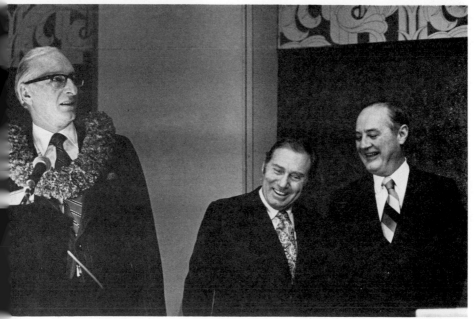

Chapter Nineteen

A Gathering of Troubles

With the accession of the pragmatists in the late 1960s, the AMA became an organization under new management. A better led, more involved board was in place now, its more assertive leadership characterized by a knowledgeable grasp of the political realities, something the AMA had needed for a long time. But the new board faced growing troubles, traceable primarily to sporadic tensions between itself and the house. While the board strained to proceed with new socioeconomic initiatives, the house clung to narrower, backhome loyalties, unsure that it wanted to move as far or as fast as the board. And although there was agreement on overall priorities, the board seemed to have only the intermittent backing of a majority in the house.

A stubborn disagreement over financing arose, creating problems that were neglected for so long that in the end they could not be solved by fiscal measures alone. When that happened, attention swung to questions of fundamental policy. What are the basic objectives of the AMA? What sort of organization should it be? How should it be structured? How should future planning be conducted? It was familiar ground; the questions were of the same soul-searching, what-did-we-do-wrong type that were angrily asked in the aftermath of Medicare.

But they arose in the 1970s with a new urgency, for finances fell to such a low that the AMA was forced to make decisions that it had been able to avoid previously. As the 1970s began, the AMA entered a period of mounting troubles; in the middle of the decade, it underwent the agony of finding solutions; in the end, going into the 1980s, it emerged successful, a leaner but more effective organization.

It did not require the gift of prophecy to predict the beginnings of a financial crunch in 1968 and 1969. The principal and immediate cause was an abrupt fall in the advertising income of the AMA publications, especially that of its flagship journal, *JAMA*. In 1967 AMA ad revenues reached $13.6 million, generating 43 percent of the association's total revenues. But they plummeted by $1.7 million in the following year and by an additional $1 million in the year after that.[1] One reason was a change in the medical journal advertising market, supported almost entirely by the pharmaceutical industry. Partly as the result of the thalidomide tragedy in Europe, Congress passed the Kefauver-Harris Act in 1963, enabling the U.S. Food and Drug Administration to tighten its regulations, making it more difficult to bring new pharmaceutical products to market quickly.

With less to advertise, overall expenditures for drug advertising leveled off. At the same time, new medical publications gained strength, sharpening the competition for the existing dollars. From a high of 17 percent in 1960, the share of the pharmaceutical advertising market held by AMA publications fell to 14.6 percent in 1967 and headed even lower, eventually shrinking to 7 percent in 1974.[2] Inflation also made inroads, sending the cost of paper, printing, and postage soaring. A comfortable $3.3 million excess of revenues over expenses in 1967 rapidly evaporated, reducing the AMA's 1969 financial position to something just above the break-even point.

Meanwhile, the AMA's other major source of revenue, membership dues, which produced $11.5 million (37 percent of total revenues) in 1967, was not taking up the slack. Possibly because it had gone for so many years (1912-49) without charging regular membership dues, the AMA had left the recruitment and retention of members to the state and county medical societies. In the process of collecting their own annual dues, some 850 local medical organizations billed for the AMA dues, and as the funds reached the state (or major county) medical societies, the AMA funds often would be temporarily invested for the benefit of the local society before being forwarded to the AMA.

To be sure, thirteen states, among them big ones like New York, California, and Illinois, had unified membership, which required AMA membership as a condition of county-state society membership. However, in the others a physician could belong to the local societies without joining the AMA. In some areas only 40 percent of the state-county society members joined the AMA; in others, 90 percent voluntarily became AMA members. It was not a situation over which the AMA exerted control. The AMA, in fact, had no staff membership department until 1972, and all the AMA did before then to promote membership was to send out a curt delinquency notice each spring to physicians failing to renew from one year to the next.

Having raised dues from $45 to $70 for 1967, after much grumbling in the House of Delegates, the AMA leadership approached the need for a further increase gingerly. A 1968 report to the house from the Board of Trustees on the financial status of the organization mentioned the impact of inflation on publication costs, the fiscal uncertainties to come, and new regulations from the Internal Revenue Service aimed at taxing the unrelated business income of tax-exempt organizations. The new tax could, of course, cut into the net advertising revenues of publications. Thus the board alerted the house to the approaching need for a dues increase, though none was sought at that time.

Two years later, however, it came time to bite the bullet. At the June 1970 meeting the board proposed that dues be raised, effective in 1971, from $70 a year to $150. An increase of this unprecedented size was necessary, the board argued, for several reasons. For one, the AMA was running in the red right at the moment, with an anticipated deficit for the year of $2 million. What's more, the board said, inflation was going to keep right on adding $2 million in annual increments to AMA expenses. The association's liquid reserves badly needed replenishing, having fallen well below the level that the house and board had agreed in 1960 to be desirable. Then there was the threat of the unrelated business tax; no one was sure how much that might be. And finally there were the demands to support new programs. Pointing to the intensified drive by labor and Senator Kennedy for national health insurance, the board emphasized the urgent need for funds to promote the AMA's Medicredit bill and to step up public affairs-public relations activities.[3]

In a separate report, the board proposed a massive communications program to stress the accomplishments of American medicine and the contributions of physicians to the health of the American people. The membership had grown increasingly angry with inflammatory criticisms of the medical profession and American medical care. In case the delegates had forgotten the demogogic hostility of these attacks—and television's relish in covering them—a noisy, bearded crowd of placard-carriers invaded the 1970 annual meeting. Doctors were complaining, with growing heat, about the

AMA's inability to counter, if not halt, the unreasoning assaults on their profession. At times they acted like a population under siege. To help raise that siege, the board was suggesting an educational-informational program that would cost up to $10 million over the next five years.[4]

The house adopted that report, but it balked at the amount of the requested dues increase. Not only was it more than three times the size of the increase levied just four years previously; the board, claimed many delegates, had not presented the sort of financial detail needed to convince them of the necessity for a dues increase that large. At the reference committee hearing, it was noted, the board proposal for an $80 increase touched off "vigorous and pointed discussion." A resolution submitted by the Michigan delegates asking that any decision be put off for six months until a more detailed financial analysis could be made was argued down. But the reference committee did not follow the board's leadership either. Agreeing with the witnesses who argued that the board had not supplied the documentation to make a solid case for the $80, the committee recommended a dues increase of only $40. If the board found that the $40 was insufficient, the reference committee suggested, it could at a later meeting of the house present additional facts and seek another increase on top of the $40.[5]

When the house took up the issue, delegates complained about the difficulty they expected to encounter in explaining the dues increase—even the $40—back home. Also hit by inflation, many medical societies—county, state, and specialty—had recently raised dues, some of them more than once. Belonging to and supporting organized medicine was getting to be an expensive proposition. More than one delegate predicted defections. Joseph P. Donnelly, M.D., said, "We will lose anywhere from 15 percent to 40 percent of the membership of the Medical Society of New Jersey, and it will be worse in New York." Delegate George Himler, M.D., of New York, where a $75 assessment to finance a new state headquarters building was coming up, said, "We are supposed to go home and sell our membership on the dues increase? I would hate to even tell them about it." Afraid at one point that the house might decide to put off all action for a dues increase until the November-December meeting, when it would be too late to have full effect in 1971, Board of Trustees Finance Committee Chairman Burt L. Davis, M.D., stressed the importance of immediate action. He told the house, "...regardless of what the amount is...set the amount today...then we, of course, will live within that budget."[6]

It was a blunder. Determined to avoid the $80 increase, many delegates seized on what Davis said, interpreting it as a board statement saying, in effect, "Well, if you don't grant the $80, we can get along with the $40." That was not what Davis meant and not what the board had in mind.

Trying to reverse the trend of the debate, Blair Henningsgaard, M.D., the Oregon delegate close to the leaders on the board, appeared at one of the floor microphones. He was angry with Donnelly and Himler and the other delegates who were wringing their hands in fear of what the members back home might say. "I want you to know," he told the house, "that the Oregon delegation was instructed by [its state society] to support the $80 dues increase. Further, $80 doesn't come any easier up there [in Oregon] than it does back...East...We [the three Oregon delegates] accept our responsibilities to acquaint a thousand members [each] of the necessity for the dues increase." He had been present when two previous dues increases had been debated, he said; he had heard the same arguments before—that membership defections would follow and that some delegates would lose their seats in the house. "However," he said, "they are still back here, loud and strong and voting every time...I just don't scare that easily."

For those who supported the reference committee suggestion that $40 be approved currently with maybe smaller increases in successive years, he had a story. He said that the president of the Oregon Medical Association had approached him that morning. "I don't really know very much," Henningsgaard reported him as saying, "but one thing I do know is that a hog will holler a lot louder if you cut off his tail one inch at a time." Henningsgaard stated the board's case forcefully, but his motion to restore the $80 figure lost by a wide margin.[7]

It was a fateful decision, for the $40 increase was not enough to get the AMA out of the red. It only reduced the annual deficit, from a little under $3 million in 1970 to a little under $1 million in 1971. The board decided that it would be futile to go back to the house with another request for a dues increase. What happened instead, according to Max H. Parrott, M.D., was a succession of deficit budgets. In a letter to the Special Committee of the House appointed to investigate the financial debacle that occurred in 1974 he wrote,

"We were forced to use liquid reserves. Every year following [1970] we advised the house of the deficit budget, and every year it was approved by the house. The board continued to be fully aware that liquid reserves were gradually being depleted and eventually we would have to ask the house for another dues increase. However, inflation and new programs were causing the state and county associations to impose dues increases at the same time. I believe the board felt a dues increase should be postponed for a while until adjustments could be made at the local level."[8]

The signals flashed back from the county and state societies in response to the dues increase were negative. Later in 1970 Montana, Nevada, and New York rescinded their unified membership policies, causing a loss of 7,873 AMA members in New York state alone. All in all, the AMA membership declined by 11,671 physicians in 1971, equivalent to a loss of $1,284,000 in dues revenue for the year. In 1972 four more states dropped their unified membership requirement—Colorado, Kansas, Mississippi, and Nebraska. Nevertheless, the AMA was able to stanch the outflow of memberships; the total of regular dues-paying members in 1972—156,854—exceeded that of 1971 by 311.

But the trouble went deeper than the dues increase. A number of physicians, some entrenched in the house, some in the AMA councils and committees, some in positions of power in their state medical societies, distrusted the new leadership and especially its initiatives in policy on socioeconomic questions. Many still believed in purist doctrine; that is, the AMA should confine itself to traditional educational and scientific activities. Others used the purist argument to mask ambitions for their own projects and programs. Still others joined the opposition because they had been hurt, or had seen their friends hurt, in the upset that brought the pragmatists to power. For a variety of reasons, many of the delegates in the house wanted to keep the board on a short leash. Depriving the trustees of some of the money they requested was seen as one way to do that.

What might have helped smooth over the rift in the early 1970s was an AMA president with a broad outlook, determined to create among physicians a better understanding of the AMA's difficulties. But the man inaugurated at the June 1971 meeting had a different agenda. A Nevada physician, President Wesley W. Hall, M.D., was elected to the Board of Trustees in 1961. He took over as the chairman in June 1966 just at the time Burtis E. Montgomery, M.D., and Parrott joined the board. Thus it was his leadership that was overturned when the Montgomery-Parrott group gained voting control in 1967 and forced Blasingame out in 1968.

Understandably, Hall had few warm feelings for the board members sitting behind him when he rose to deliver his presidential address. Convinced that the AMA was bent on a course of self-destruction, he said, "The last Constitutional Convention of the AMA was held on May 5, 1847. It is time to hold another one."[9] Actually, many of the specific constitutional changes he suggested were already under way (the admission of students and residents, for example, working for a more unified profession, and increasing responsiveness to societal problems).

Both the board and the Council on Constitution and Bylaws repudiated Hall's suggestion, pointing out that changes in the constitution could be made, and frequently were, without recourse to a constitutional convention. Hall told the council later that he had not intended to use the phrase "constitutional convention" in a technical or restrictive sense. The house, after listening to a reference committee report that fall reviewing all the accusations Hall had made, tactfully referred them to the newly founded Council on Long Range Planning and Development.[10]

It was not Hall's demand for changes that bothered the board leadership so much as his linkage of the AMA's well-known difficulties to implied mismanagement and a poor (i.e., socioeconomic) choice of association priorities. A rallying point for physicians who felt uncomfortable and suspicious over the political orientation of the men now being elected to AMA office, Hall stumped the country, addressing meetings of the state and county medical societies, giving interviews to the press, harping on the association's shortcomings and deficiencies. His attacks grew so incendiary that one of the trustees, James H. Sammons, M.D., initiated a program of trustee visits to the state medical society meetings where Hall was speaking to quench the flames. Hall's behavior not only angered the board; it puzzled them. Trustee Robert B. Hunter, M.D., earnestly trying to find out just what was bothering Hall, attempted to pin him down several times. "All he could ever convey," according to Hunter, "was an attitude of doom. He used to say, 'If you only knew, as I do, what is going on...' Wes could never really lay his hand on what it was that we had to do something about. This was a Don Quixote struggle against the windmills."[11]

Thus the AMA had the worst of all worlds. Revenues were down because of declining ad pages and membership losses. Costs were up because of inflation. A maverick president had gone on the hustings, undermining the board and leaving both the association and the federated medical societies confused. The board, having laid out the association's financial picture for the house, did not see what more it could do. The house, sensitive to membership feelings, aware of the strains felt by the local societies, and harboring reservations about the board, thought the AMA's financial needs could wait. The board, as Parrott's 1975 letter to the house committee indicated, seemed to be resigned to that decision.[12]

To be sure, better financial management was on everyone's mind. More sophisticated methods—program budgeting, for instance— were adopted. Financial communications were improved. A finance committee of the board, reestablished in 1968 after a lapse of almost fifty years, met each year with what amounted to a finance committee of the house,[13] instituted in late 1970, to review the past year's financial picture and the coming year's budget plans.*

Major measures of fiscal restraint were undertaken in 1972, including the termination of four councils (Drugs, Occupational Health, Voluntary Health Agencies, and National Security), the four committees of those councils, and two other committees (Medicine and Religion, and Medical Aspects of Automotive Safety).[14] But 1972 was only one year in the black out of the six from 1970-75. The house still passed resolutions and authorized actions without considering the costs, and only an occasional voice was raised advocating a dues increase. Like a character in Dickens, the AMA slipped toward financial calamity, aware but heedless of what was to be read on its financial ledgers.

Just who would be the legatee of all the accumulating troubles was not known at the moment. The incumbent executive vice president, Ernest B. Howard, M.D., was nearing sixty-five and had for some time emphatically made clear his intention to retire at that age. As 1973 drew to a close, the AMA, not unreasonably, began to concern itself with the choice of successor.

*Reference Committee F functions as the finance committee of the house. Like other reference committees, it holds hearings and makes recommendations at each session of the house. But it is different in that its members serve year-long terms. They meet with the board in the fall to review the upcoming budget before it is presented to the house, and they meet again in advance of the annual meeting of the house in late spring to go over the audited records of the fiscal year recently ended.

Throughout most of Howard's tenure it had been widely assumed that the next executive vice president would be the AMA's number two staff executive, Richard S. Wilbur, M.D. A Californian, Wilbur was the grandson of Ray Lyman Wilbur, M.D., president of the AMA in 1923 and chairman of the AMA Council on Medical Education from 1929 to 1946. He was also the nephew of Dwight L. Wilbur, M.D., who had been a delegate for many years, a trustee elected in 1963 and the AMA president in 1968. In addition to longstanding links to organized medicine, the Wilbur family had impeccable Republican credentials, the elder Wilbur having served as President Hoover's Secretary of the Interior. Dwight and Richard Wilbur knew the key Californians in the Nixon administration and had connections with the then Republican Governor of California, Ronald Reagan.

Among the ten candidates endorsed by the AMA for United States Assistant Secretary for Health in the newly inaugurated Nixon administration in early 1969 was Richard S. Wilbur. When that appointment did not come through,* Wilbur was open to other career offers. As a gastroenterologist in the Palo Alto Clinic, he had been active in the California Medical Association and risen to become Chairman of its Board of Councilors.** He was known to many members of the AMA board and, on one occasion, had impressed Blair Henningsgaard, the AMPAC chairman, with his forensic ability.

Since the AMA board, soon after its appointment of Howard, had urged him to "pursue a recruiting program aimed at obtaining young, energetic and highly qualified staff," it was not unnatural that Wilbur and Howard got together. A tall, self-assured man whose background impressed Howard, Wilbur accepted the offer to join the AMA staff in the fall of 1969 as the assistant executive vice president. In announcing the Wilbur appointment to the House of Delegates, Howard also identified his new assistant as "my principal deputy," adding, "I think you all know him."[15] Although Howard was not empowered to appoint his successor and although

*This appointment was a celebrated cause in early 1969. The AMA opposed the choice of John H. Knowles, M.D., administrator of the Massachusetts General Hospital, who was strongly backed for the job by the press. The choice finally went to Roger O. Egeberg, M.D., the dean of the University of Southern California School of Medicine, who was neither backed nor opposed by the AMA.

**Analagous to the AMA office, Chairman of the Board of Trustees.

the 1969 board had no power to commit a future board to a decision about a chief executive, some members of the board, many of the delegates, and Wilbur himself considered that the heir apparent had been named. The assumption was strengthened in September 1970 when, as part of a staff restructuring, Wilbur's title was upgraded to deputy executive vice president, and it was not diminished—in the public view—when he was granted a leave of absence in June 1971 to go to Washington as the United States Assistant Secretary of Defense for Health and the Environment.

But in September 1973 as Wilbur prepared to leave Washington to return to his duties in Chicago, a search committee of the board was canvassing the field as if no commitment were made—and, indeed, none had been made. The selection of the new executive vice president was developing into a controversy, a public issue, though the appointment was a well-defined prerogative of the board. At the meeting of the house that December, the New York delegates introduced a resolution calling for a committee of the house to "assist" the board in the selection. Pointing out that the search committee had already consulted house leaders on the matter, the chairman of the search committee headed off that challenge to the board's authority. Nevertheless, an air of contention hung over the matter. Surfacing again were the symptoms of unrest and distrust that, in part at least, had lain behind the action of the house when in 1970 it trimmed the board's recommendation for an $80 dues increase to $40.

Weakening the authority of the board and further deepening the feelings of distrust were the circumstances of its chairman, John R. Kernodle, M.D., who was also the head of the search committee. A former AMPAC chairman, Kernodle had won election to the board in 1968 and re-election in 1971. In June 1972 he followed Parrott as chairman. At that time he was also a trustee of a bank in the town where he lived, Burlington, North Carolina. In late 1973 he was accused of violating the banking laws by taking out unsecured loans. He denied the accusation, resigned as chairman (to be succeeded by James H. Sammons, M.D.), but retained his membership on the board and stayed on as chairman of the search committee. When indicted in January 1974 (he later pleaded guilty), he resigned all his AMA offices. Richard E. Palmer, M.D., who moved up to become vice chairman, succeeded him as head of the search committee, which then consisted of Palmer, Parrott, Raymond T. Holden, M.D., and Russell B. Roth, M.D. Those four prepared the final report and the recommendations of the search committee.

For its mid-winter meeting, March 14-17, 1974, the board gathered in Washington, as it customarily did each year at that time. It had advanced the selection of the executive vice president by one meeting, mainly to get the issue settled before it grew more divisive. All members were present. The search committee reported, describing the process by which it started with seventy names, winnowed them down to twenty-six, conducted two- to four-hour interviews with twelve candidates, and now presented five for consideration: Merlin K. Duval, M.D., dean of the University of Arizona College of Medicine and a former Assistant Secretary at HEW; Charles C. Edwards, M.D., currently the Assistant Secretary of Health and formerly the AMA's director of the division of socioeconomic activities (1963-67); Robert B. Hunter, M.D., a member of the board; James H. Sammons, M.D., the chairman of the board; and Richard S. Wilbur, M.D., the deputy executive vice president.

Before proceeding with written ballots, the board adopted ground rules. Among them: trustees under consideration (Sammons and Hunter) would absent themselves from the meeting and be ineligible to vote as long as they remained under consideration; the five candidates would be voted on simultaneously, the candidate with the lowest number of votes being dropped before the next ballot; a two-thirds majority would be required for the final decision—ten votes out of fifteen if all were present, nine out of thirteen or fourteen, depending on the absence of Hunter or Sammons or both.

The first ballots eliminated all candidates but Sammons and Wilbur, and Hunter returned to the room to make it fourteen voters for the remainder of the balloting. Then followed a succession of 7-7 votes, the deadlock lasting to the end of the day and exhausting all present. At one point, as Sammons waited for a decision outside the room in the Washington Hilton where the board was meeting, David Weihaupt, a long-time staff member, kidded him. "Jim," Weihaupt said, "I'll bet you didn't know how hard it is to get a staff job at the AMA."

By the time the board went back into executive session two days later, some minds had changed. According to Parrott, Roth had told him at dinner the previous evening that he was going to switch his vote to Sammons. Roth was convinced that Wilbur could not now win. Donald E. Wood, M.D., a trustee closely allied with Parrott, Sammons, and Palmer, went to John Chenault, M.D., another trustee, saying that he would withdraw as a candidate for vice chairman of the board and back Chenault if he (Chenault) would switch his vote to Sammons. Chenault evidently did, and the decision went in Sammons' favor on the fifteenth ballot by the necessary 9-5 majority. Feelings over the outcome ran sufficiently high that a motion to make the vote for Sammons officially unanimous, a common gesture in the AMA, was rejected. Palmer was elected the new chairman of the board to succeed Sammons, and Chenault was elected vice chairman.

Born in 1927 in Montgomery, Alabama, the new executive vice president graduated from Washington and Lee College and then the St. Louis University School of Medicine in 1951. Late in 1948, while a medical student, Sammons received an invitation from the AMA to attend its clinical meeting, which was held in St. Louis that year. This was the meeting that followed Truman's upset election and caused the AMA to gear up for a major battle over the Truman health insurance bill.

Unlike a lot of his fellow medical students, Sammons attended the meeting and was caught up in the political fervor. "I sat and listened," he recalls, "and I saw people who were up on their feet and doing things. And I thought this was a hell of an organization." As soon as he completed medical school and an internship in Mobile, Alabama, and had gone into practice in Baytown, Texas, an industrial suburb of Houston, he plunged into medical society activities.

First there were offices in the east branch of the Harris County Medical Society (Houston); then the executive board and the vice presidency of the county society. Other offices followed: president of the Houston Academy of Medicine; alternate delegate to the AMA; delegate in 1964; director and then chairman of AMPAC; president of the Texas Medical Association; AMA trustee in 1970; and finally chairman of the board. He made an extraordinarily swift journey through the chairs of organized medicine.

The rancor stirred up by the rejection of Wilbur in favor of Sammons carried over to the meeting of the house that June. Whatever prospects there might have been that interest in the board's choice might slacken were dispelled by a report of the selection in the weekly magazine, *Medical World News*. Headlined "Turmoil at the AMA," it was written by the same editor who had earlier reported, with some gusto, President Hall's disaffection with the AMA. Now the writer was close to another aggrieved physician, Wilbur. The article emphasized the "unparalleled rage and bitterness" over the recent choice of executive vice president, the "belief" by some people (unnamed) that Sammons' appointment was "in part engineered from within a federal prison by Dr. John R. Kernodle," and the "juicy benefits" parceled out to those who had voted the right way. The magazine offered the prophecy, without alluding to its own role in the possible fulfillment, that the annual meeting coming up would see "a collision between the house and the board 'establishment.'"[16]

In part, that is what happened. Picking up on actions begun at previous meetings, the house, as an early matter of business, overrode board recommendations and changed the rules so that re-election to the board became more difficult. For many years, an incumbent trustee, his three-year term at an end, ran for re-election in a single contest against whoever cared to oppose him. A personal challenge was implicit in such elections, and under normal circumstances it took a highly determined effort to unseat someone in office. To replace that "slot" system, a method of "simultaneous" voting was instituted. This called for all candidates, including incumbents, to run for all vacant full-term trustee positions simultaneously.

Here is how the new system worked. Assume an election in which there were four board vacancies and eight candidates, including some candidates for re-election. Each delegate received a ballot with the eight names on it; he was asked to vote for no more and no less than four of them. As successive ballots were taken, those nominees winning a majority of votes were elected, the one receiving the fewest votes being dropped from the next ballot.

At the 1974 meeting, there were four full-term vacancies to be filled, with three incumbents—Holden, Wood, and Chenault—among the eight or so candidates. Holden, who kept some distance between himself and the so-called AMPAC trustees and had unswervingly backed Wilbur, won re-election. But Wood and Chenault, whose role in the Sammons-Wilbur contest had been described in the *Medical World News* story, were beaten; it was an unusual, if not unique, rejection of a vice chairman.

Although those two defeats clearly registered the displeasure of the house with the way the choice of executive vice president had been handled, it is hard to read an ideological shift into the overall results of the trustee elections. As it turned out, in addition to the four full-term vacancies in 1974, there were also two part-term seats on the board to be filled, and of the five newcomers to the board (Holden, of course, was an incumbent), three were men from the AMPAC Board of Directors.* Whatever else it might have been, this was not a repudiation of political pragmatism. Incidentally, one of the unsuccessful candidates for trustee was John P. Heard, M.D., the Georgia physician who had led the PSRO militants at the previous meeting in Anaheim.

Where the house-board collision was most evident was in the election for president. For months before the meeting, no one had come forward to announce against Parrott's declared candidacy. An uncontested election for president of the AMA, though not exactly rare, is still an unusual expression of liking and respect for someone who has served the association long and well. Parrott met both qualifications.

But two days before the meeting opened, Wilbur decided that he would challenge Parrott. Wilbur quickly discovered a political base; the California delegation, the biggest in the house, supported him as a native son. All those who thought the AMA had reneged on an assumed commitment to him backed his candidacy, as did those who simply did not like the direction the board was taking generally. Challenging the leadership and calling for reforms, Wilbur accused Parrott of being part of a group "that has lost the AMA credibility and respect in Washington." This was taken as a reference to the Kernodle episode. Parrott, in turn, linked Wilbur to "a band of dissidents and disaffecteds." It was not the usual sort of AMA presidential election, traditionally polite and relatively issue-free. This one was marked by high emotional tensions, and it called into question the quality of leadership recently demonstrated by the board.[17] In the end Parrott won, but only by two votes.

That spring and summer, as Sammons, the new executive vice president, settled into the AMA's executive offices on the third floor at 535 North Dearborn Street, he was well acquainted with the association's financial plight. As a trustee since 1970, vice chairman, and, briefly, chairman, he knew that continuing annual deficits were eating into the liquid reserves; that is, the AMA's treasury notes, bonds, and stocks—the assets of the association other than those difficult to sell quickly, such as real estate, computers, office equipment, and furnishings.

*Hoyt D. Gardner, M.D., Frank J. Jirka, M.D., (both of them later presidents of the AMA), and Joe T. Nelson, M.D.

What Sammons and others were unaware of was the rate at which publication costs had begun to accelerate. In recent years, these had been rising steadily. But now the AMA's cost of printing, paper, and postage started to skyrocket, mounting, Sammons said later, at the rate of 31 percent a year. As the bills rose, the need for cash grew, and as assets were sold to cover the deficits, the loss of dividends and interest on the liquidated securities eroded income. It was a bit like watching the spool play out on a tape recorder; near the end, it goes faster and faster.

"But," Sammons remembers, "I did not know we were in quite such straits until around Labor Day when Sam Miller, the financial director, walked into my office and said we'd soon have to start borrowing money to meet payroll. Boom! Just like that. In all fairness," Sammons adds, "Sam had told both Bert Howard and me two months earlier that he did not like the way things were going. But in terms of the reality of the situation, this was a real jolt."[18]

The news, as Sammons, his fellow staff executives, and the board all recognized, had deep implications. It marked the end of the line. For the better part of five years the AMA had chosen to live off its savings rather than face hard decisions. But now, with over $10 million in liquid reserves exhausted or converted to non-liquid assets,* it was no longer possible to postpone the need for making unpopular decisions about dues increases, program cuts, and structural changes. The AMA had used its options; now it was in a corner. It had to make some radical changes.

Although he did not officially become the executive vice president until October 14, when Howard started on three and a half months of terminal leave, Sammons was, in the fall of 1974, clearly the staff man in charge at the AMA. Furthermore, he still had an unusual amount of influence with the board; after all, it had only been a few months since he had been the chairman, one of the two most powerful positions on the elective side of the AMA.

Immediately before him was the task of developing the budget for the coming year. Customarily, this is drawn up by the staff in the early fall, approved by the executive vice president, submitted to the finance committee, and then submitted to the full board in October. After that, it is discussed with the members of Reference Committee F, acting as the finance committee of the house, and finally

---

*Before the severity of its liquidity problem was recognized in 1974, the AMA used reserves to buy a $2.1 million computer and real estate priced at $364,000.

presented as a matter of information to the delegates at the clinical meeting, that year scheduled to open in Portland on December 1.

Because of the worsening finances and the depletion of liquid reserves, to say nothing of house action the preceding June calling on the board not to adopt any more unbalanced budgets, the development of the 1975 budget presented an unusual challenge. What's more, it would be an instrument that would force major issues into the open. It would confront the policy-makers with the consequences of their past actions and it would confront them with the necessity of making difficult decisions for the future. It put Sammons in the position of telling first the board and then the house how bad the financial situation was and recommending the difficult steps that would be necessary to get the AMA out of the hole.

Sammons might have chosen a more oblique approach to the AMA's central problems, but what he proposed drove right into a crowd of controversial issues. "He had the guts, the conviction, the belief," says an admiring Joe Miller, "that he could go to the board and subsequently the house with a very debatable point of view about how things should be changed. But, goddammit, that was the only way to win: take it in a straightforward way, right up front, and force all the old board-baiting behavior out in the open, change those things that had to be changed and get on about doing some other things."[19]

What Sammons proposed as a way to finance a balanced, $35.3 million budget for 1975 won the backing of the board at the October 25-6, 1974, meeting of the trustees. His plan called for house action to raise dues by $90, effective January 1, to make further cuts in the council and committee structure, to reduce the publication frequency of most AMA periodicals, to place some on a subscription basis, and to eliminate virtually all advertising from them. It was a controversial program with a complex rationale.[20]

To prepare the way for it, a letter signed by the chairman, Richard E. Palmer, M.D., and the president, Malcolm C. Todd, M.D., went out to the delegates, the state medical associations and the medical specialty societies on October 30, alerting them to the AMA's "critical financial situation." On November 12, another mailing, with the same distribution, described the 1975 budget and discussed the reasons for the proposed dues increase, the council and committee changes, the new publication schedules, and the elimination of advertising.

The reaction of the medical federation was immediate, and it varied, proposal by proposal. An informal survey done by the field staff indicated that the council and committee changes would encounter resistance; the dues increase could be expected to meet stiffer opposition; and the proposal to drop advertising from the journals—presented as something that was losing its profitability and at the same time costing the AMA "credibility"—would be met with resentment.

As the date for the meeting neared, more bad financial news arrived. The AMA finance department was now predicting a deficit for the year in the neighborhood of $3 million, rather the the $1.7 million loss anticipated in the previous forecast. In response, the board, through a telephone conference of its executive committee, voted to discharge three additional councils: Environmental, Occupational, and Public Health; Rural Health; and Foods and Nutrition. The executive committee also voted to discontinue the Council on Legislation and the AMPAC board, with the idea that the two might be combined. Further staff cuts were made, including reductions in the Washington office and the termination of the field service department. The number of AMA employees dropped from 997 in August to 932 in December.[21]

Of all the financial changes taken or proposed, none roused the delegates more than the proposal to eliminate advertising from the AMA publications. Actually, there had been sporadic carping on this subject over the years, some of the more academically oriented delegates and council members arguing that the AMA publications were "compromised" by their acceptance of pharmaceutical product advertisements. But at this juncture that view had little following. According to Joe Miller, "The same people who for years had been demeaning and criticizing the AMA's use of advertising were now among the first to express opposition to a change." The delegates objected on a number of grounds. They saw little reason to abandon a major source of revenue in a time of financial difficulties; they rejected the idea that advertising hurt the integrity of the journals of the AMA; they rejected suggestions that the presence of pharmaceutical company advertising in AMA publications compromised the AMA's legislative positions in Washington.

Another factor was involved. If the AMA said, in effect, that its medical publications had to be above all suspicion, there would be sharp embarrassment to the medical journals published by county, state, and specialty medical associations; these were also supported by pharmaceutical advertising. Partly because of the pressures from back home, the delegates were strongly opposed to Sammons' recommendation on the advertising issue.

As the board assembled in Portland, preparatory to the meeting of the house, the trustees sensed the pressures building against the advertising proposal. To clarify their position, they issued an additional report. It pointed out, first, that the 1975 budget anticipated the receipt of $8.3 million in advertising revenues; what changes were or were not made would have no effect until fiscal 1976.[22] For that reason, the immediate need for the AMA to raise cash was an issue to be considered separately from advertising policy. Then, backing away from its original position, the board agreed to a more complete study in consultation with Reference Committee F on the impact of a no-advertising policy to be developed and submitted to the house at the next meeting in June.

Nevertheless, when the house did meet, it was—as described in the headline used by *AMNews*—a "shootout." A. Roy Tyrer, Jr., M.D., a delegate from Tennessee, reflected the tone of the meeting when he told the house that he was "stunned and appalled that the organization of the nation's highest paid profession should find itself flat broke." He called for "heads to roll among AMA management."[23]

Since all the most controversial reports involved finances, and since financial matters were referred to Reference Committee F, that is where the storm clouds gathered. For most of Monday, the committee's unflappable chairman, Joseph T. Painter, M.D., presided over a long day of heated testimony. Then, starting after lunch on Tuesday, running through the rest of that afternoon and spilling over to the following morning, he presented the recommendations of his committee to the House of Delegates. It was a tumultuous three days.

As the delegates took up the Reference Committee F recommendations, their anger with and distrust of the board dominated their actions. Sammons attributes the high emotional pitch of the meeting to the delegates' recognition, at last, of their own role in the near disaster. Sammons says, "They had sat there twice a year for five years and approved the reports coming from the board saying we were deficit-spending. They had ducked the dues question in 1970, and they continued to duck it for five years. Suddenly, some of them realized what in the hell they had done. And they got mad with themselves. And they got mad with the board. And they got mad with the staff."

What made the situation worse, according to Sammons, was an earnest, well-intentioned effort by staff and the board to provide up-to-the-minute revisions of the financial data. "We were determined to give the delegates current facts, the financial status as of the latest possible moment. We did not want any question to be raised about the integrity of the information. In retrospect, I think we generated a lot of anxiety over the accuracy of the data by so many updates. What we did added to the confusion."

As the items of business came up, the delegates showed almost an eagerness to reject the proposal of the board and at times they even gave the recommendations of their own reference committee short shrift.[24] They did approve a Reference Committee F recommendation for an immediate $60 assessment instead of a $90 first-of-the-year dues increase. But they ignored the reference committee's recommendation to make a $90 dues increase effective in 1976. A new dues structure would be considered in June, they said, "contingent upon demonstration by the board of stronger economy measures and improved executive management of the association's affairs."

There were the usual forecasts of membership defections, California citing survey data indicating that the $60 assessment followed by a dues increase would cause an end to unified membership in that state and the loss of 8,000 to 10,000 AMA members. Some other delegates, like N.L. Barker, M.D., of Texas, acknowledged past mistakes. "I want you to know," he told the delegates, "and most of you were in this house four years ago when I made a hell of a boner, and I want to admit I made a boner because I really did a lot of fighting against an $80 dues increase."[25]

When the matter of the council and committee structure came up, Massachusetts offered a plan that differed from what the board and the reference committee had in mind. This substitute resolution rescinded all the actions the board had taken in recent months in respect to committee and council cutbacks; it swept aside proposals for further trimming, and it overrode the board recommendations for new publication plans, which, among other things, would have transformed three of the monthly specialty journals into quarterlies. In effect, the Massachusetts resolution called for preserving the status quo, retaining the structure of all the old councils and committees but putting their activities on hold and keeping the publishing operations intact, at the prevailing frequencies. In the meantime—and this was the central idea in the Massachusetts resolution—a special committee of the house was to be appointed to study what the resolution called "the whole situation," with recommendations to be made to the House of Delegates at the

June 1975 meeting, Adopted 142-68, it announced to the Board of Trustees, "We are going to find out the facts of the matter for ourselves."

On the board's modified recommendation that the financial impact of a no-advertising policy be studied by the board and Reference Committee F, with a report for the house in June, the delegates were agreeable. However, they made clear what their opinion on the matter was likely to be. When the reference committee recommended, rather mildly, that in the meantime advertising in AMA publications be approved "in principle," the house pointed out that "in principle" statements were not acceptable under the parliamentary rules the AMA followed. Instead, they insisted on emphatic wording that the AMA "continue its present full unrestricted advertising program pending further appropriate study."[26]

If the actions of the house did not constitute a no-confidence vote, they certainly came close to it. The delegates brushed aside Sammons' and the board's solutions to the AMA's difficulties, seizing the initiative themselves. For the trustees and senior staff members, who had seen their judgments buried in the distrust, skepticism, and finger-pointing of the house, it was an experience in frustration and despair. Joe Miller recalled later,

> It was an opportunity for all the unhappy ones to rally 'round and oppose the people who were currently in control, the people to whom they had lost battles in previous years. The Portland meeting was a happy hunting ground for that kind of warrior...Let me tell you how bad it got in the inner sanctum. One night...we'd been in session almost all day and it was well past midnight...Jim Sammons and I had been in that room with the trustees all day long and into the evening. So had a few other staff people from time to time. There was a feeling of total frustration. We'd fought and fought and fought for what we believed to be the right decisions. But everyone was fed up, disgusted by the hostility we were getting in the house. We'd never been subjected to such a degrading session in all our lives. I think it fair to say that even the strongest people in that room were ready to throw in their hand, resign their positions and go home and grow their roses. And I include myself and Jim Sammons in the group that felt just that way.

For all its rancor and antagonism, the Portland meeting eventually had a constructive outcome. First, it underscored for the members and the delegates the gravity and the urgency of the AMA's difficulties. That awareness helped break some of the old patterns, destroy some sacred cows, and open the way to some fresh thinking. During the six months between the December 1974 meeting and the 1975 annual meeting in June, the AMA subjected itself to the most intensive working review of its activities ever conducted. In this process, as the house set about discovering for itself what had gone wrong and deciding for itself what had to be done, it involved itself in the affairs of the AMA as it had rarely involved itself before. From this came a better understanding of the AMA's problems and a new appreciation of its needs.

The instrument of that gradual transformation in the early part of 1975 was the Special Committee of the House of Delegates, the one proposed by the Massachusetts delegates to look into the financial debacle. In making appointments to the committee, the Speaker of the House of Delegates, Tom E. Nesbitt, M.D., chose the current members of Reference Committee F as the delegates most knowledgeable about the AMA's finances, plus three other delegates. For that reason the special committee was also referred to sometimes as "the expanded Committee F." Its chairman was the chairman of Reference Committee F, Joseph T. Painter, M.D.

Charged with conducting a wide-ranging probe into the financial management of the association and suggesting ways out of the difficulties, the committee was initially a bit awed by the size of the job it had been handed. "There was a slight element of recrimination," says Theodore R. Chilcoat, Jr., the staff executive who served as secretary to the committee, "but mostly the concern was about whether all the facts would be there, and whether the committee could come up with a fair and explicit report."[27] Another staff man who worked with the committee was struck by the zeal with which the committee members tackled their assignment. "They were going to explore the records," Charles Macenski says, "and I mean *all* the records."

As the special committee went about its work, taking testimony, going through previous management studies, examining documents, the AMA's financial pinch started to ease. Within a few months after the Portland meeting, almost 120,000 members (out of about 170,000) sent in their $60 assessment, providing the AMA with more than $7 million in cash.[28]

The short term loans, totaling $3 million and taken out to cover part of the 1974 deficit, were repaid. An additional $2 million was earmarked to cover the anticipated 1975 deficit. The remainder of the assessment proceeds was considered a contingency fund to finance pending legal actions—the challenge to the utilization review regulations and the constitutionality of the planning act—and to see the AMA through the cash-short period that it experiences at the end of every year.

Careful financial management was still required, however. Revenues fell behind expectations, partly because advertising revenues dropped. The actions at Portland left the advertising executives of the pharmaceutical manufacturing companies confused, and they were cautious about commitments to AMA publications.

As for the AMA staff operations, there were drastic curtailments. Meetings were cancelled, appointments held up, jobs left unfilled. The editors of the publications were required to make a 20 percent cut in expenses, reducing the number of editorial pages and the use of color. Robert Moser, M.D., the editor of *JAMA*, who was having disagreements with the AMA management over other matters, refused the order and resigned. Further staff reductions made in May brought the association staff down to 824. The AMA was bandaging its financial wounds, and a long healing process lay ahead.

Chapter Twenty

The Turnaround

The AMA's financial crisis had broad dimensions and multiple origins, with at least four components contributing to the central problem. All of them required correction before a lasting, workable end to the association's difficulties could develop.

The tip of the iceberg was, of course, the prolonged lack of an adequate income base. This had caused the AMA to consume its liquid reserves, leaving it vulnerable in corporate emergencies and restricted as to options in policy matters.

There were serious problems with the publishing operation, once so successful. The basic difficulty was a lack of coordination, because the publishing responsibility was diffused over three of the AMA's eight operating divisions.

Within the management of the association, a lot of bolts needed tightening. Future planning was just beginning to be systematized. The financial reporting system was slow. The overall administrative structure made it difficult for management to exert strong central control.

At the same time, the AMA was burdened with a structure of councils and committees that was expensive, sometimes disruptive, frequently irrelevant, and geared to the pace of a more leisurely era.

The problems did not lack identification, for several outside studies as well as internal surveys conducted by committees of the house had called attention to them. But for a long time—too long, as the current crisis was demonstrating—the AMA had postponed corrective action. The December 1974 meeting in Portland threw the issues into sharp focus, that being the occasion of a head-on attempt to solve them. Though that effort was lost, the house came away aware that delay was no longer possible. At the June 1975 meeting in Atlantic City, the AMA started making the several decisions needed to lead the AMA out of its difficulties.[1]

Before the House of Delegates could take the most urgently needed step, a dues increase, the AMA had to answer questions about its future level of activity. It had three choices: it could remain as it was, horns pulled in, everything on a minimal budget; it could go back to the operational levels of early 1974, restoring to life the suspended councils, committees, and programs; or it could consider a future with new and different initiatives. What the board recommended and the house approved included parts of all those options: the continuation of current activities, the restoration of some of the suspended programs (subject to review), and the initiation of some new programs, plus the crucially needed build-up of reserves.

Implicit in the decision in favor of a dynamic rather than a static future was a dues increase of substantial proportions. In preparing for that, the staff and the board had to develop and present to the delegates a detailed financial plan. That required the careful assessment of several factors—the impact of inflation, the effect of a big dues increase on the number of members, the advertising and subscription income of the publications, the potential liability for past unrelated business income taxes, and the speed with which reserves could be replenished.

The plan that evolved was predicated on a sizeable dues increase and projected the expected operating results for the coming five years. It anticipated an excess of revenues over expenses each year through 1980, the settlement of accounts with the federal government,* and the restoration of reserves to 60 percent of annual operating expenses by 1977, to 100 percent by 1980. A graphic presentation of what was to happen year by year in the next five years showed revenues on a rising line from 1976 through 1980, topping a

---

*In addition to the unrelated business tax matter, the AMA had made errors in calculating the postage owed for parts of the controlled (i.e., free) circulation of *JAMA*. These were rectified in 1980 with the payment of $728,000. Both the postal and IRS problems arose over differing interpretations of complex regulations.

In 1974 and 1975 the AMA was infiltrated by persons affiliated with a religious cult whose personal counseling practices the AMA had once characterized as a menace to mental health. Copies of files relating to the IRS and Postal Service matters were sneaked to the press by someone who never revealed his identity but spoke to reporters, congressmen, and federal agencies by phone in such a husky voice that he was nicknamed Sore Throat, a reference to the Watergate informant, Deep Throat. A few newspapers, with Watergate in mind, aired the stolen documents, trying to build the story into a major scandal.

lower but more rapidly rising line of expenses, with an anticipated intersection of the two in 1980, after which there would, presumably, be the need to again consider dues levels.[2]

In contrast to what had happened at the 1970 and 1974 meetings,the delegates now faced the dues question forthrightly. What made that easier was not just the preparatory work done by the staff and the board but a long, preliminary report from the Special Committee of the House. This was a remarkable document. It was seventy-two pages long and bore the approval of all members of the committee. The basic outline was developed by the committee chairman, Joseph T. Painter, M.D. Exhaustive in detail, the report was written in skeletal form. There was virtually no narrative, scarcely an adjective or an adverb. It projected an unmistakable aura of clinical objectivity. Had the house instructed the special committee, "Just give us the facts," Painter and his group could hardly have executed the charge more faithfully.[3]

As a result, the emotional trip-wires that usually run through a report of this sort were absent, and, though the discussion of the report at times grew animated, the delegates kept their arguments within the facts. The impact of the report was enhanced by its distribution by mail before the meeting and by a discussion session held especially for the delegates the day before the opening ceremonies of the house. Painter and the other committee members were there to elucidate the major points, to answer questions, and to receive suggestions for a shorter, final version of the report.

The effort had a reassuring effect. The long preliminary report found the cause for the AMA's financial trouble to be much as the board had described it at Portland seven months earlier. Contrary to the suspicions of some of the delegates at Portland, it reported no misuse of AMA funds or unauthorized expenditures. In its final report, the special committee affirmed the financial needs of the AMA, calling a substantial dues increase "essential," though not specifying an amount. It recommended that AMA publications continue to accept advertising, but advocated other changes—the placing of all journals except *JAMA* and *AMNews* on a subscription basis, and the discontinuation of *Prism*, a socioeconomic monthly first published in 1973. It recommended that the council-committee structure be revised and that the house instruct the Council on Long Range Planning and Development to submit a plan for reorganization at the next meeting.

Contributing further to the policy of disclosure that the trustees and Sammons insisted upon was an executive (closed to the press and public) session of the house held on the opening day of the meeting. During this session the AMA's outside consultants discussed several matters, including the size of the association's possible liabilities for unrelated business income taxes. The AMA had for several years taken the position that income of its journals was not taxable, but the 1969 Tax Reform Act and new regulations raised the possibility that retroactive taxes plus penalties and interest would have to be paid.*

A few days later, when the time came to vote on the dues increase, the house had three proposals before it—dues of $250 a year for regular members, which was the recommendation of the board; dues of $225 a year, the recommendation of Reference Committee F; and dues of $200 a year, a proposal of the New York delegation. The feeling now ran as strongly in a positive direction as it had run negatively at Portland. Soon after debate over the three choices began, Jack Gibbs, M.D., a delegate from downstate Illinois, announced his state's full support of the board request for annual dues of $250. "Faced with unknown lawsuits, unknown tax liabilities and galloping inflation," he said, "we should be giving the maximum projected dues needed and not the minimum...Compared to the dues structure of other organizations and particularly when related to income levels, I think we have a real bargain at $250...My coal miner brother pays more dues than I do...I think we must all share in the blame for deficit spending and for the present crisis, and I hope we have the intestinal fortitude to get ourselves out of it."

In quick succession, Ohio, Michigan, Texas, Florida, Arizona, and Kansas pledged support. A. Roy Tyrer, Jr., M.D., the delegate who told the house at Portland that heads ought to roll, recorded Tennessee's support for the board recommendation, adding, "The Board of Trustees and the staff during the past six to eight months have done a superb job in shoring up the finances of the association." When the question was called, the speaker, Tom E. Nesbitt, M.D., explained that the house would vote first on the $250 proposal. If that did not win a majority, the next vote would be on the $225, and, if that failed to pass, there would be a vote on the New York proposal for dues increase to $200. When Nesbitt called for those favoring the board's $250 recommendation to stand, there was creaking of chairs

*When settled, the amount through 1974 was $7.8 million.

and a rustling of papers as delegation after delegation rose. When the delegates looked around, they saw an overwhelming demonstration in support of the $250, and they erupted into a prolonged burst of applause.[4]

Critical as a major dues increase was, that alone could not solve the AMA's cash flow problem unless physicians responded to the raise in substantial numbers. Because experience showed that a drop in the number of members invariably followed any hike in dues, the worrisome question now was: How large would the drop in the number of members be in response to the increase?

Membership development was something the AMA had long neglected. In his report to the house in June 1975, Sammons confessed, "It is amazing—downright dumbfounding—when you realize the lack of attention given by the federation to membership recruitment and retention."[5] But the cause was not so much indifference as the complexity of doing the job effectively within the federated structure of the organization. The AMA was highly dependent on—some would say at the mercy of—the county and state organizations when it came to the matter of membership. The entryway to AMA membership lay through county and state association membership, and, until 1982, it was only in exceptional cases that a physician could become an AMA member without first joining and paying the dues of the local medical societies.

And not always did the preferences, capabilities, and fiscal priorities of the local societies serve the membership interests of the AMA. Different states had different definitions of eligibility, making it hard for a physician to transfer his membership if he moved from one part of the country to another. Some county societies set up roadblocks, a two-year probationary period, for example, to discourage membership. A few made it hard for the faculty members of a local medical school or salaried physicians with an HMO to join because societies considered them to be engaged in the corporate practice of medicine.

The combined billing forms used to collect dues for the county and state societies and the AMA showed little uniformity. In some cases, especially when a local society was sensitive about the impact of a dues increase of its own, it would take the unhelpful step of noting on the combined billing form that AMA membership was "optional."

Often short of funds, local societies frequently lacked a complete record of the names of all physicians in their area, making it impossible for them to conduct a full-scale membership drive even had they wanted to do so. A survey conducted in 1979 showed that 42 percent of the state associations and 63 percent of the county societies made no effort to recruit new members. Broader factors may also have been at work, ranging from the physician's growing loyalty to his specialty (and therefore his specialty society) to a widespread distrust, prevalent especially among younger people, of institutions representing the establishment.[6]

Under the financial pressures of the mid- to late 1970s, the AMA's membership efforts took on new urgency. The staff membership department, started in 1972 with two people, was expanded to sixteen people and placed under the direction of an executive with a graduate degree in marketing. Model bylaws for membership in county and state societies were drawn up, adopted by the house, and circulated, with the hope that they might help end the vestigial obstacles to local society membership. The billing procedures were improved, with the forwarding of AMA dues put on a consistent and business-like basis. At the same time, a standard means of compensating the local societies for their work in billing for AMA dues was established. Regional meetings on membership were conducted, resulting in better cooperation in membership recruitment efforts. Joint drives were undertaken; various promotional techniques were tested. Research surveys were made, indicating among other things that small, incremental dues increases were preferable to infrequent but large raises.

The early results of the new membership efforts served mainly to underscore the difficulty and complexity of recruitment. Membership growth among students and residents was spectacular. But regular membership in the AMA, while it grew along with the growth in the size of the medical profession as a whole, remained more or less constant as a percentage of the physician universe.

Possibly the best evidence of improved membership strength came in late 1982, when the effect of raising dues from $250 a year to $285 could be measured. First of all, the request for the increase, proposed as the first of three small incremental increases to take effect over three years, enjoyed uncommonly smooth sailing when brought before the house. Then, when the results were final, the AMA found that for the first time in its history it had a year in which it raised dues and also gained members. (see Table 1.)

Despite an immediate 6.6 percent drop in the number of regular dues-paying members, the 1975 dues increase was emphatically the right decision. With the income from dues leaping from $17.8 mil-

TABLE 1.
AMA Dues-Paying Membership

	1975	1976[a]	1977	1978	1979	1980	1981	1982[a]
REGULAR	162,400	151,700	146,600[b]	1147,700	151,600	154,300	155,800	158,600
RESIDENT[c]	8,700	10,600	13,400	16,300	20,300	21,000	23,000	27,900
STUDENT[c]	8,100	9,500	13,500	15,400	20,200	21,300	22,800	26,900
TOTAL	179,200	171,800	173,500	179,400	192,100	196,600	201,600	213,400

[a] Dues were increased in these years.

[b] In 1977, when California rescinded its policy of unified membership, the AMA lost 5,507 members in that state, the total of AMA members in California dropping from 22,295 in 1976 to 16,788 in 1977.

[c] Medical student dues: $15 a year; resident dues: $35 ($45 in 1982 and after).

lion in 1975 to $36.6 million in 1976, the long string of annual deficits was broken. Reserves accumulated rapidly, and the AMA's net worth climbed from a low of $12 million in 1974 to $86 million in 1982. Almost overnight, the AMA transformed itself from an organization in financial trouble to one in comfortable circumstances.

Although the dues increase authorized in 1975 assured the AMA's financial viability, the achievement of enduring good health also demanded radical change in the association's publishing operations. Historically, almost from the beginning, these had been successful, supporting the AMA virtually unassisted from 1912 to 1949. During the 1950s and possibly into the early 1960s, the net revenues from publishing exceeded the income from dues. But in the 1970s the operation slipped into the red, and for 1974 the AMA reported a loss from its periodicals in excess of $4.2 million.

Unlike the need to raise dues, a course of action that was easy to identify, the AMA's way out of its publishing difficulties was not all that clear. To appreciate the complexity of the factors involved, one must remember that the AMA's basic reason for being in the publishing business was not profit. The medical journals were published to serve the profession's informational needs—especially the physician's requirements for the authoritative evaluation of new data, new medicines, new methods of treatment, new observations. Educational programs and the dissemination of information are, in fact, among the functions that distinguish a professional organization from others. In addition, the AMA had over the years found, like other organizations, that a publication on general association activities was needed, not for revenue, but to keep the membership involved, interested, and informed. Thus, when it came time to make decisions on the frequency, continuation, and distribution of its periodicals, the AMA could not apply the orthodox editorial and financial criteria that a commercial publisher might use.

Further complicating publications decisions was the necessary involvement of the House of Delegates. The American Medical Association periodicals owed their existence to actions of the house, and actions of the house were therefore necessary before significant changes could be made. To make matters even more complex, the distribution of some publications was required in the bylaws, which read, "Member dues shall include the right to receive *JAMA*, *Today's Health*, and *American Medical News* and such other publications as the board may from time to time authorize."* To effect a bylaw change, an amendment has to lie over until the next day and requires a two-thirds vote to be approved.

Administratively, the AMA publishing operation presented another anomaly: there was no publisher. There were editors and advertising sales executives, people in charge of circulation and production. But there was no professionally experienced executive to draw together and coordinate the many disciplines that underlie a successful publishing operation. Why this curious reluctance to consolidate a large and financially critical operation under a single executive? One reason was that things went along smoothly for a long time without a publisher. The other stemmed from unhappy memories of Morris Fishbein, M.D., and the way he used his position as a *de facto* publisher to buttress his personal power.

As Sammons and other top staff executives surveyed the publishing scene near the end of 1974, all they could see ahead were liabilities. In a report to the special committee of the house in 1975, Sammons wrote, "The publishing program comprises 42 percent of the total AMA budget. Moreover, it is this portion of AMA pro-

---

*Until late 1972 the bylaws specified the choice of one of the ten AMA specialty journals to each dues paying member as a benefit of membership. Early that year the house adopted a board recommendation placing the specialty journals on a paid subscription basis. The decision was reversed at the 1972 clinical meeting, but the bylaw change leaving the distribution of the specialty journals up to the authorization of the board was made anyway.

gramming that is most subject to inflationary pressure, to enormous and sudden variances in expenditures. At the same time, the income produced by this program is not only declining but is the most unpredictable of all AMA revenue sources. This huge program is also the one in which it is most difficult to make cost reductions. Obviously, the rising cost and falling revenue of a dominating program must have an adverse effect on other AMA programs, and—in the long run—on the very ability of the AMA to function."[7]

Later, speaking long after the event, Joe Miller stated the danger more bluntly. "The AMA's publishing activity, if not conducted properly, can devour the whole organization in a short period of time."

Of the fourteen major publications to which the AMA was committed in 1975, eleven were medical journals, their content technical and scientific. The articles published, by and large, were articles submitted by physicians or other scientists and reviewed before publication by experts in the appropriate field. Only rarely, and then in restrained tones, did the journals take up a matter that could be considered legislative or political.

Among the scientific publications, the oldest and most prestigious was *JAMA*. Published weekly, its cover graced with a four-color reproduction of a handsome work of art, *JAMA* was edited more to meet the needs of the practitioner than those of the academician. It then had a weekly circulation of 240,000. The other ten medical journals were specialty journals, published monthly, with circulations that ranged from 9,800 to 65,000.* Some of the specialty journals were well regarded in their fields; others suffered by comparison with their competitors. About 35,000 non-members subscribed to *JAMA*, a lesser number to the specialty journals. The AMA medical journals accepted advertising, virtually all of it from pharmaceutical manufacturers for prescription drug products. As a group, the ten specialty journals lost something over $1 million in 1974; *JAMA*, down from its 1967 high in the number of advertising pages, had incurred some financial losses during the preceding five years.

Dating from April 1, 1923, the AMA published a monthly health magazine for consumers originally called *Hygeia*, and renamed

---

*The *Archives of Dermatology*, the *Archives of Environmental Health*, the *Archives of General Psychiatry*, the *Archives of Internal Medicine*, the *Archives of Neurology*, the *Archives of Ophthalmology*, the *Archives of Otolaryngology*, the *Archives of Pathology*, the *Archives of Surgery*, and the *American Journal of Diseases of Children*.

Today's Health in December 1950. Its purpose was the health education of the public, a typical issue containing how-to advice on personal health, straightforward discussions of various diseases, warnings against common health hazards, and exposures of quackery. In 1974 it had a paid circulation of 295,000 and modest advertising revenues from a limited range of consumer products. Because it implied a medical endorsement of advertised products, *Today's Health* was cautious about what advertisements it would accept. It rejected ads for many "health" products because the claims made were considered to be exaggerated, unsubstantiated, or meaningless.

Today's Health was a benefit-of-membership publication, so designated in the bylaws after 1959 when the house decided that it should be sent free to members, presumably for reception room display. Physicians, however, were often irritated by it, especially in its efforts to appeal more broadly to younger readers. For thirty years, as a matter of fact, physicians had questioned whether the AMA should be in the business of trying to publish a consumer magazine at all. Wasn't it the AMA's job to communicate with doctors?

The magazine had great public relations value. Its articles were often reprinted in *Reader's Digest*, its comments picked up by newspapers. During 1974, there was a half-hour *Today's Health* television show carried by more than fifty stations, usually on Sunday mornings. But the magazine's readership was too small and its readers too diffuse demographically for it to grow into an important consumer advertising medium. The cost of getting renewals and new subscriptions was rising, and the requirement to supply the membership with unreimbursed subscriptions erased what slim margins of revenue over expense there might have been. For a number of reasons, it was vulnerable.

In 1958, the year Blasingame took over as executive vice president from Lull and modernized the organization, the AMA began publication of a medical newspaper. Appearing first on September 22 that year as a sixteen-page, fortnightly, tabloid-size paper, *American Medical Association News* sought to fill a perceived gap. "The AMA believes it has done a good job in keeping its members informed of scientific developments," Blasingame wrote in a signed column on the first editorial page. "In the non-technical area, however, there is much to be done. This is the assignment of *AMA News*." The lead editorial stated that the paper did not intend to become a house organ but that it would report the AMA's many and varied activities. Furthermore, the editorial said, "The medico-economic and socio-economic fields of medicine are becoming more complex each year. The interest of Congress in matters directly and indirectly related to medicine is growing." The maiden issue carried a column of Washington news called "On the Legislative Front," and there was a scattering of ads for cars, office equipment, and other non-pharmaceutical products. Not until 1971 did the *AMNews* accept drug advertising.

The AMA's effort to found a medical newspaper succeeded. It went to a weekly publication schedule in January 1965 and altered its name to *American Medical News* in 1969 to reflect a less organizational stress on its news coverage. One editor stated the new policy this way: "I tell my staff [of nineteen] that they are required to report all sides of an issue. That is the reporter's first rule. But the paper is owned and published by the AMA, and it has the right to have its views advanced on the editorial page."[8] For a while in the early 1970s, *AMNews* was sent free not just to the members but to all physicians and medical students.* Readership compared favorably with that of other "non-scientific" medical publications, and advertisers were looking on *AMNews* with growing favor.

Of all the periodicals, the one in the weakest financial position was *Prism*, a monthly magazine intended, as its prospectus stated, to be a "forum for discussion of those social, ethical and political issues in which American medicine finds itself increasingly involved." It was elegantly designed and respected by many physicians as the *Fortune* of the medical publication field. Others, conditioned by the austere graphics of most medical publications, thought it overdone, objecting specifically to the unusual 11 × 11 inch format used during its first year and a half of publication. Because the articles repeatedly dealt with sensitive topics and took a view of the issues that was broad (and much too liberal, many physicians thought), *Prism* was considered controversial.

Developed without the benefit of serious marketing studies, *Prism* sprung from a variety of hopes and expectations that permeated the AMA in the early 1970s. Conscious of the problems the AMA was having in getting dues increases, some AMA leaders looked with interest on any potential new source of revenue. The advertising director in those days, sensitive about the shrinking

---

AMNews and *Prism* were controlled circulation publications. That is, they were sent free to those physicians whom the AMA wanted to reach, either for reasons of policy or advertising sales. Part of *JAMA*'s distribution was also controlled circulation.

performance of *JAMA*, envied the success then being enjoyed by *Medical Economics* and *Medical World News*, both medical magazines but neither a scientific medical journal. Jabbing a finger at the publications, he used to say, "That's what the doctors are reading these days." Actually, there was an opening in the AMA publication line-up. The journals were scarcely covering the socioeconomic issues at all, and *AMNews*, being a newspaper, had space limitations and short deadlines.

Important as those factors might have been, the major force behind *Prism's* start was the growing interest in national health insurance legislation and an intensified interest among physicians in socioeconomic matters. The respected American Society of Internal Medicine, a large association of internists that focused its attention on legislative and socioeconomic matters and left scientific questions to the American College of Physicians, thought the current socioeconomic issues merited a more penetrating and dispassionate discussion than they were getting. Accordingly, they explored the idea of a new socioeconomic publication but came to the conclusion that the AMA was better equipped to launch one. They strongly urged the AMA to do so. Many others in medicine wanted to see a magazine on socioeconomic issues, not a propaganda organ to "tell medicine's story" (which would have been the attitude of the AMA in 1949 or 1965), but an equable, authoritative, informative publication. In December 1971, as the AMA staff was getting a first dummy ready to test on potential advertisers, the house passed a resolution indicating its interest in such a publication.

Prism, as many magazines do, had a slow start after its first issue in April 1973. In early 1975 *Prism* dropped its unorthodox format, adopted originally to enhance its graphic appeal and to make it stand out from the welter of other controlled circulation publications that physicians received. The switch to orthodox size helped advertising sales. But although readership studies indicated strength, *Prism* was $2 million a year away from being a self-sustaining operation.

By the time the delegates got to the publications question at the June 1975 meeting, they had been exposed to a formidable accumulation of facts and advice. In addition to the detailed report submitted by the special committee, reports on the publications were given by three outside consultants at the closed session on the opening day of the meeting. A representative of Cambridge Associates reviewed the findings of their study of reader and advertiser opinions of the various publications. An executive from the AMA's auditors, Arthur Young & Company, talked about the production, distribution, and financial aspects of the publishing operation. And finally, Edward W. Barrett, head of the Communications Institute, a former *Newsweek* editor, and a former dean of the Columbia University School of Journalism, offered some broad editorial judgments of the publications.

Reflecting later, he recalled how impressed he had been with the size of the publishing operation, "...a whole damned publishing empire," he said. He thought the newspaper "well-handled for its purpose" and felt that the magazines ranged from "fair to excellent...not a real dud in the collection." He did, however, recommend that the AMA cease publication of *Today's Health*. He liked *Prism*, as "a recognition of social change," and hoped that it could be continued as a quarterly.[9]

Out of the 1975 annual meeting came several actions and declarations that led to revisions in the AMA's publications policy. First of all, accepting the recommendations of the special committee, the house reaffirmed the position it had taken at Portland, endorsing "aggressive advertising promotion." In regard to *JAMA* and *AMNews*, no changes were recommended; in fact, said the house, they were to be "provided with the resources necessary for the continued maintenance of these publications at the highest levels of excellence and service to the membership."[10]

In respect to the other publications, the actions of the house require some interpretation. Briefed by the outside publication consultants earlier and then hearing some of the trustees emphasize the need for flexibility, most of the delegates became aware of the complexities of shutting down a publication, selling one, altering frequency, or changing from benefit-of-membership status to paid subscription. Final publishing decisions, it came to be recognized, just could not be handled by a quasi-legislative body of two or three hundred physicians meeting twice a year. The house had recommendations to make, but at the same time it acknowledged there was a difference between "recommend" and "direct."

Following the conclusions of the special committee, the house recommended to the board that the ten specialty journals be put on a subscription basis, the price level sufficient to make them self-sustaining. If some could not survive on that basis, talks were to be opened with appropriate specialty societies regarding possible sale, transfer, or joint operation. It was the recommendation of the special committee that *Prism* be discontinued. The committee report said nothing specifically about *Today's Health*, but since other recommendations called for all publications but *JAMA* and *AMNews* to be put on a subscription basis, the presumption was that physician members were no longer to receive the magazine free. The report of Reference Committee F recommended that the AMA discontinue both *Today's Health* and *Prism*.

When the house took up the future of these two publications, the difficulties inherent in winding down the publication of a periodical were underscored. The contractual obligations in advertising and subscription sales were discussed along with the possible sale values. In the case of *Today's Health* questions arose as to its benefit-of-membership status specifically stated in the bylaws. Changing that would require a two-thirds majority vote.

Beneath all the wrangling and arguing that ensued it was clear that many if not a majority of the delegates wanted the end of *Prism* and *Today's Health* as a trade-off for their support of a dues increase. As he often did, delegate Joseph P. Donnelly, M.D., stated the matter bluntly. "I represent about 8,000 physicians in New Jersey," he said, "and I have to listen to them more than to these publication experts...*Today's Health* and *Prism* are something we can no longer afford, and the sooner we get rid of both of them, the better... When I go home and tell the members we just raised their dues ...their first question will be, 'Well, what did you do about the publications?'"

In the end, the house voted to remove *Today's Health* from mention in the bylaws as a benefit of membership; its management and survival were left to the board's judgment. The house did recommend to the board that *Prism* be discontinued. But the house gave the board the discretionary power its members asked for. Trustee Jere W. Annis, M.D., wanted to be sure. "I just want it to be clear in your minds," he said to the house, "and I want it to be clear before tomorrow because as I interpret your action...I still have the responsibility to cast my vote on that board to continue or discontinue *Prism*. I would, if I think it is a feasible thing, keep it for a while or, on the other hand, if we can dispose of it to better advantage, then I feel that is what I am going to do.

"I believe that is what you said."[11]

The delegates indicated their agreement with Annis' interpretation by applause. Thus the publishing operation, which had been regarded as a joint house-board responsibility, now became a responsibility of the board in its fiduciary capacity. Now equipped with broad authority to make decisions regarding publications and clear as to the wishes of the house, the AMA could tackle the real business at hand: the complicated and difficult job of restoring the publishing operation to fiscal health.

AMA staff executives later agreed that the first remedy proposed—the one made at the Portland meeting that would have taken the AMA out of the advertising business—would have been a mistake. "We were then and are now bound to the democratic process," Miller said in explanation. "We could not act like a commercial publisher because dozens of people and dozens of policy positions, by the house and the board, were all involved in the decisions that had to be made. We just couldn't go to them and simply say, 'The way we've been running the publishing operation is crazy.' It took a lot of hard knocks and a period of trauma to cause everyone to better appreciate the reasons for some of the changes that had to be made."[12] Between the clinical meeting at Portland in 1974 and the annual meeting at Atlantic City in 1975, there was enough trauma for everyone concerned, and the AMA did finally make decisions that enabled it to reverse the calamitous financial direction its publishing operations had taken.

As a first move, and at the strong urging of the Arthur Young & Company consultants, the AMA overcame its long-standing reluctance to have a publisher. It created a new position—Group Vice President for Publishing—and launched executive recruiting efforts to fill it. The new publisher was to have responsibility for all the functions: production, purchasing, advertising, market research, promotion, subscriptions, circulation, and even editorial, except for the scientific journals.

While the search for a publisher proceeded, staff task forces embarked on lengthy reviews of all the consultants' studies, attempting to reconcile the business-oriented recommendations they contained with the desires of the house and the management philosophies evolving as Sammons' administration took hold. At an early stage, it was decided not to pursue a proposal made first in 1970 that would establish the publishing operation in a separate corporation, an idea which offered advantages as well as disadvantages.

Late in the year, the new group vice president for publishing joined the staff, Thomas F. Hannon. An executive in his forties at the time, Hannon had had a successful career with the Vance Publishing Company and Conover-Mast, both profitable publishers of books and trade magazines. He quickly caught up with the profusion of offers and proposals the AMA had received from outside publishers and the variety of options that had to be sorted out. He played a major role in the difficult, final decisions that had to be made in this period.

In overhauling its publishing operation, the AMA's first order of business was to gain control over and limit the major sources of expense. Part of doing this involved the possible sale of money-losing properties, and to help, an outside broker/consultant was brought in. *Prism* found no potential buyers, and a decision was made to end publication with the January 1976 issue. However, an effort was made to carry on its editorial function through *Impact*, a special, monthly section published until 1981 as part of *AMNews*. *Today's Health* received more than twenty offers, and it was sold in March 1976 to Family Communications, Inc., the publisher of *Family Health*, which had been a competitor. The terms of the sale called for the payment of $200,000 over several months, with the purchaser assuming the liability for $1.4 million in prepaid, unfulfilled subscriptions.

As for the specialty journals, a number of choices had to be considered. One outside publisher proposed handling them all under a management agreement that would leave only the responsibility for the editorial content with the AMA. For a time this was seriously considered, but the proposal fell through. Then marketing and promotion tests were undertaken to see if the specialty journals could be successfully published on a subscription basis.

Meanwhile, discussions were held with some specialty societies to explore sale or merger possibilities. The idea of changing some of the specialty journals into quarterlies was dropped when it became evident that the new frequency would affect the editorial content and turn them into research-oriented rather than clinician-oriented publications. In the end, one of them, the *Archives of Environmental Health*, was sold in December 1975 to the Reed Education Foundation, located in Washington, D.C. No cash was included in the transaction, but the purchaser assumed the liability for the unfulfilled portion of some 3,500 prepaid subscriptions.

Eventually, the remaining nine specialty journals were retained and edited as before by outside physicians who, as editors, were responsible to the AMA's director of scientific publications. The journals were kept on a monthly basis, and the board authorized dues-paying members to receive one of them free along with *JAMA* and *AMNews*. In some cases the AMA insisted on revisions in editorial format, and in all of them an effort was made to enliven the graphics. "We spruced up the covers to generate a little excitement," Hannon recalls. "At that time it was important to let everyone know that we were still alive and committed to staying in the advertising side of the publishing business."[13] In a few cases, the editorial boards of the journals, which were autonomous, registered objections.

In March 1976 the AMA Board of Trustees found it necessary to assert its authority over the journals in a policy statement. The trustees reminded all concerned that the editor of each journal was appointed by the AMA and that, while he could choose his editorial board, the AMA, as publisher and owner, had complete and sole responsibility for the size of the publication, sale, acceptance of advertising, frequency, format, layout, subscription rate, distribution, and financial management.[14] One editor-in-chief, feeling a loss of authority, resigned.

Another aspect of the drive to control publishing expenses was a decision to tighten up on non-periodical publishing costs. These arose from a stream of pamphlets, brochures, booklets, and even books that was hard to limit. In past years the stream had flowed from the AMA's profusion of committees, councils, and semi-autonomous departments. There were prices on most of these publications that were often unrealistic, as were the estimates of expected sale. To effect a new policy requiring that the costs of such materials be self-liquidating, Hannon brought in a marketing director to develop reliable profit/loss estimates before the print orders were given out. That brought the flood under control and turned what had been a money-losing proposition into a moderately profitable activity. The AMA developed the capability of successfully merchandising medically-oriented books to the profession, especially such technical and authoritative offerings as *Current Procedural Terminology* (an updated, uniform terminology code for medical procedures) and *AMA Drug Evaluations*, a compendium evaluating some 1,300 drugs that, in its 1980 edition, had a sale of 36,000 copies at a price per copy of $54.

Partly to continue a *Today's Health* function—the health education of the public—and partly to test a possible new source of revenue, the AMA started a consumer book program under Charles C. Renshaw, the former editor of *Prism*, in 1977. Using its medical and editorial resources, the AMA developed manuscripts while an outside book publisher handled the printing, promotion, and sale. It proved to be a successful way for the AMA to get helpful, accurate medical information before the public while minimizing the high risks of book publishing. The risks were assumed by the publishing house; the AMA played the role of author, receiving compensation through publisher advances and royalties. Two of the first five books were especially successful: the *AMA Handbook of First Aid and Emergency Care* and the *AMA Family Medical Guide*.

Slowly at first, but with increasing rapidity after 1979, the financial performance of the publishing operation turned around. Many factors contributed to the improvement: the simple fact of the consolidation of functions under a publisher; the application of more business-like thinking; the upgrading of the sales staff; and a growth in the number of new pharmaceutical products coming to market, especially after mid-1981. Of great importance also was a publishing decision to provide ways by which advertisers could reach special segments of the total physician market through *AMNews* and *JAMA*. Starting in 1980 with *AMNews* and in 1983 with *JAMA*, both publications offered demographic advertising editions that reached a carefully tailored audience of practicing physicians in these categories: general practice, family practice, osteopathic physicians, internists, and cardiologists. Because so many drugs are frequently prescribed by the roughly 90,000 physicians in those categories, that segment of the physician population is highly desirable to many pharmaceutical advertisers. The new demographic capability made the AMA more effective in selling against commercial magazines that are tailored specifically to reach just that audience.

Helped by the new circulation options, the AMA publishing operation recovered the competitive edge that it lost early in the 1970s. From a low of $8.2 million in 1975, AMA advertising revenues (with three fewer publications) rose to over $20 million in 1982 and to $23.7 million in 1983. At the same time, the publications raised their share of the pharmaceutical advertising market from the 1974 low of 7 percent to 17 percent. It was a decisive comeback.

After the Heller study of the AMA's management problems in 1958, the association organized itself into half a dozen operating divisions, each with a large degree of autonomy, each reporting to the executive vice president. By the early 1970s the divisional system had grown to comprise eight major administrative units: the Divisions of Scientific Affairs, Scientific Publications, Medical Education, Medical Practice, Public Affairs, Communications, and Management Services, plus the Center for Health Services Research and Development. A sharp improvement over the disarray that preceded it, the system still had drawbacks, for it encouraged independent action by the divisions and made coordinated action difficult.

It was particularly hard for the divisional structure to correct for a condition that was inherent in the nature of the AMA: a vague perception of end-product on the part of employees. Those who work for an automobile manufacturer or an airline have a clear idea of what the company is doing, and it is therefore easy for them to understand the relationship between what they do and what those in another department do. But in an association like the AMA, as one employee put it, "nothing goes out the door," and, lacking a clear perception of corporate output, association employees tend to immerse themselves in their own disciplines and became isolated from one another. Under the divisional system it was easy for the various administrative units to do their own thing. Thus, when a project called for the efforts of more than one division, it often moved with uncertain speed. Like a convoy in wartime, the pace was determined by the slowest performer. It was easy for things to get bogged down at the AMA.

Ernest B. Howard, M.D., recognized the problem when he served as the executive vice president, and he appointed two assistant executive vice presidents to inject a higher degree of coordination into the system. From 1970 to 1974 the "medical" divisions—Scientific Publications, Scientific Activities, and Medical Education—reported to William R. Barclay, M.D., while the "socioeconomic" divisions— Medical Practice, Public Affairs, Communications, Management Services, and the Center for Health Services Research and Development—reported to Joe D. Miller. The supervision of the assistant executive vice presidents helped coordinate the projects and programs that crossed division lines. Nevertheless, the divisional system with its emphasis on semi-autonomous divisional directors required an unusual amount of coordinating. Managing it from the top absorbed time and effort.

The need for restructuring the staff organization had concerned the AMA for almost ten years. Immediately after the Medicare battle, the House of Delegates, of which Sammons was then a member, focused a great deal of attention on the AMA's organizational structure and especially its capabilities for future planning. Although most of the interest centered on proposals to alter the council-committee-Board of Trustees relationships, the way in which the staff was structured also came under question.

The background, which is sometimes difficult to follow, begins in 1967 with the appointment of a Committee on Planning and Development headed by George Himler, M.D., a delegate from New York. Submitted to the house at the November-December 1969 meeting, the Himler report gave the delegates a panoramic view of the medical issues of the day. Fifty-six pages long, it did all the things a planning analysis usually does. It defined long range goals and objectives, discussed current trends and legislation, looked toward the future, and examined the organization's ability to meet the challenges. But the report suffered in being a highly personal document. One member of Himler's committee, John H. Budd, M.D., submitted a polite but strongly worded minority report saying that the viewpoints and recommendations in the report differed sharply from his own ideas and what he believed to be the sentiments of the house. He found a great deal of the basic tone "unacceptable," and he said some of the proposals would, if adopted, lead to "far-reaching and epochal changes in the philosophy, policy, responsibility, scope of activity and commitment of the AMA."[15] Himler, for instance, suggested sharing the policy-making function of the AMA with a coalition of physicians, nurses, dentists, osteopaths, hospital representatives, and insurance executives in a proposed new National Academy of Health Professions. This, he said, would be the most effective way to secure socioeconomic data and formulate policy on health and medical issues in the future. The house paid little attention to that proposal, or most of the others for that matter, generally agreeing with Budd's position and his objections to the "air of apology and self-denunciation" that he felt characterized Himler's description of the AMA's actions preceding Medicare.[16]

But one thing did come out of the Himler report: a Council on Long Range Planning and Development, which was formally established through amendment of the bylaws at the June 1970 meeting. The new council was variously regarded. Some delegates thought it would strengthen the AMA by bringing on structural change and forcing the association to pay more attention to factors that would affect policy in the future. Others saw the council as another challenge by the house to the authority of the board. That touchy conflict was reflected in the original composition of the council. The board chose four members—two trustees and two at-large members of the AMA; the speaker of the house chose four—two delegates and two at-large members of the AMA; the president of the Student American Medical Association picked the ninth member from student AMA members.

Suspected at first of having little more than a political motivation, the council had difficulty establishing itself as the focal point for AMA planning activities.[17] The definition of AMA objectives and the adequacy of its resources, programs, and organizational structure to achieve them were widely considered to be functions of the board. Certainly the board felt that way.

Responding to the calls for reform and a constitutional convention made by President Hall in 1971 and 1972, the new council conducted open meetings for members in six cities to hear those with reforms to suggest. The effort seemed to be something of a waste of time, for many of the complaints were based on misconception or lack of information. The most commonly sought change, the direct election of state delegates to the AMA, was a matter squarely up to the state medical associations, not the AMA.

But the council gained stature after a professional consultant on planning, the Battelle Institute, was brought in to give the council some professional direction.[18] Battelle persuaded the AMA to start a new staff department, the Office of Planning, which eased the jurisdictional conflict between the council and the board. The trustees' decision-making powers were reaffirmed; the council's usefulness in spotting trends, analyzing outside factors that would affect medicine in the future, evaluating proposals, and developing recommendations was stressed. Working closely with Battelle, the council submitted a major report to the board and house that won approval at the June 1973 meeting as the design for a long range planning system.

In the following year, as the financial skies started to darken, the first cycle of the planning process designed by Battelle was completed. At that time, the AMA had developed the notion that it should split the planning effort into two areas: operational or staff planning; and critical issue planning, which was council-related business. The management staff focused first on operational planning, and this became known as program planning. It was also responsive to Sammons' urgent request for a way to get a firmer grip on the staff operation. At one meeting of those working on the development of the planning system, Sammons okayed the progress to date but added, "I need a management system too. We have to have a handle on the whole thing."[19]

Sammons felt uneasy, jeopardized by the pockets of autonomy that still operated within the AMA. Especially in the case of staff departments with links to long-standing councils and committees, he suspected that financial directives were being fudged and delayed, that maybe financial commitments were being made without prior authorization. Circumstances dictated a sort of tight, central control that the AMA had not found necessary before.

As the dimensions of the financial crisis widened, Sammons made his first moves to restructure the AMA staff. In September 1974 the two assistant executive vice presidents, Miller and Barclay, were promoted to deputy executive vice president to strengthen their authority, and Whalen M. Strobhar, who four years earlier had succeeded Miller as the director of the public affairs division, was promoted into a newly created position with the title of assistant executive vice president. The post included responsibility for a few functions that had been under the executive vice president for some time—staff services to the board and the house, and the administration of the AMA Education and Research Foundation. But Strobhar's new assignment encompassed a great deal more than that.

Reporting directly to Sammons and working from an office adjoining his, Strobhar had charge of what was, in effect, a new administrative unit within the AMA. It was a headquarters staff, and it was established to do a number of things, with emphasis on supervision of the many staff task forces appointed at this time to deal with various aspects of the crisis and on a careful oversight of financial performance. The new administrative unit also coordinated several interdivisional projects, leaving less opportunity for the bureaucratic isolation that could complicate and delay them. A few months after Strobhar's appointment, the newly named Office of Finance, as well as the Office of Planning, was placed under his jurisdiction. By expanding Miller's and Barclay's authority and especially by creating the new headquarters staff under Strobhar, Sammons dramatically strengthened the central management of the AMA. He was starting to find the management "handle" that he said he was looking for.

In a March 19, 1975, memorandum to the finance committee of the board, Sammons stepped back for a moment to summarize the administrative measures he had taken up to that point in response to the AMA's financial exigencies. He mentioned a budget committee "within the Office of the Executive Vice President" (i.e., Strobhar's operation) to review financial reports and projections on a monthly basis and more frequently when indicated. He alluded to what were called Key Indicator Reports, submitted on a weekly or biweekly schedule to monitor daily cash flow, size of payroll, status of membership, advertising revenue, travel expense, and editorial and production costs. He listed a number of staff committees set up to review such things as salary increases, hirings, and requests for printed materials. "The result of these multi-faceted efforts to control costs," Sammons concluded, "was a realized savings from budget of $711,932 for the first quarter, fiscal year 1975."

In July 1975, just after the house had raised dues for fiscal 1976, it was time for the staff to start the preparatory work on the 1976 budget. As the division directors were already aware, the process this time would rely on a new planning philosophy. Up to this point, when so much independent responsibility was vested in the individual division directors, they drew up their budgets for the year ahead with little guidance from senior management. They did not, for example, receive specific direction as to what the upper limits might be on dollars or personnel. They might have to justify a major increase in the level of their activity or argue hard for a new program or project. But within such limits there was considerable latitude for the exercise of judgment.

Partly a result of the financial crisis, partly a reflection of Sammons' preferences as to management style, and partly in response to the recommendations of the new Office of Planning, the AMA approach to its budgeting process changed abruptly. The new system shifted a far greater degree of initiative onto the senior managers, Sammons, Miller, Barclay, and Strobhar.

"What we designed," says Bruce Balfe, who headed the Office of Planning, "was a planning and budgeting system that called for going back to square one every year. We assumed that the AMA was not in business to support the existence of so many divisions with so many departments but to carry out certain programs."

In operation, the system began with top management making the early decisions: what the AMA would have available to spend on programs in the year ahead; what programs needed emphasis or de-emphasis to reflect board and house policy, or to keep AMA activities attuned to external, societal trends; and then, finally, what allocation of dollars to make for the program. After that, the division directors proceeded with their plans to implement the programs.

"Senior management now focused on the programs," says Balfe. "It started to manage programmatically. The divisional budgets became an outgrowth of the program decisions, not the other way around, which was what we had done previously. It was quite a departure."

The new budgeting system corrected what the Battelle consultants considered a major flaw in the AMA's operations. As the 1973 Battelle report noted, "Planning should be a two-way street, with guidance and information from the senior units of an organization flowing from the top down, and information, suggestions and specific programs flowing from the bottom up. There tends to be a bottom-up bias in the Association."[20]

With the new emphasis on "top-down" management, Sammons, in the fall of 1975, moved to make even deeper changes in the organizational structure of the staff. His proposals, stated in a memorandum to the Board of Trustees for its consideration and approval, drew from consulting studies done by Arthur Young & Company, which had pointed out in its recent management letter, "Quite a few national associations and health care organizations have changed to a corporate form of executive management organization to clarify the organizational pattern of authority, span of control and functional program identification." Such an approach, the memo continued, would provide more clearly for the delegation of responsibility for the total operation of the AMA from the "governing and policy-making bodies to its chief executive officer."[21]

At its meeting late in August, the board approved the staff reorganization as proposed by Sammons. Miller's and Barclay's titles changed from deputy executive vice president to senior vice president; Strobhar retained his title of assistant executive vice president. Five new group vice presidencies were created, the positions filled by executives already on the staff, with the exception of the Group Vice President for Publishing, to which Thomas F. Hannon was appointed three months later. At the same time that Hannon was recruited, the AMA upgraded its financial operation and hired an outside financial executive, Jan W. Erfert, to expand and modernize its operation. "Dr. Sammons wanted a new level of professional management in finance," according to Erfert. "He was looking for someone to develop and put in place a new system of checks and balances and internal controls. He wanted someone who could tell the AMA where the organization was going rather than where it had been."[22]

By late 1976, when it was time to make his report to the House of Delegates, Sammons could say,

> The AMA is quite a different organization from what it was two years ago....The point that needs emphasis is not the achievement of a better financial condition so much as the change in underlying financial management that made it possible. Sharp changes have been made in the way the AMA now handles its finances, with emphasis on more detailed, thoughtful planning; zero-base budgeting—which means, basically, a rejustification of all programs each year; tighter day-by-day controls; and realistic, monthly reporting of financial condition. This new system of financial management evolved from a thorough study done by the AMA auditing firm, Arthur Young & Company. It is a departure from the way things used to be done; it should prevent the sort of crisis that arose two years ago; and it should provide a basis for an even closer rein on finances in the future...In terms of fiscal control and staff management's capacity to manage AMA finances, dramatic progress has been accomplished.[23]

Although there were subsequent modifications in the AMA's internal structure—notably one made in 1981 that revived the title of deputy executive vice president and put the AMA's business-oriented functions under one and its policy-oriented functions under another—the shift to tighter, more centralized management in 1975 set the administrative philosophy that the AMA followed during the rest of that decade and well into the next.

Of all the changes that resulted from the 1974-75 upheaval, none broke with tradition more abruptly than the revision made in the AMA's council and committee structure. From the beginning, for over a century, this was an essential part of the way the AMA did business. It was a point of origin for policy; it was a part of the association's decision-making process; it was the system by which the AMA addressed most issues, gathered opinions and, above all, developed consensus.[24]

Many of the councils and committees could, of course, point to proud accomplishments, and many of them continued to meet a genuine need. But, on the other hand, many had outlived their usefulness and, to perpetuate themselves, focused their attention on matters of narrower and narrower interest. Some of the older and more powerful councils had extended their influence into the staff structure, establishing independent and strongly rooted fiefs. Because some were councils and committees of the board, while others were councils and committees of the house, they played a part in the mutually destructive feuding that went on. Useful as they were as forums for the airing of diverse opinion, the councils and committees tended to produce compromise positions rather than leadership. They were slow to act. At a cost of somewhere between $1 million and $2 million a year, they were expensive to maintain. And they were certainly numerous. The *Proceedings* of the 1965 annual meeting listed thirteen councils, sixty-five committees, six joint committees (with other organizations), and one subcommittee.

At least as early as 1968 there was evidence of a desire to cut back. A resolution adopted by the house in June that year asked the board to make recommendations as to the consolidation or "even abolishment" of councils or committees "whose reason for creation may no longer exist."[25] Little came of that, however; there were sixty-nine councils and committees in 1969 compared to the sixty-eight identified at the time the resolution was adopted a year earlier. Terminating a council or committee does create breakage. Especially in a small, democratically structured organization where people know each other, termination can be a bruising exercise, testing personal relationships and causing hurt feelings. It usually takes a combination of circumstances to bring about change.

It is safe to say that the AMA leadership had mixed feelings about the councils and committees. There was general agreement that there were too many but no agreement at all on which ones, specifically, to drop. The duality of attitude within the AMA is apparent from a brief examination of a management study done in 1969 by the firm of Cresap, McCormick and Paget.[26] At the time of Blasingame's departure, the board chairman, Burtis E. Montgomery, M.D., talked about "the complex operational needs" of the AMA, a demand for "other managerial skills," and the need for "an analysis of the AMA operations." Whatever the motives, Cresap took on the task, designing a three-phase study. When the house met that June, Cresap had completed a report on the first phase, which was distributed to the delegates.

The newly appointed executive vice president, Ernest B. Howard, M.D., took exception to what Cresap had to say, maintaining in a critique sent to the board that the consultants, accustomed to analyzing the operations of for-profit corporations, simply had no understanding of something organized as the AMA was. "The consultants," Howard charged, "seem unfamiliar with the structure of a federation and are therefore confused by it." The report, he suggested, was filled with "comparisons of chalk with cheese." Moreover, he said, "Cresap concludes that the AMA is inefficient in a number of areas because it does not function as a corporation...the councils and committees are somewhat disturbing, in that they parallel no groups extant within a corporation...the House of Delegates, as the consultants see it, is the Riddle of the Sphinx."[27]

Despite Howard's point, which had a certain validity, the Cresap report had two criticisms of the councils and committees that could not be dismissed as misunderstandings. First of all, argued Cresap, the role of the councils and committees was confusing, contributing to "the absence of a clear delineation of responsibility for policy development." That some councils reported to the house and others to the board made the matter even more complicated. In reply, the board said it certainly had no intention of changing anything. "The council and committee structure of the association is complex," it acknowledged. "This system has been considered by the house on numerous occasions and the house has not chosen to change it. The Board of Trustees accepts this ruling. The need is to recognize the unique nature of the AMA, its positive attributes as an organization, the widespread diffusion of participation, the grassroots, federated character... "[28]

In its other criticism, Cresap called the number of councils and committees "excessive." The board accepted this point, saying, "The basic criticism of the duplication, overlapping and absence of identifiable priorities is valid. This matter is well known to the Board of Trustees and the House of Delegates." But, the board added, it did not want to destroy the democratic qualities of the council-committee system by imposing "efficiency" on it. The whole duplication problem would improve, the board promised, as soon as the new system of project-oriented budgeting went into effect.[29] Emphasizing its strong negative reactions to the Cresap report, particularly what it had to say about the council-committee structure, the board not only took no action but terminated the arrangements with Cresap before it could move on to phases two and three of its proposed study.

By late 1972, though, it was a different story. Financial pressures had mounted and, faced with another deficit year, the board abruptly discharged ten councils and committees, all of which were councils and committees of the board.[30] Objections arose, the loudest from a few members of the disbanded Council on Drugs.

Over recent years, this council had managed to make itself unpopular—with members of the board, the house, and the staff department of drugs. Board Chairman Max H. Parrott, M.D., recalls, "The council had been trying for three years to develop a formulary. They spent about $3 million on the project, and it hadn't gotten off the ground. I was a member of a board review committee which wanted to get the council moving more quickly on the first edition of *AMA Drug Evaluations*. We ramrodded through a three-man editorial panel to end the way they took a council vote on every damn sentence in the book as it was being developed."[31]

Worse, there were people on the council who were very rigid in their attitudes about combination drugs—what the council called "irrational mixtures." When the first edition of *AMA Drug Evaluations* did appear in 1971, it was full of "not recommendeds" for what it termed "irrational mixtures." Many of these drew complaints from the pharmaceutical manufacturers (who had already had to meet the FDA safety and efficacy standards) and from practitioners who found combination drugs (those that contain more than one active ingredient) convenient, practical, and efficacious. Parrott remembers that the first edition set off "a big yow-yow" in the house. John C. Ballin, Ph.D., the staff director of the Division of Drugs, thought that the council was more of a hindrance than a help. "There were some good people on the council," he says, "and some who were marginal."

The trouble was that they were not really giving the staff what it needed for the second edition: scientific input. For that, the AMA staff people were having to rely more and more on outside consultants. "It was difficult to write a book," said Ballin, "and do all the research and then have the council sit and nitpick. And that's what it did. The members tinkered with the editing and the spelling and the grammar instead of concentrating on supplying us with the scientific information we needed."[32]

Unmistakable as the financial pressures were as a factor in the council-committee restructuring in 1975, the changes also have to be understood in another context. Over time, as the profusion of councils and committees broadened, it came to symbolize what many AMA leaders perceived to be a lack of well-defined objectives, a feeling expressed from time to time that the AMA was not structured properly and did not really know where it was going. In 1967 when the house voted to establish a permanent Committee on Planning and Development (the Himler Committee), it hoped "to get the subject of better planning on the table and keep it there."

The only existing declaration of mission, in Article II of the constitution, called for the AMA "to promote the art and science of medicine and the betterment of public health." In the words of a consultant at the time, that was "as big as all outdoors." Through the new committee, the board hoped to initiate the first and perhaps critical step in the development of long range plans for the association—namely, the clarification of objectives. The Himler report disappointed those hopes, and for a while so did the reports of the Council on Long Range Planning and Development. But with the Battelle study, adopted as administrative policy by the house at the 1973 annual meeting, progress began.[33]

In addition to Battelle's urgings of "top down" management, the Office of Planning argued for management on a program basis and called for planning efforts at the policy level, that is, by the Board of Trustees and the Council on Long Range Planning and Development. This process began with the identification of a limited number of AMA "missions," each a category of activity as well as what might be considered an ongoing association goal, or "mission." As developed by the council, approved by the board, and adopted by the house in 1973, they were:

- direct service to the public;
- scientific service to physicians;
- promoting the effective delivery of care;
- assuring quality;
- representing the profession; and
- strengthening the AMA as an organization.

The next step in the planning process was the formation of six Mission Groups, each of which included a trustee and a representative of the Council on Long Range Planning and Development. Their job was to review the work of the councils, committees, and staff departments and to amalgamate their unit plans into mission plans. These, in turn, would go to the board, which was charged with drawing up an annual "AMA plan" for submission to the house. Inevitably, as the members of the Mission Groups went about their assignments, they came to conclusions about the way the councils and committees fitted into the AMA's operations. In making preliminary recommendations to the board at its October 1974 meeting, the council, whose members had served on the Mission Groups, suggested sweeping changes in the council-committee structure. Unlike the 1972 changes, these were not motivated by financial considerations but by a desire to see the work of the councils and committees merged into the framework of goals and priorities as expressed in the planning process. The recommendations went to the board with a vigorous endorsement from Sammons and his senior management staff.

"AMA should be reviewed," the council report to the board said, "with a view toward operating with a relatively small number of permanent committees directed toward broad areas of concern. As a particular problem or issue arises which calls for a special study, an ad hoc committee should be appointed for that purpose and should be given a specific charge and a specific time frame. These could operate under the auspices of the board or one of the permanent committees."[34]

Alarmed by the scale of the deficits that loomed before it in late 1974, the board welcomed the recommendation. It served to support a major action the trustees took that October, a recommendation prepared for the house that in order to bring the 1975 budget into line the AMA should discontinue two councils and eighteen committees of the board and, additionally, eleven committees that reported to councils of the house. As described in the preceding chapter, that recommendation was swept under at the Portland meeting, and a special committee of the house was appointed to decide, among other things, what should or should not be done about the council-committee structure.

In developing its recommendations for the June 1975 meeting, the special committee conducted a thorough analysis of the AMA's structure, operation, and programs. It broke down the allocation of dollars in three different ways: according to the six missions; according to a list of six priority items identified by the board and house in Portland (e.g., alleviation of the problems of professional liability); and according to five broad categories of activity (e.g., medical education, scientific activities, etc.). What the special committee was exploring were ways by which the AMA could reduce the size of its council-committee structure, eliminate the dual lines of responsibility (some to the board, some to the house) and bring council-committee efforts into harmony with the missions and priorities of the association as a whole.[35]

In its final report, the special committee recommended, and the house adopted, recommendations that the councils and committees (with the exception of the advisory committees of the Council on Medical Education) marked for deletion the previous October and November remain inactive and without budget, that the material the special committee had developed on structural reorganization be turned over to the Council on Long Range Planning and Development, and that that council submit a reorganization plan for the AMA to be considered at the next meeting of the house.[36]

Included in the material given to the Council on Long Range Planning and Development was a copy of a presentation that Sammons had made in April to the special committee. A section with the subhead, "Staff vs. Committee Approach to Programs," outlined his thinking on what the future role of the councils and committees should be. He told the committee:

> The choice of whether a particular activity should be pursued by staff or by a committee, is not cut and dried and does not present a mutually exclusive set of choices. Virtually all activities currently conducted by councils and committees could be handled by the staff through the use of appropriate consultants to advise on matters that require professional judgment. By the same token, almost any staff activity could be expanded to include a role of some kind of committee activity...the needs of the organization determine the kinds of mechanisms that will be needed. If the AMA is likely to be faced with an increasing number of 'quick decision' situations, as many of us feel will be the case, then something other than the traditional committee approach will be needed. This was one of the factors that led to management's recommendation to the board that, in many cases, ad hoc committees and ad hoc consultants should be used in the future instead of permanent committees.[37]

The Council on Long Range Planning and Development, the special committee of the house, the board, and Sammons were all thinking along the same lines: that the profusion of councils and committees should be pruned down to a few councils—maybe five or ten— with powers to appoint ad hoc committees or call in consultants as special needs arose. The example they used to illustrate how successful this method of operation could be was the experience with the staff of the Division of Drugs after the discharge of the Council on Drugs in 1972. "It should be clearly understood," said a board report a few months after that decision, "that the termination of a standing committee, for example, [the Council] on Drugs, does not mean that the AMA has withdrawn from that area of concern." The report suggested that the staff, with the help of consultants, could function effectively, completing succeeding editions of *AMA Drug Evaluations* as well as meeting the AMA's other obligations in the field without the existence of a council. In this case, and presumably others, the council was redundant.

Assembling in the hotels that line Waikiki beach shortly after Thanksgiving 1975, the delegates looked forward to a relaxed meeting. The anger and recriminations of Portland had passed. The really tough decisions had been made in Atlantic City the preceding June. Of the internal issues that had been raised just a year before, the only one that now remained to be settled was the future of the council-committee structure.

A consensus had developed in the months preceding the meeting that was strongly supportive of the proposals for radical change. Accordingly, when the key recommendation from the report of the Council on Long Range Planning and Development was read to the house—"that the AMA function with as few standing councils as possible and use committees with specific goals and limited time-frames to address specific issues whenever possible"—there was not a word of discussion before it was adopted. Approving related recommendations, the house reduced the whole AMA structure—sixty-seven councils and committees at the time of the Portland meeting—to just eight councils. Without debate, the house at one stroke altered the form and revised the operating methods of a hallowed AMA institution.[38]

But one controversial matter still had to be resolved: would the eight surviving councils be councils of the house or councils of the board? The old jealousies between house and board were not dead. The recommendation of the Council on Long Range Planning and Development envisioned councils "of the AMA" elected by the house but reporting to the board. To many of the delegates this meant councils "of the board." An amendment to have the new councils be elected by the house and report to the house, clearly creating councils "of the house," opened up the conflict. For once, the power struggle was out in the open for all to see.

In the end, it was George Himler, M.D., of New York who had the compromise language that his fellow delegates could agree on. His amendment called for councils "of the AMA" elected by the house but reporting "through" the Board of Trustees. One of the board members, Jere W. Annis, M.D., who had been arguing the board's case to have the councils report to the trustees, wanted to know the difference between reporting "to" and reporting "through."

Himler was ready for the question. He said,

> I think we cannot invest authority in one or the other; we have to work out a working relationship with both. This we have failed to do over time, and this is why I introduced [this amendment] in this manner.
>
> Perhaps [the idea] is a little vague, but nevertheless this gives you a framework which the board and the house can finally reach some agreement on. I think they both ought to accept this. Neither one is getting what it fully desires, and I think neither one probably should.
>
> I don't know if that answers your question, Dr. Annis, but that is the way I feel about it.[39]

The house gave him an enthusiastic round of applause and adopted his wording. Although the AMA made one additional deletion, dropping the Council on Continuing Physician Education in 1981 when the AMA recognized the increased role of the specialty societies in this area, the council-committee structure as adopted in 1975, with its house-board alignment as modified by Himler, has proved to be workable and durable.

It is hard to overstate the importance of some of the decisions made during the 1974-75 crisis. In some cases, of course, the impact is easy to understand, just as the necessity for making the decisions was obvious. That would apply to the assessment, the dues increase, and the changes made in the management of the publications. Those decisions were not complex; but they were difficult—because of the political undercurrents within the AMA. But some of the other things done in those two years had a more subtle and lasting impact on the association, especially in respect to its policy-making process.

The rebuilding of the AMA's financial reserves had special significance, liquid reserves being to a corporate management as tactical reserves are to a military command. Reserves accomplish two things: they protect against unforeseen, adverse developments, and they permit the flexibility needed to maneuver, to act quickly, to exploit opportunity. Sammons was insistent on the importance of reserves when he made his presentation to the special committee in

April 1975. "Any dues increase," he said, "must be large enough to buy the speedy re-establishment of an adequately funded liquid reserve. As executive vice president of the organization, I must state plainly that we need at least $20 million in liquid reserves, and I shall do everything I can do to accumulate it as soon as possible."[40]

The prompt restoration of liquid reserves enabled the AMA to commit itself to several important, lengthy, and expensive legal actions at this time. Had the association's finances remained strained, it would have been difficult to contest the actions as vigorously as it did. These actions included a long dispute with HEW over utilization review regulations, the complaint of anti-competitive practices issued by the Federal Trade Commission in late 1975, and an antitrust suit alleging a conspiracy to monopolize health services brought by chiropractors in 1976.

This case, referred to usually as the Wilk case, initially resulted in a jury verdict favorable to the AMA and sixteen co-defendants in 1981. An appeal was argued in 1982, with a decision against the AMA in late 1983. The case was sent back for retrial.

Quickly improved reserves also made it possible for the AMA to respond to the menacing medical liability situation by starting the American Medical Assurance Company. This wholly-owned subsidiary was initiated by action of the House of Delegates in 1975, at a time when the commercial insurance companies were either abandoning the medical liability field or raising premiums to levels that staggered the profession. In many states, physicians formed their own insurance companies, and, when sources of commercial reinsurance grew tight, the AMA launched its own company to assist the physician-owned companies. The AMA's investment in this subsidiary, originally $5 million, stood at nearly $11.5 million in 1983.

The AMA also committed some of its growing reserves, for investment purposes, to the accumulation of additional real estate. It expanded its holdings in the neighborhood of its Chicago headquarters to ten acres and entered the Washington market with the purchase of two properties there. One of them, a 12-story office structure that the AMA built and completed in 1982, houses the association's Washington office on its top two floors. The other involved the purchase and renovation of an office building on E Street, across from FBI headquarters and adjacent to Ford's theater.

But of the many decisions made in that period, none changed the AMA more radically than the revision made in the council-committee structure. In the 1940s and 1950s, the activities of the councils and committees predominated. With the exception of those who worked on the publications and in some other departments, the staff worked at their direction. "A lot of the decision-making," in Joe Miller's opinion, "was then strictly seat-of-the-pants stuff. And if you asked yourself, 'What is the AMA?', the answer was, 'The sum of all those independent, autonomous activities.'"[41] That changed slowly, more rapidly after 1958.

"Most of the fiefdoms had been eliminated by the time I came in," Sammons recalls. "But we still had a top-heavy superstructure. The thing that let us get rid of it was the money problem. The pressures of reorganization in 1974 and 1975 changed the system completely, and that would have been impossible without the financial crisis. The change in direction, in management, in the way policy is developed, is a landmark in the history of the AMA. Retrospectively, the financial crisis, in my view, turned out to be the best thing to have happened to the AMA in fifty years."[42]

With the elimination of so much of the council-committee structure, it is easy to conclude that a great deal of physician participation in the AMA was eliminated too. That is not true, for the board and the surviving councils have made extensive use of ad hoc committees and consultants. For example, the most important contribution the AMA made to the socioeconomics of medicine in the late 1970s and early 1980s undoubtedly came from the National Commission on the Cost of Medical Care, one of the ad hoc appointments. According to Sammons, the AMA would not have been able to find the resources for that commission had the association still been supporting the previous council-committee structure.

Another example of the AMA's revised method of operation was the new Council on Scientific Affairs. Through the use of ad hoc advisory panels, this council involved hundreds of physicians in the development of the fifteen to twenty reports it generated annually, and its assessment of diagnostic and therapeutic technology. These provided analyses of current medical and technological subjects with the help of recognized experts in the field. Operating this way, rather than through a profusion of semi-permanent, narrowly focused committees (e.g., the former Committee on Cutaneous Health and Cosmetics), the AMA made its scientific activities far more relevant to the needs of its broad membership.

With a more central direction imposed on the work of the AMA through the various staff reorganizations as well as the restructuring of the council-committee system, the role of the staff in the policy-making process expanded considerably. "We created a new environment," Miller observed in 1981. "The birth of an idea can now take place anywhere—within the staff, in the house, in a council, in the board. After it has been kicked around and received endorsement officially, then it comes to the staff in the form of work orders, so to speak. The way we are organized now, we can put together the battle plan. We can make sensible decisions on timing and on the amount of resources to spend. We can coordinate things. We can go back and suggest modifications if they seem to be called for. We now have an understanding of the AMA as a whole, not as a number of pieces."

What about Sammons' view of his role as the executive vice president? Before his election to the office, he certainly had the chance to study it from a variety of perspectives—as a dues paying member, local medical society president, delegate, trustee, state medical association president, and chairman of the AMA board. Moreover, he had long exposure to the management styles of his two predecessors, Blasingame and Howard. "Sometimes," he said in a 1980 interview, "I think my role is somewhere between being another full-fledged voting member of the board and being an objective, dispassionate arbitrator of all the various viewpoints that come before the board. Staff does not get in trouble by pushing something too hard or too fast. It never gets in trouble when it says to the board, 'Now, do whatever you want. But here are the facts of the case and here are our recommendations, which we are prepared to defend.' The problems come when the staff fails to stand up and state candidly what its beliefs are."

A strong executive himself and a believer in a centralized staff operation, Sammons recognized a boundary between staff initiative and policy-making. That is not to say, however, that the two processes remained walled off from each other. Because it is the one element within the AMA whose involvement in issues and events is continuous, the staff can frequently see places where there is a need to modify existing policy or adopt a new position. Using its own capabilities to assemble data and marshal arguments, the staff can go to appropriate councils or to the board to present a case for a policy change. Thus, the staff, while not making policy, has become significantly more active in its formation.

To distinguish the role of policy-makers from that of staff members, a nautical analogy has sometimes been used, with one group equated to the owners of a ship, the other to the crew. The analogy is useful up to a point. The crew is, supposedly, the operational group, committed to a destination chosen by the owners, knowledgeable about the ropes and wise in the ways of the sea. But the crew is essentially executing a strategy set by the owners.

Asked if he would accept that description as a way to distinguish the functions of the staff from those of the board and the house, Sammons offered a modification. "It is a policy decision, a decision of the house or the board, to say, 'We want to go from Point A to Point B.' But the *way* you get from A to B," he said, "how you get from one place to the next, that is a management decision. That is a responsibility of the staff."

Part IV

Interfaces

The AMA and Education

If you look at the pie chart that the AMA financial staff prepares each fall to make its annual budget presentation for the House of Delegates, you will notice a wedge that carries the label, "maintain educational standards." One of the eight principal categories into which the AMA divides its activities, it is, at something over $8 million, neither the largest nor the smallest item in the budget. But from the perspective of history it is a particularly important one, for it was to upgrade American medicine and improve public health that the AMA was formed in 1847.

Since then, the AMA has pursued those goals with praiseworthy achievements in many fields—nutrition, public health and safety, pure foods and drugs. But it is in medical education that the AMA's *pro bono publico* efforts have accomplished their most dramatic results, and it is largely through its insistence on high standards of medical education that the AMA has helped raise the quality of American medical care. Although it was clearly a pioneer in demanding excellence in medical education, the AMA did not accomplish its goals single-handedly; in no other profession or occupation have the members participated so actively in the training of their future colleagues, and nowhere else have so many professional organizations intervened so forcefully in the development and monitoring of educational standards. While responsibility for them has come to be shared, the AMA nevertheless retains a leadership role.

Though hardly noticeable to the individual himself or herself, the AMA's mark on the medical educational process can be sensed at every stage of the physician's long educational journey. The influence, in fact, begins to be felt even before entrance into medical school, at about the time a prospective medical student starts examining the entrance requirements. The student will generally find that he or she will have to complete most if not all of college, with a curriculum that includes a minimum number of science courses. Actually, the requirements vary from medical school to medical school, and by no means does the AMA set them. However, in part at least, they take the shape they do because of something the AMA did years ago.

Around 1900, only a few medical schools required any college at all, and most of them did not even demand that those entering complete high school. That began to change around 1905 when the AMA Council on Medical Education developed and published in *JAMA* what it considered a minimum and an ideal standard for medical education.[1] Up to that point only five of the 160 medical schools then existing in the United States required any college-level exposure to the biological and physical sciences before admission. But with the council's early reforms, more and more medical schools set their requirements higher, and leading schools demanded at least one college year in 1914, two in 1918. By the 1940s, nearly all the medical schools required completion of three years of college, and today about 95 percent of entering medical students have their B.A. or B.S. degrees.[2] Although the admission standards recommended by the AMA have been less stringent than those of most medical schools—the AMA standards are minimums—the knowledge level at which a medical school education begins has risen steadily from the time the Council on Medical Education started making its first recommendations.

If you consider as a unit the course of study that the student follows up to the point of licensure today, you will find that it conforms generally to the ideal standard drawn up by the Council on Medical Education in 1905. There have been important changes, of course, and responsibility for various parts of the curriculum has shifted. Yet in broad outline, medical education today reflects the principles expressed in these 1905 "ideals:"

- college-level study of the basic sciences—physics, chemistry, and biology;
- two medical school years in the laboratory sciences—such as, anatomy, physiology, microbiology, pathology, pharmacology;
- two medical school years in the clinical branches of medicine—surgery, obstetrics, pediatrics, internal medicine, and others "in close contact with patients in dispensaries and hospitals;" and
- one year of graduate education in a hospital.

The concept of American medical education derives from many sources. Philosophically, it is indebted to the emphasis on graduate education in the nineteenth century German universities, the reliance on hospital teaching in the British system, and the prevalence of preceptorship training in American colonial and frontier societies.[3] In practical terms, it owes a debt to the Johns Hopkins University School of Medicine, founded in Baltimore in 1893. Because of the way it was able to merge the best elements in those three traditions and because of uniquely high standards of student admission and faculty credentials, Hopkins soon established itself as the nation's premier medical school. It was therefore logical that the Council on Medical Education would carefully consider the Hopkins curriculum when it developed its statements of minimum and ideal standards for all schools in 1905. That is not to say that the AMA sought to replicate Johns Hopkins on a national scale. Rather, it was trying to define and establish essentials that would insure at least "acceptably" educated physicians. The AMA was interested in a basic framework general enough and flexible enough to allow the schools themselves to innovate, respond to regional needs, and develop individually.

The early guidelines were not an end but a point of departure for a series of increasingly rigorous educational criteria. In 1907 the council drew up a ten-point standard of medical school inspection. Among other things, it called for an examination of laboratory facilities and instruction, dispensary facilities and instruction, and hospital facilities and instruction. In 1909 the report of a committee of 100 physicians appointed by the council was adopted, describing a 4100-hour medical school curriculum that might serve as a model for schools wishing to upgrade their standards. And in 1910 came the first "Essentials of an Acceptable Medical College," a device used again and again by the AMA in the process of elevating standards. There were twenty-five original "essentials," covering such things as admissions standards, faculty qualifications, library facilities, grades, record-keeping, and attendance. The Essentials said further that a medical college should own or control a hospital so that students could come into "close and extended contact with patients under the supervision of the attending staff." The Essentials were revised eight times in the next forty-one years, to be superseded by the "Functions and Structure of a Modern Medical School" in 1957. This was revised in 1973; the word "modern" was dropped from the title. Then in 1976 the AMA and the Association of American Medical Colleges jointly developed a supplementary document, "Guidelines to Function and Structure of a Medical School."

A lay person glancing through these documents will come away impressed by the heavy stress put on practical, non-classroom experience. The various essentials deal not only with the availability of dispensaries and hospitals for teaching purposes, but also with the availability of laboratory animals and "sufficient dissecting material to enable each two students to dissect at least a lateral half of a human cadaver." The American medical student is exposed to the practicalities of medicine early, and it is this emphasis on first-rate clinical facilities and early clinical experience that distinguishes an American medical education from that given in other countries.

In order to base its evaluation of medical school curricula on first-hand information, the AMA has long relied on a program of on-site inspection visits. The first of these, actually a tour of all the 162 medical schools then existing in the country, was carried out in the 1906-1907 school year by various members of the Council on Medical Education, often in the company of its long-time secretary (1905-31), Nathan P. Colwell, M.D. A second tour was done during the 1909-1910 school year by Colwell and Abraham Flexner of the Carnegie Foundation for the Advancement of Teaching. This tour, on which the famed Flexner Report was based, included 131 schools then operating in the United States and, at their request, the eight Canadian Schools.* Through the Council on Medical Education, the AMA continued its program of site inspections of the schools until 1942. That year the council joined with the Association of American Medical Colleges (AAMC) to form the Liaison Committee on Medical Education and continue accrediting programs on a joint basis. For many years the two organizations had duplicated some of each other's work; the AAMC surveyed medical colleges periodically to see if they met the qualifications for membership, which in many instances paralleled the council's criteria.

In 1952 the liaison committee received federal recognition when the United States Department of Education needed an organization to designate approved medical schools so that veterans could use their G.I. Bill benefits to attend them. In 1968, the Department of Health, Education, and Welfare, through its Office of Education, certified the liaison committee as the official accrediting agency for undergraduate medical education. It was also recognized by the

*The medical education standards of the United States and Canada have been virtually the same ever since.

National Commission on Accrediting, the predecessor of the Committee on Postsecondary Accreditation, a private organization.

In 1983 the liaison committee consisted of six members representing the AMA's Council on Medical Education, six representing the AAMC, one Canadian member representing the Committee on Accreditation of Canadian Medical Schools, and two members of the public. In addition, on a non-voting basis, there were two medical students and one participant from the federal government. The expenses were shared equally by the AMA and the AAMC, and the staff responsibility and secretaryship alternated each year between the two sponsoring organizations.

Working with the liaison committee and making their reports to that committee, ad hoc site visit teams conduct regular surveys of the educational program at about twenty-five medical schools every year. The teams usually consist of four people, two designated by the Council on Medical Education (who tend to be teachers or clinicians), and two designated by AAMC (who tend to be medical school administrators). The process actually begins well in advance of the site visits, when the team reviews a self-study report that the schools are asked to complete several months before the site visit. Developed by the liaison committee in 1976, the self-study report consists of an elaborate and detailed set of forms basically asking the school to describe what it is trying to do and how it intends to accomplish its objectives. Faculty, students, administrators, and others are involved in the self-study process. The forms and narrative provide information not only about overall, long-term goals but also about the physical plant, the governing structure, and finances.

Having studied this material, the team makes a three- to four-day visit, talking at length with the department heads, senior and junior faculty members, and student groups, and examining the physical facilities—the laboratories, the libraries, the audio-visual centers, and the programs at affiliated hospitals. By studying objective data and quizzing students at random, visitors find it relatively easy to learn how well academic subjects are being taught. According to Leonard D. Fenninger, M.D., who retired in 1984 as the AMA vice president for Medical Education and Scientific Policy and a frequent site visitor in the past:

> The difficult part of a site visit is evaluating the educational experience the students are having with patients. That is really the crux of the whole business. You can find lots of documented evidence in

laboratory exercises and lecture schedules. You can look at the credentials of the teaching staff. You can walk through a lab and see students
working. But on the other hand, if you want to find out what the
students are learning clinically, I know of no way to do this other than
by going on rounds with the students and reviewing charts with them.

On the final day of the visit, the site team meets with the dean of
the school being surveyed and discusses the findings. The dean has
this opportunity to discuss what he or she might think are invalid
conclusions, bring up facts that may have been overlooked, and
correct errors. Following that, the site team and the dean meet with
a top administrator of the university of which the medical school is
a part to review the nature of the principal findings and the recommendations the site team plans to make.

Soon thereafter, the secretary of the site team writes a report
reflecting the views of the members. A confidential document,
it contains a description of the school's resources and programs,
observations on its strengths and weaknesses, suggestions for improvement, and recommendations regarding the accreditation of
the school's educational program. Often running to more than a
hundred pages, the reports usually include the recent accreditation
history of the school, tables of data, organizational charts, and
financial statements as well as the review of the site visitors. A draft
copy goes to the dean, who may circulate it to his staff for correc-
tions and comments. After that, the site team secretary prepares a
final version of its report, which is sent to individual members of
the Executive Council of the AAMC and members of the Council on
Medical Education for their comments. The liaison committee then
receives its copy of the report for action at its next meeting.

The liaison committee has a number of options. It can, of course,
decide to remove a school's accreditation. But that rarely happens.
Accreditation, though voluntary, is considered so important by the
schools that warnings of deficiencies usually get action. After 1948
there were no unaccredited schools until 1979, when one opened in
Puerto Rico. In cases where several substandard conditions are evident, the liaison committee can, and occasionally does, grant accreditation with probation and requests progress reports on what
is being done to correct serious deficiencies. What usually happens, though, is accreditation for varying lengths of time, up to
a maximum of ten years, depending on the problems the school
is encountering.

In addition to the approximately twenty-five regular site visits per year, about ten additional surveys are made. These are either limited and consultive surveys done at a school's request usually to deal with specific or short-range problems, and surveys conducted yearly to establish initial accreditation for new schools that have not yet graduated their first class.

Having completed a course of undergraduate education in which the AMA has shown enduring interest, and having received the M.D. degree, the young physician almost always proceeds directly to the first year of graduate training, after which he or she becomes eligible for licensure. This is another rite of passage that might be different without past actions by the AMA.

For much of the nineteenth century, medical licensure, where it existed at all, was a haphazard procedure. It was performed in a variety of ways—by practicing physicians for their apprentices, by professors after a course of lectures, by state medical societies, by the medical schools (including the dubious ones), and in some states by licensing boards.[4] From the time of its founding the AMA urged that the licensing function be separate from the educational process, and during the last two decades of the century it called for the wider establishment of state licensing boards, empowered to decide on qualifications and conduct examinations. Helped when the AMA delegates persuaded local medical societies to back the appropriate legislation, the concept of licensure by independent state medical boards took hold. In time, most of the states came to a general conclusion that three criteria for medical licensure should be met: graduation from an approved, recognized, or accredited medical school; a year of graduate work in an approved program in a hospital; and the successful completion of an examination.

Although a contemporary doctor would regard those accomplishments as minimal, American physicians enter a profession whose scientific stature is widely admired, and when they start taking care of patients they find those patients have an extraordinary confidence in their qualifications. During the early decades of the twentieth century, before the reforms initiated by the AMA took effect, that was not the way it was.

The AMA's motives for reforming undergraduate medical education have been variously ascribed.* Some journalists and a few

*See chapters one and twelve.

historians[5] have stressed economic factors to the exclusion of others, insisting that the deprecation of "overcrowding" in the profession by some AMA leaders proved a desire to create and maintain a scarcity of physicians, thereby (presumably) insuring high fees. These analysts like to point to the supposed leverage the AMA established over the schools, reinforcing the argument that what the AMA really wanted to accomplish was a reduction in the number of schools and physicians. The schools needed the approval of the Council on Medical Education because the students sought the approved schools, and the reason the students did so was that more and more of the state licensing boards required graduation from an approved school as a condition of licensure. Thus, the reasoning goes, through the prevalence of higher licensing requirements—something the AMA was strongly encouraging—the AMA was able to control medical education. The argument offers a certain tidiness for those who like to explain human behavior in terms of Adam Smith, but it omits other and more significant factors.

While undoubtedly responsive in some degree to the calls of self-interest, physicians are more strongly motivated by their pride in being a doctor and their sense of professional responsibility. That is a view held by many physicians, and strongly held by C. H. William Ruhe, M.D., who has spent more than forty years in medical education, part of it as the Dean of Admissions at the University of Pittsburgh School of Medicine, part of it, before retirement, as the AMA senior vice president for Medical Education and Scientific Policy. He says,

When the AMA was established in 1847, the idea was to form an organization that would improve at least two things: the ethical conduct of practitioners and the quality of education in medicine. Doctors were saying, "My God, look at medicine! We've got all kinds of people out there practicing and calling themselves doctors. And they're a disgrace. Let's form an association and set up some standards."

That *can* sound like someone trying to save his skin or fatten his purse, but I don't think so. Pride is involved; so is the physician's desire to stand out and excel. The whole idea of a profession is to improve performance. Being part of a profession means something to a lot of people—lawyers, engineers, architects and physicians especially. And it is one of the criteria of a profession to have a mechanism by which to judge the standards of entry into the profession, the quality of professional education and levels of performance and ethical conduct.[6]

In Ruhe's opinion, it was the concern over professional standards, not a desire for economic advantage, that underlay the drive for higher educational standards.

If the physicians' professional concern ran that deep, it is fair to ask why the AMA did not act sooner than it did. Certainly conditions warranted action well before 1905. Actually, the AMA did call for reform measures early, taking the position that licensing and education should be separately conducted (1866) and later successfully advocating universal establishment of state licensing boards (1883).

That no further actions occurred until they did may be explained by several factors. Medicine was a relatively young science until well into the second half of the nineteenth century, and it was not until the advances in bacteriology and other sciences—and acceptance of the germ theory of disease—that people showed a strong interest in their physician's scientific qualifications. Then there was the state of the AMA itself. Before 1901 it was not nearly as effective an organization as it became when it reorganized itself into a broadly representative, formally structured federation whose actions carried a more convincing legitimacy. Finally, there was the role of *JAMA*. Under George H. Simmons, M.D., appointed to the editorship in 1899, *JAMA* took on a fresh vigor. When Simmons compiled the data from all the state examining boards and began in 1905 to identify the medical schools whose graduates had the highest failure rates on their licensing examinations, the publicity directed at those schools was, in the word of the day, pitiless.

It must be remembered, too, that the AMA's major reform measures took place when a number of other institutions were being reformed. This was the decade of the muckraker—of Ida Tarbell and her exposure of Standard Oil, of Lincoln Steffens and *The Shame of the Cities*, of Upton Sinclair and *The Jungle*, of Samuel Hopkins Adams and his magazine series, "The Great American Fraud," on patent medicines and quackery. Committed to a popular campaign of trust-busting, Republican President Theodore Roosevelt was assailing those he called "malefactors of great wealth." The states were instituting such reforms as initiative, referendum, and recall and providing for the direct election of United States Senators by voters rather than appointment by the state legislatures. The Pure Food and Drugs Act was passed, along with early laws to protect the environment.

It is difficult to ignore the presence of the Progressive Era in American history, for this was the context in which the upgrading of medical education took place. AMA policy in this instance coincided with the strong sweep of public opinion, and the combination was difficult to oppose. The time was right for reform, and that must be taken into account when the motives underlying the AMA's drive to reform medical education are interpreted.

Hardly had the Council on Medical Education organized its efforts to lift the standards of undergraduate education than the matter of graduate medical education presented itself. Although somewhat similar programs existed earlier, often designed more for the benefit of the hospital than the training of the participant, the internship (one year of general, hospital-based training) and the residency (succeeding years of hospital-based training in one of the specialties) became part of formal American physician training only after the start of the Johns Hopkins Hospital in 1889 and the Johns Hopkins University School of Medicine in 1893. By 1910, spurred on by the Hopkins example and the Council on Medical Education's ideal standard, over 70 percent of graduating medical students were seeking internships.[7] The word comes from the French *interne*, common to medicine in France in the nineteenth century.

Since the internship was just as much a part of a physician's education as the four undergraduate years, the Council on Medical Education extended its jurisdiction to include internship programs. The council recognized the need to identify hospitals that conducted acceptable internship programs in 1912* and published a list of approved internships in 1914. The first "Essentials of Approved Internships" followed in 1919. A year later, partly in recognition of the Council on Medical Education's expanded role in medical education programs conducted in a hospital setting, the AMA changed the council's name to the Council on Medical Education and Hospitals.**

*Pennsylvania became the first state to require an internship for licensure in 1914.

**The other reason was that the AMA, through the council, published a list of registered hospitals; that is, those it considered to be ethically run and capable of providing satisfactory patient care. In 1951, the AMA joined the American College of Surgeons (which had been inspecting the medical facilities of hospitals), the American College of Physicians, and the American Hospital Association to found the Joint Commission on the Accreditation of Hospitals. The reference to hospitals was dropped from the Council's name in 1963.

To set educational standards for the pre-licensure years, the AMA put in place a system of standards that operated on three levels. First, at the point of entry, there were academic minimums. Next, there was surveillance of the medical school and internship programs with continuing scrutiny of the curricula. And finally, there was independent evaluation of the end-product, administered by the state licensing boards. In developing the standards for graduate medical education, the AMA arrived at a similar three-tiered structure, but its establishment, in contrast to the relatively speedy creation of the undergraduate procedures, was to present a more complex challenge.

Specialization in medicine has been present from the beginning.[8] It was acknowledged by the AMA in 1859 when it divided those attending the educational sessions of its annual meeting into scientific sections. As new diagnostic and therapeutic techniques developed, the need to communicate and share new knowledge grew. Thus, between 1864 and 1888, six American specialty societies were founded, first by the ophthalmologists, then the otologists (ear specialists), followed by the neurologists, the gynecologists, the laryngologists, and the pediatricians. Several others were started in the nineteenth century, and there are more than 700 today. In early times, the qualifications for membership were minimal, in some cases as little as the completion of a single six-week graduate school course. Nevertheless, membership in a specialty society made it easier for a physician to assert his status as a specialist. But shortly after 1910, starting with the surgeons, medicine began actions that would give the term specialist a more exact meaning.

Leading surgeons at this time thought that too many operations were being performed by physicians who were not qualified to do them. What they wanted was a defined curriculum of graduate medical education in surgery for physicians desiring to become surgeons, and then a method of recognizing those qualified to do surgical work. Led by Franklin H. Martin, M.D., a man well known and recognized in the field, the surgeons decided that the best way to achieve their goal was to found a specialty society along lines quite different from the specialty societies that then existed in other branches of American medicine.

In 1912, they started the American College of Surgeons, modeled after the Royal College of Surgeons in England. Both the names and the concepts of the organizations were similar, the American College of Surgeons requiring its candidates for membership to undergo an extensive program of academic and practical training as specified by the college. As was the case with the Royal College, membership in the American College of Surgeons was intended, *by itself*, to identify someone qualified in the field of surgery.

Accordingly, in 1914, a physician who wanted to become a fellow in the American College of Surgeons had to complete an internship, serve three years as an assistant, give evidence of visits to a number of surgical clinics, and submit abstracts of 100 cases, in fifty of which he performed the operation, and in fifty of which he acted as the assistant. Once he had hurdled the membership barriers, the physician could put the letters F.A.C.S. after the M.D. following his name, announcing that he was a Fellow of the American College of Surgeons and thereby informing other physicians and prospective patients of established credentials as a specialist in surgery.

Four years later, partly to counter a competitive threat from optometrists, the ophthalmologists sought to formalize their specialty status. But when the two specialty societies, the American Ophthalmological Society and the American Academy of Ophthalmology and Otolaryngology, joined with the AMA Scientific Section on Ophthalmology to do so, they found a different means to the end. Distrustful of government, they did not want to rely on licensure as their mark of specialty competence, and they were wary of academic degrees as well because of the wide variations in the quality of the education provided at different educational institutions. Nor did they have much enthusiasm for launching another medical society, as the surgeons had recently done.

Instead, the three ophthalmological organizations combined to create a joint examining board to map out an educational program, appoint examiners, and conduct examinations. It was made up of people nominated in part by the AMA, in part by the specialty societies. The board was to grant a diploma to those who completed the program and met other requirements. Thus in 1917 the first certifying board in American medicine was incorporated—the Board of Ophthalmic Examinations, known after 1933 as the American Board of Ophthalmology. The two specialty societies agreed that in the future they would accept for membership only those holding diplomas from the board—diplomates, or, as they were more commonly called, board-certified ophthalmologists.

Meanwhile, the AMA was looking broadly at the whole field of graduate medical education. Before World War I it was not uncommon for an American physician to go abroad for graduate study, often to Edinburgh, Berlin, or Vienna. But just before the war began, growing attention started to focus on the opportunities available in the United States. The quality of graduate medical education here was uneven, ranging from eight-year surgical residencies at Johns Hopkins down to four-week courses conducted by proprietary (for-profit) medical graduate schools. No decisions had been made as to what sort of institutions should sponsor graduate medical education. Programs were being conducted in a variety of settings: universities, hospitals, and independent graduate schools. There was no decision either on where specialist credentialing should come from, despite the decisions of the surgeons and the ophthalmologists.

In 1913 the Council on Medical Education appointed a committee under Horace D. Arnold, M.D., dean of the Harvard Medical School's graduate program, to look at the quality of teaching at other postgraduate institutions; there were then some five or six university schools and about a dozen independent schools, such as the New York Postgraduate School and Hospital. Another committee, headed by Arthur Dean Bevan, M.D., the council chairman, and Louis D. Wilson, M.D., of the Mayo Foundation, was appointed in 1919 to survey the field again and come to some conclusions as to what was needed in graduate medical education. This committee's report, transmitted through the Council on Medical Education and adopted by the House of Delegates in 1920, found a large demand for graduate courses. About 6,000 physicians a year were taking short courses of study (four to six weeks), and about 4,000 others desired longer programs (two years or more). But the facilities, the report said, were "inadequate." The demand was legitimate but should not be met by the proprietary institutions. "It would be desirable," said the report, "for 15 or 20 strong university medical departments to consider the development of graduate medical departments." The need for more and better opportunities for hospital-oriented training was stressed.[9]

Later that year, to help the development of standards for residency programs in selected fields, the Council on Medical Education appointed fifteen committees "to recommend what preparation was deemed essential to secure expertness in each of the specialties"—internal medicine, pediatrics, neuropsychiatry, orthopedic surgery, dermatology and syphilology, surgery, ophthalmology, otolaryngology, urology, obstetrics and gynecology, public health and hygiene, anatomy, physiology, pharmacology and therapeutics, and pathology-bacteriology. In 1923 the council issued a document titled, "Principles Regarding Graduate Medical Education;" in 1927 the first listing of hospitals approved for residency training in various specialties appeared; in 1928—inevitably—came "Essentials of Approved Residencies." It sounded like an echo of what the AMA had done in undergraduate medical education beginning in 1905, but the differences were profound.

Despite the initial call for fifteen or twenty "strong university medical departments" to get involved, graduate medical education expanded around residency training programs conducted by the hospitals, many of them hospitals affiliated with medical schools and universities, but many of them free-standing or unaffiliated community hospitals. A unique and highly fragmented system of graduate medical education evolved. Instead of being concentrated in less than 100 medical schools, graduate medical education was eventually dispersed among nearly 2,000 hospitals—institutions that were dedicated primarily to providing medical care for sick people. Under an educational system that placed the emphasis on learning by doing, the wide involvement of the hospitals was inevitable. Although this was to make the standard-setting and monitoring difficult, the AMA did not appear to be particularly concerned over the hospitals' growing educational role. In the process of approving internships, the AMA had developed confidence in the teaching qualifications of the hospital staffs.

The significance of the fifteen committees appointed to develop the guidelines for the early residency programs in particular specialties in 1920 should not be overlooked. Their function duplicated one of those of the first examining boards, and they became the precursors of the thirteen additional examining boards that sprang into existence between 1930 and 1937.* This confirmed a strong new influence in American medical education.

In contrast to undergraduate medical education, where it was to prove easy to bring the two principals together into a joint accrediting organization—the Liaison Committee on Medical Education— the pursuit of a smoothly functioning, cooperative effort in graduate medical education was more elusive. One divisive factor was the number of different organizations that could legitimately demand a voice in the decisions. There was the AMA, which included mem-

*The second certifying board was established in 1924 by the otolaryngologists (ear, nose, and throat specialists). They generally followed the ophthalmologists' concept.

bers from all specialties, and which had written the Essentials and published an annual list of the residency programs it approved. There were the specialty examining boards, fifteen of them in the late 1930s. As the organizations that determined the questions for the candidates on the certification examination, each of them had a great deal to say about the educational experience the residents underwent. Then there was the American College of Surgeons, intent on the quality of training being given in the surgical specialties. There simply was no overall system of accreditation and monitoring during most of the 1930s.

To make the situation more difficult, there was a diversity of viewpoint regarding the whole purpose of specialty training and board certification. One school of thought held that the specialist should be very special indeed and believed that certification should be for an extremely high degree of excellence. Some of the specialty societies took that position, arguing that specialists should be a small elite, with the profession as a whole consisting predominantly of generalists. But other specialties, notably the surgical specialties, took an opposite view. The purpose of certification in their opinion was to recognize physicians who had successfully completed a rigorous specialty training program and satisfied academic requirements. This approach was far less elitist and restrictive, and contemplated a profession in which specialists could easily become a majority. Although individual programs ran smoothly, the general state of graduate medical education was one of turmoil, with conflicting claims as to where the accrediting authority belonged and opposing philosophies as to how far the specialization of the profession should proceed.

By 1940, however, the accreditation situation had improved. Ten of the specialty boards were cooperating with the Council on Medical Education in approving residencies. More significantly, the American Board of Internal Medicine and the American College of Physicians (respectively, the certifying board and the specialty society for internal medicine) and the AMA Council on Medical Education formed a joint committee to accredit residency programs in internal medicine. Interrupted by World War II, it was reactivated afterward and named the Residency Review Committee in Internal Medicine. The surgeons followed suit soon afterward, and during the 1950s a growing number of Residency Review Committees was established, each with positions for appointees from the AMA Council on Medical Education, the relevant specialty certifying board, and often the specialty society as well.

What evolved by the end of the 1950s was a three-tiered system for graduate medical education that was parallel in function to what the AMA had established for undergraduate medical education. There were qualifications for entry: the M.D. degree and the completion of an internship. Through the Residency Review Committees, there were standards for the educational programs and a surveillance procedure to monitor them. And finally, through the specialty board examination, there was an independent evaluation of the end-product. The Residency Review Committees, seventeen of them in 1960, theoretically provided a means by which both general and special interests could be served. It was a workable mechanism, but one that did not solve all of the problems.

As the profession continued to change from one dominated by generalists into one in which specialists constituted a growing majority, both patients and physicians were asking with increasing insistence: Whatever happened to the family doc of revered memory? To many people, especially those in large urban communities, he had almost vanished. Around 1910 there had been one general practitioner for every 600 people; now, fifty years later, there was only one for every 3,000.[10]

The explosive growth of knowledge in the biomedical sciences was greatly responsible, but so were the preferences of the patient. More and more frequently, he or she was taking family medical problems to a pediatrician, an obstetrician/gynecologist, or an internist. The recent crop of medical school graduates had also contributed to the trend. The general practitioner was someone the students scarcely encountered, either in the classroom or the teaching hospital, and when students started formulating career plans, they naturally turned to their specialist teachers as models. There was, moreover, the matter of prestige. Specialists, frequently accused of elitism, were condescending toward the general practitioner. "He provides medical care within the limits of his competence," they said.[11]

No one, least of all the AMA, was happy about the trend. While some physicians worried about what would happen if everyone became a specialist, others were asking, "How, exactly, do you define a 'general' physician?" The medical journals were full of pleas and plans to elevate the general practitioner—preceptorships, chairs, professorships, and residencies. In 1963, at the fifty-ninth

Congress on Medical Education, one of the five major topics was, "Family Practice—Impending Crisis."

The problem, however, went deeper than the mounting concern over specialization and the consequent fragmenting of the profession. Those close to medical education sensed an absence of broad leadership, a lack of direction to the conglomeration of forces that made up the nation's system of graduate medical education. Specifically, they believed one of the most serious problems to be the preponderance of a narrow, specialty-oriented viewpoint that was affecting the pattern of graduate medical education and was at least partly accountable for the situation in general practice. The Council on Medical Education considered the situation so serious, and so difficult politically, that it urged the Board of Trustees to appoint a blue ribbon committee of predominantly non-medical people to develop a solution. Something on the order of a second Flexner Report was what the council had in mind.[12]

The result was the Citizens Commission on Graduate Medical Education, a panel of twelve appointed by the AMA Board of Trustees. Starting work near the end of 1963, it was to provide, as the Flexner report had, an *external* examination of medicine, conducted objectively in the public interest. Its report was to be submitted to the board, but it was also to go "simultaneously and in the same form" to everyone concerned with graduate medical education and to the public at large. Included on the commission were three physicians, five Ph.D.s, a retired Justice of the United States Supreme Court, the executive director of the American Association for the Advancement of Science, and the presidents of two universities, one of whom, John S. Millis, Ph.D., of Western Reserve, served as the commission chairman.

Meeting most frequently in Chicago, the commission operated as a committee of the whole, that is, without a great deal of staff work and without separating into subcommittees. The commission studied reports and position papers; it listened to representatives of the teaching hospitals, the medical schools, the specialty societies, and the examining boards. Walter S. Wiggins, M.D., the AMA staff secretary of the Council on Medical Education, served as a consultant. His presence was important, for more than any other one person he had supplied the early initiative that led to the establishment of the commission, and he wrote the internal AMA memo that laid the basis for its agenda.[13]

At this same time, other organizations were addressing some of the same problems as the commission and moving in sometimes similar directions. Acting on the recommendations of an outside committee headed by Lowell T. Coggeshall, M.D., vice president of the University of Chicago, the Association of American Medical Colleges altered its structure to bring in the specialty societies and the teaching hospitals, thereby opening the way for the universities to extend their responsibility for graduate medical education. The American Academy of General Practice reversed its long-standing opposition to specialty status for family practitioners,* and at its December 1966 meeting the AMA House of Delegates adopted the report of an Ad Hoc Committee on Education for Family Practice which declared that "medicine needs a new kind of specialist, the family physician who is educated to provide comprehensive personal care."[14]

Although the AMA did not adopt all of the specific recommendations of the citizen's commission, it did take several actions that were in harmony with broad ideas embodied in the Millis report. These included the creation of the new specialty, family practice, with a three-year residency and diplomas issued by an examining board. It also included the recommendation to eliminate the internship, based on the premise that the clerkship in the final years of undergraduate education furnished enough clinical training of a general nature. Graduate medical education, it was argued, should be a planned, unified, progressive continuum in one of the specialties. The Millis report also urged a deeper involvement in graduate education on the part of the universities.

Those recommendations all bore fruit. An American Board of Family Practice was incorporated in 1969. At its November-December 1970 meeting, the AMA House of Delegates approved the incorporation of family practice residencies into the residency review process. At the same time, the house said that after July 1, 1975, freestanding internships would no longer be approved. A closer linkage between the universities and the residency programs developed, though it is difficult to quantify. More and more residencies are conducted in university-affiliated hospitals, but the degree of

---

*Instead of a residency, it had insisted on programs of continuing medical education. It was, in 1948, the first specialty society to require that as a condition of membership.

affiliation can vary. In many cases, the ties from the hospital teaching program back to the university are stretched long and thin.

The Millis commission's final recommendation, however, stirred a major controversy. This called for a powerful new commission on graduate medical education: "A central body with greater authority" was the way the commission described it; "one deeply concerned with all graduate medical education and possessed with enough knowledge, prestige and authority to secure more unified planning and better articulation of the parts."[15] The commission was worried about "fragmentation," too much attention being given to the individual concerns of the specialties, and not enough attention being given to the broader needs of society.

Specifically, the recommendation suggested a ten-member commission to include not only medical educators and practitioners but also people from the related sciences and other non-medical fields. It specified that three members should be chosen from candidates nominated by the AAMC and two from candidates nominated by the National Academy of Science. The remaining five positions might be filled by nominees from other distinguished organizations, with all the final appointments to the new commission to be made by the AMA Council on Medical Education. This still left a great deal of the authority over graduate medical education where it was, with the Council on Medical Education.

To see what might be done about the commission idea, the AMA brought together a group representing other medical organizations with responsibilities in graduate medical education. Included were the AAMC, the American Board of Medical Specialties, the Council of Medical Specialty Societies and the American Hospital Association. This group in turn appointed an ad hoc subcommittee of five, one from each of the organizations, to sift through the welter of reaction and response and develop proposals for the parent organizations to consider.

Even at this early stage it was clear that this part of the Millis report was not going to be accepted without major alteration. It was apparent that non-medical representation on the proposed commission—if it ever came into being—would be far less broad than the Millis commissioners had suggested. It was also clear that a commission appointed by the Council on Medical Education alone was hardly in the cards either. Too many other organizations now had a piece of the action, the AMA having recognized their claims by inviting them to participate in the discussions regarding a possible new commission for graduate medical education.

In its comments at the end of 1968, the Board of Trustees, through a report adopted by the house, recommended that the Council on Medical Education should continue its exploratory activities and that the commission concept be given "further multilateral consideration," with the AMA serving as the logical one to "develop the necessary cooperative relationship."[16] Conciliatory as the words sounded, they hardly disguised the power struggle that the Millis report had touched off. If it were not already visible, it came out in the meetings of the ad hoc subcommittee during which, over the next nine months, little agreement on anything was achieved.

The person at the center of the developing storm was C. H. William Ruhe, M.D., who in 1967 had succeeded Walter S. Wiggins, M.D., as the AMA staff secretary to the Council on Medical Education. Ruhe had also become director of the Division on Medical Education. "I was deeply disturbed by what was going on," he recalls, thinking back to 1969. "The direction things were taking ran counter to the whole intent of the Millis study." Ruhe was getting worried that some of the other organizations might get together without the AMA to take over segments of the review process in graduate medical education. The AAMC had just established a Council of Teaching Hospitals, and the medical schools were doing their best to encourage students to take residencies in these teaching hospitals. Possibly, Ruhe feared, the AAMC might gain jurisdiction over the residencies in the teaching hospitals, leaving the AMA to monitor standards in the community hospital programs.

At the same time the American Board of Medical Specialties suggested to Ruhe that that organization, representing the specialty boards, and the AMA might want to join in forming a liaison committee on graduate medical education roughly analogous to the one for undergraduate medical education. Why not? A key factor in the accrediting of graduate medical education was the concept of the Residency Review Committees, made up largely of AMA and specialty board representatives. "I could see medicine becoming balkanized," Ruhe thought at the time.

Sensitive to the atmosphere of divisiveness that prevailed throughout 1969, Ruhe, with the backing of the Council on Medical Education, advanced a plan in February 1970 that won acceptance, at least in principle, from the four other parties to the discussions. This was a proposal to expand the membership and function of the

Liaison Committee on Medical Education. Instead of being a joint committee of the Council on Medical Education and the Association of American Medical Colleges, it would be enlarged to include several additional members representing the American Board of Medical Specialties, the Council of Medical Specialty Societies, the American Hospital Association, and the public. And instead of confining itself to undergraduate medical education, its charter would now extend to graduate medical education too.

What Ruhe really had in mind, however, went beyond this and considerably beyond anything the Millis commission envisioned. His thoughts are recorded in a March 2, 1970, memo addressed to "Participants in Meetings on the Proposal to Establish a Commission on Medical Education"—the five-organization group created by the AMA in late 1968 to develop proposals out of the Millis report for their parent organizations. In an early section of Ruhe's proposal to expand the original liaison committee he stated a basic philosophy. "Medical education," he wrote, "is a continuum from premedical preparation through the continuing education of the practicing physician and is intertwined with education for the allied health professions and services...To have separate bodies to deal separately with these problems without relation to each other would defy the concept of the continuum and would inevitably lead to divergent policies." Accordingly, he continued, "There should be a single, overall, authoritative body to determine policy and establish standards for the entire field of medical education."[17] He anticipated that the expanded liaison committee would take over as that single, overall, authoritative body with four subcommittees working under it, one each for the accrediting of undergraduate, graduate, continuing, and allied health education.

The proposal, to say the least, was a radical one, for in one stroke it would disperse the AMA's long-standing, carefully developed, and generally respected authority over medical education. True, the AMA shared responsibility for undergraduate medical education with the AAMC. But in graduate medical education, continuing medical education, and allied health education, virtually all of the responsibility and financial burden was the AMA's.

Despite the Ruhe proposal's far-reaching implications and (many thought) challengeable assumptions, the Council on Medical Education accepted it at its March 12-14, 1970, meeting, including the perception of medical education as a continuum. "The parts of physician's education cannot be sectioned off," Ruhe believed. "If you make a major change at the undergraduate level, for instance, it affects the process later, often necessitating a change at the graduate level. It is not a compartmentalized process, and I did not think the various groups involved in the accrediting should be setting policy independently of one another."

The Council on Medical Education did, however, modify one section of the proposal (Section VI), the one with the plan for the four subcommittees that would oversee parts of medical education under the expanded committee's supervision. Instead, some general wording was substituted. Except for that, Ruhe's concept of a new medical education superstructure won the Council on Medical Education's endorsement.

That is not to say, however, that the issue was settled. During the rest of 1971 a number of procedural difficulties had to be resolved. Frequent battles erupted over the number of seats each of the participating organizations was to have on the new liaison committee. At the beginning of 1971, the AMA Board of Trustees, which had expressed considerable uneasiness earlier over the "free-standing" authority of any new joint commission, reasserted its reservations. Relations between the board and the Council on Medical Education—still a "council of the house" and at least technically independent of the board—were cool. During a meeting with the council, the board raised questions as to why the AMA should share its current authority over medical education while continuing to supply the major part of the financial support for the accrediting process. Graduate medical education was costing the AMA about $2 million a year, the accrediting of continuing medical education another $850,000. There was, therefore, a sensitivity over the costs and, in time, it became a factor in moving the AMA toward an accreditation process shared with other organizations.

But in March 1971 when the board received a copy of the working arrangements for the new and expanded liaison committee, it tabled discussion. Uncertain as to what the Board's intentions were, the Council on Medical Education decided to call a halt to things too; the whole matter was stalled for lack of consensus.[18] Meanwhile, the American Board of Medical Specialties renewed its overtures to the AMA to break away from the other organizations and start a bipartite liaison committee on graduate medical education. The AAMC issued a paper, which it insisted was merely a "draft," suggesting that the medical schools had a "corporate responsibility" for residency training in school-affiliated hospitals. This was interpreted as notice that insofar as the AAMC was concerned the specialty boards and the AMA could confine their accrediting activities to programs conducted by hospitals not affiliated with medical schools. With all parties headed in different directions, the idea of an expanded liaison committee was dead, at least for the time being.

Clearly, something had to be done. Fired by the number of organizations claiming an interest in graduate medical education, pressure had now mounted too high for the Council on Medical Education to say, simply, "We'll keep on doing the accreditation by ourselves." Late in 1971, the AMA Board of Trustees established a negotiating committee to break the impasse; it consisted of two members of the board and three from the Council on Medical Education. The negotiators were to meet with the other organizations to develop a joint committee on graduate medical education.

At first, the AAMC refused to meet with the negotiating committee, but it changed its mind soon after the AMA indicated it might proceed without it. In Washington on January 25, 1972, the negotiators from the five organizations involved all agreed, subject to ratification by each parent organization (which was forthcoming), on a Liaison Committee on Graduate Medical Education* with seats apportioned as follows:

- 4 American Medical Association
- 4 Association of American Medical Colleges
- 4 American Board of Medical Specialties
- 2 Council of Medical Specialty Societies
- 2 American Hospital Association
- 1 federal government
- 1 public

The concept of a superstructure—the role that the expanded liaison committee was once expected to play—also came into being at the January negotiating session.[19] This took the title of the Coordinating Council on Medical Education.** Its function was "to review all matters of policy relating to undergraduate and graduate

*In 1981, membership parity for the sponsoring organizations was established, and the name was changed to the Accreditation Council for Graduate Medical Education.

**In 1980 the coordinating council was disbanded, its sponsoring organizations too often unable to compromise on differences about policy matters. It was replaced by the Council for Medical Affairs, consisting of appointees of the same parent organizations. It functions largely as a forum with no connection to the joint accrediting councils.

medical education and to make recommendations to the parent professional organizations concerning them." Seats on the coordinating council were distributed as follows:

- 3 American Medical Association
- 3 Association of American Medical Colleges
- 3 American Board of Medical Specialists
- 3 Council of Medical Specialty Societies
- 1 federal government
- 1 public

What had now emerged was variously regarded as progress and blunder. Though the results were far from what the Millis commission originally had in mind, it could be read as an improvement that graduate medical education (and medical education in general) appeared now to have more broadly based oversight committees, presumably with broader concepts of responsibilities. With the institution of the coordinating committee, the Council on Medical Education realized its desire for a way to achieve an interrelationship in the work of the various accrediting bodies. The new Liaison Committee on Graduate Medical Education was clearly one of the subcommittees conceived in Ruhe's original proposal. Another of the subcommittees would take form as the Liaison Committee on Continuing Medical Education in 1977.

Yet there were those within the AMA who thought a major mistake had occurred, that the AMA had yielded unnecessarily to outside pressures and was proceeding on shaky assumptions about medical education. Some AMA leaders agreed with the view that medical education was a continuum and therefore needed a coordinated accreditation process to assure an overall viewpoint in the standard-setting decisions. But others, including Ruhe's successor Leonard D. Fenninger, M.D., disagreed, arguing that the essential continuum in medical education arose in individual students, who chose a large proportion of the programs they participated in, sought out the teachers they admired, and pursued a lifetime of education in a variety of physical settings at different stages in their personal development. As for sharing the accreditation function with other organizations, some agreed that the AMA had little choice but to widen the membership in the accrediting bodies. Others thought the AMA had made concessions when it really did not have to, maintaining that the AMA, with its diverse and inclusive membership, already reflected a broad viewpoint, obviating the need for others to be represented in the accreditation system.

Despite the conflict in viewpoints in graduate medical education, an accommodation has endured. The Accreditation Council for Graduate Medical Education (four members from each of the five parent organizations, plus a public representative, a resident representative, and a federal government participant) has the overall responsibility for the standard-setting process. How does it now function?

Technically, the medical residency casts the young physician in a dual role. He or she is both an employee of a hospital, expected to perform services, and a student, present to benefit from a formal educational experience. In outdated physician memoirs and countless fictional portrayals, the relationship between the two roles has been badly distorted, the "student" virtually ignored, the "employee" shown as a youthful medical graduate, given awesome responsibilities and left largely alone to learn the harsh realities of medicine with only occasional help from other, more senior residents. Serviceable as the stereotype has been for commercial drama, it bears little resemblance to the real world, especially the world of today.

The fact is that a formidable medical hierarchy affirms the "student" role, insuring that the residency accomplishes its purpose: the graduate education of physicians. The objective is defined in the AMA *Directory of Residency Training Programs.* "During the graduate phase," it reads, "the knowledge and skills acquired in medical school are expanded through the progressive assumption of personal responsibility for patient care in supervised, clinical, educational environments which provide opportunities to learn about their biological, emotional, and social problems. As residents progressively gain more knowledge and skill, they are provided more latitude to make decisions and treat patients, but always under supervision."

Since residency training is organized by specialty, much of the AMA's standard-maintaining function rests on the work of residency review committees—one for pediatrics, one for dermatology, and so forth—twenty-four of them altogether. They have responsibilities in the forty-eight medical disciplines for which there are approved residency programs. Some of the residency review committees obviously deal with more than one discipline; the review committee for psychiatry, for example, has responsibility for programs in both psychiatry and child psychiatry. In the forty-eight disciplines, or categories of approved programs, there are a total of about 4,700 individual programs (conducted by about 1,500 institutions) in which about 70,000 residents are enrolled. The residency review committees vary in size, ranging from six to twelve members. Generally, they are made up of appointees of the AMA Board of Trustees and appointees of the relevant specialty certifying board. Some of the committees have, in addition, appointees from the relevant medical specialty society. Each residency review committee focuses on the quality of education in its own specialty.

The committees examine the fundamental components of training that should be present in the programs, delineate program requirements, and outline criteria that reflect the educational prerequisites for a resident's eventual board certification. These are referred to as the Special Requirements of a residency program and, of course, they differ specialty by specialty. At the same time, there are General Requirements, broader in nature, that are applicable to all programs and cover such things as the capability of the hospital teaching staff and the availability of resources to make an effective program possible.

The Special and General Requirements are combined in the Essentials for residencies in each specialty. New or revised Essentials require review and recommendation by the residency review committees' sponsoring organizations. In the AMA's case, the Council on Medical Education passes judgment on the Special Requirements, but the General Requirements, as statements of broader policy, require adoption by the House of Delegates. Subsequent approval of the Accreditation Council for Graduate Medical Education is also required.

The Essentials define the standards by which programs are or are not accredited. Some programs are accredited by the accreditation council after recommendation by the residency review committee. Others, where the accreditation council has delegated authority, are accredited by the residency review committees.

Although accreditation is voluntary, as it is in undergraduate medical education, the process establishes and effectively maintains a high standard for vocational education and training for residents. The programs are reviewed periodically, about every five years in the case of established ones. Altogether, some 1,400 programs a year are reviewed. An on-going program may have its accreditation renewed or, if deficiencies are found, it may receive a probationary accreditation. If the deficiencies are corrected, a program can be restored to full accreditation; if they are not, probationary accreditation may be continued, or accreditation withdrawn altogether. In the course of a year, something like 300 adverse actions are taken.

What do the residency review committees look for when they examine the records and reports on a program? John C. Gienapp, Ph.D., director of the AMA Department of Graduate Medical Education, believes the first thing is the range of cases presented to the residents. "Does a surgical resident get four cases requiring a particular surgical procedure a year, for example, or does he get ten? Does he only stand around when the difficult operations are done? If residents never do anything complicated, the review committees tend to assume the residents are not being given enough responsibility. Is a fifth-year surgical resident still doing a lot of gallbladders and appendectomies? Or is he handling aortic resections and thoracotomies?"

The committees also look at the availability of medical "material," that is, the variety of cases that come before a resident. Is that resident exposed to patients with the less common diseases? Review committees also spend time examining the "balance" in a residency program. "You have to do enough clinical medicine to be good at it," says Gienapp. "But in addition, you have to reflect on the clinical work, and that involves didactic conferences, teaching sessions, and the like. If you get a tremendously busy clinical service and the residents have a heavy clinical load, you might find that there is no time for reflection and thought. And that is not good education either."[20]

To make its evaluation, a residency review committee relies mainly on documentary information. The hospital submits, among other things, a self-study report that is its own description of a program. This may be supported by various records, statistics, analyses, and so forth. Hospitals, for example, usually list how many surgical procedures are performed by staff physicians, how many by residents. The review committees are also assisted in their findings by reports from site visitors. Sometimes these are special appointees, usually physicians with relevant specialty credentials. But the AMA also maintains a full-time field staff under Gienapp especially to survey residency programs. It consists of two staff members with Ph.D.s in education and seven with medical degrees.

It should be emphasized that the site visit procedure in graduate medical education differs sharply from the procedure used in the inspection of the medical schools. In the case of the residency programs, the surveyors are primarily fact-gatherers—reporters— whereas the teams that visit the medical schools are asked to form broad judgments on the basis of what they see and hear. By contrast, the residency site surveyor's job is largely to verify facts and figures submitted by the director of a residency program. This may involve interviewing people on the hospital staff and residents themselves, but nonetheless the staff surveyors are restricted in the reports they develop for the residency review committees to objective, non-judgmental fact. The specially appointed inspectors operate under different rules. They are expected to offer personal judgments.

Although the profession has long agreed that a physician, in order to keep his clinical judgment in peak form, should stay abreast of new medical knowledge, the efforts by the AMA to encourage and improve medical education for physicians in practice have been difficult. The overall purpose is simple enough: the safe and effective translation of scientific advances into patient benefits. But other aspects of the concept of a lifelong educational process are unexpectedly complex. One major problem with any sort of monitoring program is the lack of institutional focus; continuing medical education can originate from thousands of sources and be conducted in numerous ways. It is provided by medical schools, hospitals, local, state and specialty medical societies, the AMA, and the manufacturers of medical equipment and drugs. It can take the form of academic courses, clinical demonstrations, seminars, lectures, conferences, symposia, and workshops. Self-administered assessment tests, audio and video tapes, correspondence courses, and even the conscientious study of medical journals rate as legitimate forms of continuing medical education. Diverse and episodic, carried on by mature "students" often working alone, continuing medical education is difficult to quantify.

Because it can take so many different forms, philosophic differences have arisen over whether continuing medical education should be voluntary or compulsory, and disagreements as to its effectiveness are plentiful. The profession is largely skeptical, for example, that requirements for continuing education can be used to identify a physician who delivers substandard care because he fails to keep up. The profession shares that public concern, but asks: Who is to say what sort of new knowledge it is that the practitioner needs to increase his competence? In order for a course of continuing medical education to result in improved patient care, a physician must identify, usually on the basis of careful self-assessment, some areas of his own practice and some areas of his own knowledge where an improvement can be made. Ironically, it is probably the physician who is practicing safe and effective medicine in the first place who will do this, not the isolated, wayward practitioner whose methods are out of date.

When it first decided to upgrade the state of continuing medical education, the Council on Medical Education set out on a familiar path. In 1952 it launched an extensive, two and-a-half-year survey of the field, with a full report published in 1955. The report noted the growing interest in and demand for continuing education, and suggested that fifty hours a year might be a reasonable amount of time for a physician to devote to it.[21] The report served as the basis for a guide for sponsors of programs that the House of Delegates adopted two years later and called "the first step in a long range program that will be of assistance in the improvement and increase" of continuing medical education. In 1967 the council began to accredit the institutions offering courses (not the programs), and 1970—inevitably— the "Essentials of Approved Programs in Continuing Medical Education" emerged. Among other things, these urged that where possible "participative" instruction, that is, live clinics and bedside rounds, be favored over "standing lectures."

As it started to develop standards, the Council on Medical Education kept in mind the broad features of the monitoring systems developed for undergraduate and graduate medical education. In this case, there was no point in control over entry. But guidance relating to educational content could be given and the on-site evaluation of the educational institutions, usually by volunteer visitors, was feasible. Accordingly, accreditation procedures were put in place. To measure the end product, no academic equivalent to the licensure or certification examinations was practical. Might some sort of equivalent be developed or invented?

In the mid-1960s, Ruhe and the Advisory Committee on Continuing Medical Education started talking about various incentives that could be offered for at least recognition purposes. Initially, there was talk about reviving the Fellowship category of AMA membership, bestowing the title Fellow of the AMA on those meeting some sort of standard accomplishment in continuing medical education. Fellowship struck the committee members as a possibly confusing term, and another suggestion of Ruhe's, for a Physician's Recognition Award, was recommended and eventually adopted by the house.

Instituted in 1968, the Physician's Recognition Award attests to the completion of 150 hours of continuing medical education over three consecutive years. A minimum of sixty of the hours must be in an accredited program in a subject directly related to the physician's professional medical activities. A course in psychiatry, for example, would count for an internist, but one in financial management would not. However, a physician in hospital management could properly take credit for a course in finance. During the first fifteen years, the AMA issued over 300,000 awards.

With the coming of the 1970s, continuing medical education became the focus of a major medical controversy. In response to the Millis commission recommendations, the AMA agreed in 1972 to give up its exclusive accreditation of continuing medical education and share the responsibility in a Liaison Committee for Continuing Medical Education with six other organizations: the Association of American Medical Colleges, the American Hospital Association, the American Board of Medical Specialties, the Council of Medical Specialty Societies, the Association for Hospital Medical Education, and the Federation of State Medical Boards. There was, in addition, to be one representative each from the public and the federal government.

Disagreements soon developed, however, and the meetings of the committee, which was not actually formed until 1977, grew steadily more sulphurous. One group of committee members, inclined toward the theories of professional educators, sought to formalize continuing education by establishing rigid standards and requirements. Should accreditation be confined to programs that could demonstrate improvements in patient care? Should testing procedures be developed, something equivalent to licensure in undergraduate medical education or board certification in graduate medical education?[22] The AMA representatives on the committee sharply dissented, perceiving a crucial difference between the educational quest of the medical student and the needs of a practitioner. While a rigid structure of learning might be acceptable to the medical student, it would not, they believed, be effective for the mature, more responsible physician in practice. In contrast to the student, willing to do everything necessary to gain entrance to the profession, practitioners were motivated to seek answers to specific problems they wanted to solve or to meet needs that they considered unmet. The philosophical dispute ran deep. Arguments arose on other points as well, among them the role, authority, and competence of the state medical associations in accrediting their own state programs.

At the same time, there was a fundamental dispute as to the extent of the committee's authority.[23] All parties had originally agreed that policy matters should be referred to the sponsoring organizations. But what exactly constituted policy? There was no definition. More and more frequently, issues that the AMA representatives considered policy and wanted to present to the board or house were judged by the others to be within the committee's authority. When the AMA found itself being outvoted on what it considered policy matters, the AMA resumed the accrediting activities it had transferred to the committee when it was created, re-establishing its former accreditation procedures and its own committee. For a time, two accrediting bodies existed. In 1981 the original sponsoring organizations joined again, this time to form the Accreditation Council for Continuing Medical Education, with an agreement that recognized the role and authority of the state medical associations. There was also a firmer agreement on how policy matters would be handled; changes in Essentials, for example, would be considered policy decisions. The accreditation council is staffed by the Council of Medical Specialty Societies,* rather than the AMA, which by agreement had done the staff work for the original committee. The accreditation council is now the body that develops the Essentials and Guidelines, monitors the programs, and does the accrediting, except for what are considered intrastate programs. These are accredited by the separate state medical organizations.

Since 1937, when *JAMA* first started the annual listing of available opportunities in continuing medical education, there has been remarkable growth. One index is the number of physician registrations for continuing medical education courses sponsored just by the medical schools. From 21,131 in 1955, the total climbed to 100,822 in 1967, and to 665,882 in 1979.[24] Besides the early and sustained interest of the AMA, several other factors help explain the expansion in continuing medical education programs of all kinds. Most significant was the enormous progress in biomedical research and the

---

*The executive vice president of the council is Richard S. Wilbur, M.D.

attendant growth in technical knowledge that characterized the immediate post-World War II years.

Then later, in the 1960s, there was in addition a strong public demand, reflected in the press and the actions of many medical societies, for greater "social accountability." A new factor came into play in the 1970s as continuing medical education was made mandatory by more specialty societies, by several state medical societies, and by twenty-five states as a condition of recertification, membership, or re-registration of license. Of the nineteen states that had such requirements in operation in 1983, eleven accepted the Physician's Recognition Award as satisfying the requirements. Of the thirteen state medical societies requiring continuing education of their members, all but two relied on the recognition award.

The roughly 500,000 physicians in the United States do not, of course, deliver medical care to the American people unassisted. Judgments vary as to just how many helpers they have, but the AMA Department of Allied Health Education and Accreditation has estimated a ratio of twenty other health professionals to each physician, and that may be as authoritative a figure as any.[25] Much of the assistance is, of course, indirect, supplied by men and women in statistical, clerical, data processing, administrative, and managerial jobs. But there are equally impressive numbers of people, including 1.6 million active nurses, who are more directly involved in medical care. Among these are members of twenty-six allied health professions whose training standards are of interest to the AMA.

Some of the occupational names are familiar: emergency medical technician-paramedic, physician's assistant, respiratory therapist. But others are as arcane as anything in medicine: cytotechnologist, electroencephalographic technologist, perfusionist.* Because of their linkage to physician performance, the profession, through the AMA, started taking a close interest in the quality of the training these workers received.

The establishment of a recognition and accreditation process for the allied health professions started slowly. In 1933 two organizations came to the AMA seeking its collaboration in setting up training standards for two classes of allied health workers. One was the American Society of Clinical Pathologists, a medical specialty

*Respectively, professionals who make microscopic examinations of cells, measure electrical impulses of the brain, and regulate the flow of liquids through a heart/lung machine during surgery.

society whose physician members wanted advice and assistance in developing training programs for technologists to assist them in laboratory work. The other organization was the American Occupational Therapy Association, an established allied health group whose members wanted the AMA's help in developing educational standards for programs in their field. A bit later, the American Physical Therapy Association came to the AMA for the same reason. The results in 1935 and 1936 were the familiar Essentials for approved programs in occupational therapy and physical therapy, and for medical technologists in pathology laboratories. In each case it was a joint undertaking: the AMA Council on Medical Education collaborated with the allied health groups, the concerned medical specialty societies, and educators in the various fields, and the final drafts of the Essentials were submitted to the AMA House of Delegates for adoption.

These Essentials did not try to standardize things too rigidly. They did not, for instance, specify entrance requirements or the duration of the curriculum. By relying on general statements as to what the graduating student was expected to know and to be able to do, the Essentials left a great deal, including admission requirements and length of study, to the discretion of those conducting individual programs. Basically, it was a new application of the same philosophy of flexibility with which the Council on Medical Education had approached physician education for many years.

Between 1937 and 1967, except for a spurt during World War II, the allied health professions grew at a leisurely pace. Five additional occupations were recognized. Their Essentials were carefully and collaboratively developed, adopted by the AMA House of Delegates, and used as the basis for accreditation by the Council on Medical Education. But with passage of the federal health manpower bills, beginning in 1963, the federal government signaled a new, massive expansion of the health care system. Medicare and Medicaid fueled sharply increasing demands, and fresh energy surged through the allied health care field. To deal with the new issues, the AMA established a Council on Health Manpower in 1968. A council of the board rather than the house, the new council was regarded by some observers as an effort by the board to limit the jurisdiction of the academically oriented Council on Medical Education over allied health care matters.

The pressures to expand the allied professions raised two important questions. The first was the danger of too many new allied health professions. The AMA had, of course, no power to impose limits, but if a group wanted an educational program that was recognized and accredited by the AMA, it had to deal with the Council on Health Manpower and the Council on Medical Education. On the initiative of the Council on Health Manpower at the November-December 1969 meeting, the House of Delegates adopted "Guidelines for the Development of New Health Occupations." By raising questions as to need, duplication, and so forth, the document performed the valuable service of setting criteria for the entry of new occupations into the AMA's accrediting process. The expansion was generally orderly, the number of professions with training programs accredited by the AMA rising from eight in 1967 to twenty-six in 1983. The number of individual training programs climbed from fewer than 200 in the 1940s to more than 3,000 in 1983.

The other question that arose was the appropriateness of leaving the accrediting power so fully concentrated in the hands of the AMA. Recognizing the need for the advice and counsel from the allied professions and from the educational institutions concerned with the training of its members, the Council on Medical Education recommended in 1967 the formation of an allied health advisory committee. This was soon expanded by the addition of a panel of consultants from the allied health organizations. An independent study was recommended to explore formation of a more broadly representative alternative to the accrediting function of the Council on Medical Education.

The council, then responding to the Millis report urging a similar step in graduate medical education, agreed that there should be joint approach to accreditation.

In 1976 the Committee on Allied Health Education and Accreditation was established. It differs from the other liaison committees in that it is a committee of the AMA. The AMA finances it and furnishes the staff support. However, in its general structure and function this committee is much like the other accrediting committees. Under it are seventeen program review committees that conduct site inspections and recommend the granting, denial, probation, or renewal of accredited status. The full committee reviews and acts upon the review committee recommendations, and reviews and makes recommendations on the Essentials. The Essentials require the approval of the sponsors of each review committee and of the AMA Council on Medical Education.

The Allied Health Committee has fourteen members, all appointed by the AMA Board of Trustees. Two are ex-officio members of the Council on Medical Education and two are members of the public. One member is a student in one of the programs or a recent graduate. The other nine are chosen from nominees made by the many organizations engaged in this diverse field. They may include people from hospitals (which conduct nearly half of the training programs), junior/community colleges (which conduct over a quarter of the training programs), four-year colleges/universities (which conduct about 15 percent), the allied professions themselves, the medical specialties, and educators with no direct connection to allied health. Representation of the allied health professions is rotated.

Of all the strains put on the AMA's structure of educational standards, none raised a more difficult challenge than the influx of graduates of foreign medical schools. The migration began modestly enough in 1950, soon after Congress enacted an exchange program for students interested in coming to this country for graduate work in many fields.* Among those taking advantage of the new opportunities were growing numbers of foreign medical graduates, known as FMGs. Arriving on newly established exchange visitor visas, they received a particularly cordial welcome from the institutions that provide graduate medical education in the United States—the hospitals. At the time, hospitals were anxiously looking for help. Immediately after World War II, they had expanded the number of residencies to accommodate young American physicians just released from military duty. But as the war veterans moved on, the hospitals found themselves offering more internships and residencies than could possibly be filled by the graduates of American medical colleges. They clasped the arriving foreign doctors in a warm embrace.

The immigration quickly swelled to proportions no one had anticipated or intended. During the first academic year in which the new legislation had an impact, 1950-51, 2,072 internships and residencies were filled by FMGs. This was 7 percent of the total positions offered. The number climbed to 9,935 ten years later, 22

---

*There were two earlier influxes of foreign-educated physicians, one in the late 1930s resulting from Hitler's racial policies, another immediately after the end of World War II in Europe. By and large, those refugee physicians had completed their education. The FMGs, by contrast, were younger men and women seeking intern and residency training.

percent of the total, and to 16,307 in 1970-71, 26 percent of the total.[27] In 1972, 14,476 physicians in the United States received their initial licenses to practice. Of this number of additions to the medical profession, 46 percent were foreign medical graduates.[28]

The intent of the original legislation was, of course, at distinct variance from the actual result. The original idea was to increase international understanding and friendship by having young people come here for a period of advanced study and then return home to apply their new-found knowledge. In other fields, most of the exchange students did that. But in medicine, for a variety of reasons, much of the flow was one-directional. An estimated 75 percent of physicians who arrived on exchange visitor visas were able to adjust them to permanent resident visas and stay in this country, many to become citizens.[29] As a result, FMGs* now constitute about 20 percent of the United States physician population.[30]

It is not quite correct to say that the United States deliberately set out to drain some 100,000 physicians from the medical educational systems of foreign countries for service here. Although that is what happened, the migration is attributable less to calculated policy than to the workings of ordinary human desire. So-called "push factors" were at work on physicians abroad—conditions in their own countries that encouraged their departure. In many cases, the economy was just too poor to support the number of people graduated by the medical schools. For many, the prospects for a medical career in their homeland seemed bleak. There were, in addition, "pull factors" from this side: the chance for first-class training in a medical specialty, for example, and all the traditional considerations that have made America the land of opportunity. Many foreign physicians came to this country for precisely the same reasons as millions of other individuals.

Yet if the United States had wanted to raise the number of physicians here by a program of importation, it could scarcely have improved on what it accomplished—unintentionally—through its immigration policies. The changes began near the end of World War II. The man who argued the cause of student exchange programs most forcefully was Senator J. William Fulbright of Arkansas, who had benefited from being a Rhodes scholar himself. The United States Information and Education Exchange Act, which became operational in 1949, formalized and extended Fulbright's earlier

---

*Note should be made that the FMG statistics include American citizens who have graduated from foreign medical schools.

ideas, but it was the Exchange Visitor Program established in this legislation that changed the nature of the inflow and made it possible for the FMGs to receive training here.

There followed a sequence of additional legislation and rulings, all of which made it easier for a physician to enter the United States. Some entered on visas, which usually led to naturalization. Others entered on exchange visitor or other temporary visas and converted them to permanent residency status. The Fulbright-Hays Act of 1961 broadened the student exchange program and further liberalized immigration policy. Legislation in 1965 ended the quota system based on national origin, thus leading to a sharp increase in the number of physicians from Asia. India and the Philippines then became the principal contributors to our present total of FMGs. In 1965, the Department of Labor ruled that a shortage of physicians existed, thereby voiding requirements that certain physicians furnish proof of an employment or educational opportunity before a visa could be granted or adjusted. Legislation in 1970 virtually eliminated the remaining obstacles to switching from exchange visitor status to permanent residency status, including the requirement that physician exchange visitors spend two years outside the United States before coming in again on a permanent visa.

From the beginning, the Council on Medical Education was concerned about the impact of the immigration on the quality of American medical care. Its policy for admission to an internship required graduation from a United States (or Canadian) medical school that met all the AMA standards and received accreditation from the Liaison Committee on Medical Education. Since no comparable system of accreditation existed in any foreign country other than Canada, there was no assurance that the FMGs entering U.S. internships and residencies in such growing numbers had educational qualifications similar to those of the graduates of American medical schools. An essential control mechanism, the standard for entry into graduate education, was therefore missing. Many established physicians feared that a two-class system of medical care would develop, one delivered by American medical school graduates and FMGs properly prepared for graduate work in accredited institutions, the other by FMGs either unable to enter the graduate programs or unable to perform well enough to stay in them.

The critical question was how to measure the qualifications of the incoming FMGs for entrance into accredited residency programs. The applicants for visas came from more than 100 countries, from hundreds of widely scattered medical schools of disparate quality. The AMA started out trying to evaluate the schools, hoping to develop a list of foreign medical institutions offering an education that could be considered comparable to that offered here. The objective was to draw up something like a roster of "approved" foreign institutions, graduation from which might be equated broadly with graduation from an accredited American school. Standards were developed, and the Council of Medical Education proposed to the House of Delegates that an evaluation program be undertaken. The list would be useful in the licensing process as well.

At its June 1949 meeting, the House of Delegates authorized the council to draw up such a list, and medical educators were appointed to make site visits to the foreign medical schools. In 1950 the council and the AAMC started publishing the list. Initially, thirty-nine medical schools were listed; fifty if the University of London's twelve hospital-based medical schools had been considered separately. All but three of them were in Western Europe.

But the listing program satisfied almost no one. It was woefully incomplete, partly because visits to all the schools were so difficult to schedule, partly because of the large number of new schools. To a great extent, too, the list was irrelevant, for large numbers of the incoming physicians did not come from Western European schools. Even so, the list was severely hedged with warnings; it did not carry anything like the authority that domestic accreditation did. In 1954 the House of Delegates started asking for a new system, one to evaluate the graduates, not the schools.[31]

The results were, first, a new organization, incorporated in 1956, called the Educational Council (later Commission) for Foreign Medical Graduates, and, second, starting in 1958, some new procedures. These included a review of the credentials of incoming foreign graduates to make sure they had successfully completed the course of study required in the nation where they received their undergraduate medical education, and an examination to qualify them for internships or residencies at accredited American hospitals. The new commission included representatives from the AMA, the AAMC, the American Hospital Association, and the Federation of State Medical Boards. It was in a position to make the examination virtually mandatory. By accepting FMGs who did not have certification from the commission, a hospital could find the accreditation of its residency programs in jeopardy.

Quickly established as a way to evaluate FMGs, the examination was organized in two parts. The first was a test of English—comprehension of spoken English, sentence structure, and vocabulary. The second included a test in the sciences, a few questions in the basic sciences (chemistry, biology, etc.), 80-85 percent of them in the clinical sciences (pediatrics, obstetrics, etc.). These questions, prepared by the National Board of Medical Examiners, were among those used in tests that American medical students usually took at the end of their second and fourth years of medical schools.[32]

By the mid-1970s, widespread opposition had arisen to the influx of FMGs.* Most of the complaints reflected views from abroad. Why, it was asked, couldn't the United States itself educate a sufficient number of physicians to fill its own needs? Why should the poorer countries make such a contribution to America's supply of physicians? In 1975, the Coordinating Council on Medical Education issued a report, adopted by the AMA House of Delegates, that said, in effect:

- the United States should educate enough doctors to fill its own needs;
- exchange visitor physicians should receive training of specific benefit to their nation upon their return home;
- foreign governments and those conducting American educational programs should make advance agreements before an individual visitor's visa was issued; and
- in general, the stay of an FMG should be limited to two years.[33]

Soon afterward, federal policy, which for so long had encouraged the immigration of foreign physicians, started to change. In 1976 and 1977, amendments to the Immigration and Nationality Act toughened the entry requirements for alien physicians by establishing a Visa Qualifying Examination that was considered more difficult than the established test. The new one placed as much emphasis on questions in the basic sciences as in the clinical sciences. Congress overruled the Labor Department on the existence of a physician shortage, and suddenly it became more difficult to upgrade

---

*At the same time the number of American citizen FMGs, most of them unable to gain admission to American medical schools, was growing significantly. Between 1970 and 1980 the percentage of American citizen FMGs taking the examinations rose from less than 3 percent to nearly 20 percent. See *The Changing Role of the Foreign Medical Graduate in the Practice of Medicine in the U.S.* (Philadelphia: the Educational Commission for Foreign Medical Graduates, 1981): 27.

an exchange visitor visa into a permanent immigration visa. A group appointed by the Secretary of Health and Human Services called the Graduate Medical Education National Advisory Committee recommended in its 1980 report on physician manpower that "the number of foreign medical graduates entering the U.S. yearly...should be severely restricted."[34]

What was happening, of course, was that the health manpower bills passed in the 1960s were at last having their effect, causing a sharp upturn in the number of United States medical graduates. As the size of the graduating classes of American medical schools rose (over 15,000 graduates in 1980 versus 8,300 in 1970), the immigration of FMGs began to slacken.[35]

Generalization about the whole FMG experience is dangerous, for a great deal of mythology surrounds the subject. Some statistical data are unreliable or incomplete, and there is always an inherent unfairness in making broad assessments about any group as heterogeneous as the FMGS. Unlike American medical graduates, who are the product of an educational system with reasonably consistent standards, the FMGs come from a variety of systems, different from ours, different from one another. There are, moreover, cultural gaps of varying width. FMGs from English-speaking countries, for example, find the transition into the American medical system far easier than FMGs from, say, the countries of Asia.

There is no denying that the exchange visitors program disappointed the hopes of its early backers. While it may have stimulated student exchange, that intended objective was overshadowed by its unintentional service as an immigration vehicle. And FMGs who did return home often took back a highly sophisticated medical training that was irrelevant to comparatively simple native needs. This was a special problem with students from Third World countries; the United States was, in effect, training jet pilots for nations that could barely afford automobiles. Nor did the FMGs ease the manpower problems of rural America, as many hoped they might; one year, only 1 percent of the FMGs receiving medical licenses received them in the ten states with the lowest physician/population ratios.[36] The cultural and educational differences have been too difficult for many of those given visas for permanent residency, and 10,000 FMGs, according to the estimate made in the coordinating council report of 1975, have failed to qualify for unrestricted licensure, continuing to function, especially in institutional settings, with repeatedly renewed temporary licenses or none at all.[37]

For various reasons, including cultural differences and possible test inequities, FMGs have more trouble with United States examinations than American students do. During 1968-72, on an examination given widely for licensure, FMGs had a failure rate of 50 percent compared to a failure rate of 15 percent for American graduates. Even on specialty board examinations, after completion of the long residency, FMGs do not average as well as their American counterparts. The failure rates on one set of examinations was 50 percent for FMGs and 13 percent for American graduates.[38]

On the positive side, the presence of FMGs unquestionably prevented a serious manpower crisis in the 1950s, 1960s, and early 1970s. Created by the growth of private insurance and the passage of Medicaid and Medicare, the demand for medical services soared in those years, and the availability of the FMGs was the salvation of many hospitals. Thousands of FMGs have successfully blended into the American medical system, in a variety of ways. To a greater extent than American medical school graduates, they favor careers in research, medical school teaching, and full-time hospital staff work. On a percentage basis, they have not gone into private practice in such numbers as American medical graduates.[39] But they have won more than their share of academic honors. During the years of 1966-80, eighteen American physicians were awarded the Nobel prize in medicine and physiology. Of that group, ten were graduates of American medical schools, one was a graduate of a Canadian school, and seven were FMGs.

The AMA and Science

From the early 1940s on, at the various times when the House of Delegates worried over the political direction the AMA was taking, how well founded were the fears that its traditional scientific role was being downgraded? Were the scientific programs, as some implied, sacrificed to finance the AMA's legislative battles, to develop AMPAC, and to expand the AMA's presence in Washington?

Certainly the AMA's scientific functions changed. They changed in character, and they shifted into a different administrative structure. But even during the worst of the financial crunch in 1974 and 1975 the AMA did not reach the point where an either/or decision had to be made, and it is more accurate to say that the AMA's socioeconomic and political strengths developed in addition to, rather than in place of, its scientific role. Activities classified as scientific now constitute something like 40 percent of a typical annual budget.[1]

"Science" is a word that evokes pictures of original achievement: Galileo at his telescope, Darwin among the tortoises of the Galapagos, Fleming observing the growth of mold in a Petri dish. That, of course, is the dramatic part of science, and, for a time, the AMA participated in it through the operation of a biomedical research laboratory. But science includes activities other than research and exploration, and it is on such supportive work that the AMA has concentrated most of its energies: appraisal of new observations and clinical techniques, evaluation of new medicines and devices, dissemination of verifiable new knowledge and information, investigation of claims, warnings of danger, exposure of fraud.

The scientific activities of a medical organization are important to a physician. Unable to verify new theories or observations alone, he or she must frequently rely on medical societies and their journals. Science is at the core of medicine, even its ethics. For example, the AMA Principles of Medical Ethics for many years carried a statement beginning: "A physician should practice a method of healing founded on a scientific basis."

Few would argue with that concept today. But in the nineteenth century there was less agreement on just what was scientific in medicine, for the great advances in bacteriology and immunology, which occurred in Europe in the 1880s and 1890s, were slow to gain acceptance here. At the turn of the century many who called themselves doctors still believed that there was only one disease and only one cause of fever.

Medicine of that day was flanked by healers of many persuasions. At the center were the regulars or, as they were also called, the allopathic (conventional) physicians; these doctors, by and large, constituted the AMA. Around them were what were referred to as cultists or sectarians. They believed in an assortment of causes and cures for disease, which included these:

• Homeopathic physicians thought that "like cures like," that a sick person should be treated with a medicine that would induce the same symptoms in a healthy person. The doses they administered were infinitesimally small. When the Council on Medical Education made its 1906 survey, it visited the twenty homeopathic schools in operation, among the best known being one in Philadelphia named after Samuel C. Hahnemann, the German physician who articulated the original homeopathic theories. The institution later renounced homeopathy and survives today as a respected, accredited medical school.

• Eclectics applied single remedies to pathologic conditions with little attention to the diagnosis of the disease. Following theories voiced by Wooster Beach, a medical school graduate who opposed heroic therapy, they worked with herbal remedies. But because they were also willing to use mineral medicines derived from arsenic and mercury, they became known as eclectics. There were ten eclectic schools in 1906, all inspected as part of the survey made by the Council on Medical Education that year.

• Osteopaths, following the theories of Andrew T. Still, M.D., the founder of osteopathy, believed that the normal body could adequately defend itself against diseases. Still argued that these arose because of derangements in the musculoskeletal system; early osteopathic practice particularly demanded a lot of manipulative work. As discussed in an earlier chapter, osteopathy later broke with Still's theories.

• Chiropractors believed that diseases could be cured by the adjustment of the vertebrae. Chiropractic started in 1895, so the legend goes, when Daniel David Palmer, a Davenport, Iowa grocer, adjusted the spinal column of a local janitor and supposedly cured him of deafness.

• Naturopaths did not employ drugs but relied on such natural elements as water, heat, and massage for the cure of disease.

By pressing for tougher licensing laws and instituting educational reforms, the AMA accomplished a great deal in the first part of this century to protect the public from inadequately trained physicians and from healers whose theories and practices had no foundation in scientific fact. Quackery, though sharply curbed by the AMA's battle for scientific medicine, did not disappear. Human nature probably assures it of perpetuity; according to Voltaire, quackery dates from the moment the first fool met the first knave.

Soon after appointing the Council on Medical Education to reform the medical schools, the AMA established the Council on Pharmacy and Chemistry and embarked on an equally vigorous campaign to rid the country of unscientifically formulated medicines. In 1905, when the campaign began, drugs were sold without restriction. Until 1914, even narcotics could be purchased as easily as nail polish is today. Fraudulently branded and deceptively advertised products flooded an unregulated market. For "female weakness" there was Lydia Pinkham's Vegetable Compound; for men there were such things as Sporty Days Invigorator. Additional hazards to the public health were vividly stated by the journalist, Samuel Hopkins Adams, the first article of a series published in *Colliers* beginning October 7, 1905. The articles were later collected in a booklet, "The Great American Fraud," and distributed by the AMA. Adams began his series:

> Gullible America will spend this year some $75 million in the purchase of patent medicines. In consideration of this sum it will swallow huge quantities of alcohol, an appalling amount of opiates and narcotics, a wide assortment of varied drugs ranging from powerful and dangerous heart depressants to insidious liver stimulants and, far in excess of all other ingredients, undiluted fraud. For fraud exploited by the skilfulest of advertising bunco men is the basis of the trade. Should the newspapers, the magazines and the medical journals refuse their pages to this class of advertisement, the patent medicine business in five years would be as scandalously historic as

the South Sea Bubble, and the nation would be the richer not only in lives and money but in drunkards and drug fiends saved.

Even when legislation, strongly advocated by the AMA,[3] was passed in the following year, the abuses did not vanish. The federal Pure Food and Drugs Act of 1906 said nothing about the safety of medicines or their effectiveness. All it did was require that ingredients be identified and that they be unadulterated.

The AMA Council on Pharmacy and Chemistry, having established a chemical laboratory to assist in its work, turned its attention first to the sort of medicines developed for use by ethical physicians. At the time, a number of remedies already enjoyed official status, meaning that they were listed in either the *U.S. Pharmacopoeia* (a publication established by federal statute) or in the *National Formulary*, a publication of the American Pharmaceutical Association. The two books identified and described the most frequently used medicines, those whose safety and appropriateness had been established by custom and experience. The AMA council did not concern itself with those official remedies but set up an approval procedure for new medicines.[4]

If a manufacturer intended to advertise a new remedy in consumer publications or if he refused to disclose its ingredients, his product was automatically excluded from consideration by the Council on Pharmacy and Chemistry. But if he would make the composition of his remedy known, do nothing to promote it to the public, submit samples, state the therapeutic claims he intended to make, and give evidence of the drug's efficacy (i.e., effectiveness), then it was eligible for the review process. The AMA chemical laboratory would analyze the material, verifying that the ingredients were as stated, in the proportions as stated, with nothing present other than what was stated.

A special subcommittee of experts appointed by the council would go over the analysis, the evidence of efficacy, and the claims of therapeutic value. They would make a recommendation to the council, itself made up of people with excellent credentials in medicine, pharmacology, bacteriology, and chemistry. After examining the report critically, the council would either give or withhold approval. If the findings were negative, they might be reported in the pharmacology section of *JAMA*. If positive, the product was accepted and a short description of it appeared in a regular feature of

JAMA called "New and Nonofficial Remedies." At the end of each year, these comments were collected in book form, and soon *New and Nonofficial Remedies* became the authoritative source of information on new drugs for practitioners.

Another early publication of the council was *Useful Drugs*, a selection and description of the better known and more valuable drugs listed in the *U.S. Pharmacopoeia* and the *National Formulary*. The accomplishments of the new council, though accepted slowly, had great value for physicians and their patients. For the first time, there was a scientific screening of new medicines and a source of objective information about them. There were long-range implications as well, for the activities of the Council on Pharmacy and Chemistry foreshadowed what the Food and Drug Administration would start doing some thirty-five years later to assure the public of the safety and efficacy of drugs for labeled indications and claims.

Besides new remedies, the council also promised to investigate old ones of doubtful usefulness, employing the capabilities of the chemical laboratory and publishing its findings in *JAMA*. Out of this evolved a new staff operation, the Propaganda Department, headed by Arthur J. Cramp, M.D., who came to *JAMA* as an editorial assistant in 1906 but soon took over the new department. It was renamed the Bureau of Investigation in 1925, headed by Cramp until his retirement in 1935.[5] Cramp combined the findings of the chemical laboratory and the reports of the council with investigative work of his own to create a regular section of *JAMA*, at first headed simply "Pharmacology," but after 1911 called "Propaganda for Reform." His targets for investigation included nostrums (remedies for which the ingredients were kept secret), patent medicines (which supposedly had patented formulas), non-approved proprietary medicines (whose names were registered) and other substances that upon scientific investigation were found to be useless, deceptively advertised, or dangerous. In reports of sometimes considerable length, Cramp also exposed individual quacks, miracle cures, and medical scams of every description.

He then collected the *JAMA* reports into books. One of them, *Nostrums and Quackery*, appeared in three volumes and at least ten editions between 1907 and 1936. The other, *Propaganda for Reform in Proprietary Medicines*, dealt with unaccepted remedies and was designed more for the profession than the public. Actually, a considerable amount of reforming had to be done within the profession, because physicians on the fringes of ethical medicine then often endorsed dubious products.

Heavily reliant on the prestigious Council on Pharmacy and Chemistry, the AMA's reform drive had, in time, wide impact. It not only provided the profession with a reliable guide to new medicine; it also alerted physicians to the useless or sometimes fraudulent qualities of others. This was really the first attempt to establish standards for new medicines and remedies marketed to the public. The Propaganda Department also generated a rich store of information for reform-minded journalists, and their stories, supported by the information published in *JAMA*, shamed many newspapers and magazines into rejecting the advertising for the nostrums and quackeries so righteously exposed in the editorial columns.

Mindful of the success of the Council on Pharmacy and Chemistry, the Board of Trustees in 1925 established a Council on Physical Therapy. Largely as a result of World War I, physical therapy had made great strides in this country and had become a recognized part of medicine for the first time. That brought forth a variety of new devices, everything from artificial limbs and hearing aids to sunlamps and diathermy equipment. Much of it had genuine therapeutic value; some of it was useless and deceptively advertised. The new Council on Physical Therapy took its lead from the Council on Pharmacy and Chemistry, investigating the worth of new products and using *JAMA* to inform the profession of its findings.

Meanwhile, the Council on Pharmacy and Chemistry found itself drawn into the approval of food products. This reflected a previous interest of the House of Delegates in the quality of the nation's milk. Early in the century, it had urged municipal regulations for the sanitary condition of the milk itself and tuberculin tests for the dairy herds to guard against bovine tuberculosis. Now, a more immediate concern was arising in the role of food products in health care. More and more food companies wanted to place ads with health claims in AMA publications. Since these had to clear the Council on Pharmacy and Chemistry (as did ads for pharmaceutical products), the council established two review committees in 1929, one for medicinal foods, one for non-medicinal foods. (They were combined into a Committee on Foods under the Board of Trustees in 1930, which became a council in 1936.) The subcommittee on non-medicinal foods proposed in 1929 that some sort of

AMA emblem be authorized for promotional use by the manufacturers of accepted products. The council, which included Morris
Fishbein, M.D., among its members, also thought it was a good idea,
and the AMA inaugurated the Seal of Acceptance program. If one
of the participating councils (Pharmacy and Chemistry, Physical
Therapy, Foods, and later a Committee on Cosmetics) accepted a
product and the claims made for it in advertisements for use in
AMA publications, then the manufacturer could display the AMA
Seal of Acceptance on the product packaging and use the seal in
advertising placed elsewhere. Often useful in stimulating new advertising in AMA publications, the idea was to cause trouble later.

The Seal of Acceptance program, which might have qualified the
AMA as a "consumerist" organization in the 1960s and 1970s,
absorbed most of the energies of the three councils and one committee that participated. For that reason it tended to obscure the
other aspects of the work undertaken by those bodies—educational
reports directed to the profession, informational activities for the
benefit of the public, and the general advancement of that particular segment of medicine with which the councils and committees were concerned. The Council on Pharmacy and Chemistry
(changed to Drugs after 1956) maintained a valuable informational
service for physicians by continuing *New and Nonofficial Remedies*
and other publications. The Council on Physical Therapy (Physical
Medicine from 1944 to 1949, then Physical Medicine and Rehabilitation) worked energetically to educate the profession on the rapid
progress being made in this field, especially after World War II. The
Council on Foods (and Nutrition after 1940) used the pages of *JAMA*
to conduct a successful educational program for the profession on
the subject of nutrition, developing a survey book on vitamins in
1939, when vitamins were still something of a curiosity, and a
Handbook of Nutrition in 1943, with a second edition in 1951. Both
of these books were generously excerpted in *JAMA*.

The Council on Food and Nutrition was one of the first groups to
encourage the enrichment of bread, flour, and cornmeal to prevent
vitamin deficiency diseases—beriberi and pellagra in the early
days, iron deficiency anemia later. The widespread use of vitamin
D fortified milk (to prevent rickets) and iodized salt (to prevent
endemic goiter) is due largely to the pioneering work of the council.
As the processing and packaging of food grew more sophisticated in
the 1930s and 1940s, the council led the way in urging that the

nutritional values of the original food (of vitamin C in orange juice, for example) be identified and preserved.[6]

Though they were not involved in the Seal of Acceptance program, other councils and committees contributed to the AMA's scientific activities. A Council on Industrial Health (Occupational Health after 1960) was created in 1937, mostly out of the AMA's concern over the rising incidence of skin and respiratory diseases. A monthly specialty journal, *Occupational Medicine*, was first published in 1946. The council drafted the essentials for a residency in occupational medicine a year later. In 1951, the Board of Trustees established a Committee on Mental Health (a council after 1955) to improve treatment of the mentally ill and to improve the mental health of the general public. Alcoholism became an urgent topic on the agenda. The AMA worked for improved standards of treatment, ways to evaluate clinics, and better instruction on the subject in medical schools. It persuaded the insurance companies to regard alcoholism as a disease.

Starting in the 1920s, the Bureau of Health Education beamed health education material to the public by radio, sent out weekly health bulletins to 5,000 newspapers, established close liaison with the National Education Association, and promoted Keep Fit programs. The monthly AMA consumer magazine, *Hygeia* (*Today's Health* after 1950) served as a vehicle by which the Seal of Acceptance councils could communicate with the public. The magazine later started a regular feature on cosmetics, "The Look You Like," and a column, "Let's Talk about Food;" articles dealing with quackery and fraudulent medical devices frequently appeared.

Successful as the Seal of Acceptance program was—it served as an especially effective weapon for the Council on Pharmacy and Chemistry—the Board of Trustees brought it to an end on February 15, 1955.[7] Some of the councils and committees themselves wanted out because the program had reached a point where it was taking energies away from more valuable pursuits. The Council on Physical Medicine and Rehabilitation estimated that 90 percent of its work was taken up by the appraisal of apparatus.[8] The Council on Foods and Nutrition had to manage the administrative details concerning 2,400 brands of vitamin D milk, each of which had to be evaluated three times a year.[9] An editorial in *JAMA* the week the end of the program was announced pointed out, "It has been so time-consuming that there has been little time left for attention to other important work." At the same time, there was speculation over the financial impact of the program. Representatives from the advertising staff of *JAMA* told the board that discontinuing the acceptance programs would boost advertising revenues (which rose steadily during the 1950s, more rapidly after 1955); the salesmen for *Today's Health* estimated a 40 percent drop in their advertising revenues if the seal were eliminated.[10]

Valid as all those considerations might have been for terminating this particular sort of watchdog function, the board was also heeding what the AMA lawyers were saying. In September 1953, two brothers, Edward W. and Richard W. Boerstler, brought a lawsuit against the AMA after receiving a rejection of their claims for a therapeutic lamp they proposed to advertise in AMA publications. Although the suit was settled, it caused the attorneys to examine the legal exposure arising from the Seal of Acceptance program. It was not so much the type of case raised by the Boerstlers that gave the lawyers a chill; it was the threat of personal injury suits. "The public," recalls the AMA's former general counsel, Bernard D. Hirsh, "assumed that every product that bore the AMA seal had been tested by the AMA in AMA laboratories by AMA scientists and that the product was guaranteed by the AMA. We had visions of horrendous cases over injuries resulting from products which turned out not to be perfectly safe. Even if you test a product adequately, something can happen. Think of the lawsuit you'd get if some little kid lost an eye because something went wrong with an AMA accepted device."[11]

The decision of the trustees led the three councils and the one affected committee to reappraise their role and chart new directions for their efforts. The Council on Drugs radically changed its evaluation program, expanding it to provide the profession with information on a wider variety of products. During the Seal of Acceptance period, its principal output consisted of monographs in *JAMA* on new, nonofficial, and accepted remedies, which were compiled annually into *New and Nonofficial Remedies*, a compendium, really, of only AMA accepted products. Now released from the acceptance function, for which the need had diminished because of the growing activities of the federal Food and Drug Administration, the council broadened its scope of review to include a wider variety of drugs. Before, it was saying, "Here are new products we accept." Now it was saying, "Here are new products and comments as to why some are excellent, some effective only under limited conditions." *New and Nonofficial Remedies* became *New and Nonofficial Drugs,* which differed sharply from its predecessor in that it included discussion of many products that did not have the council's endorsement. In the 1965-67 edition the title was shortened to *New Drugs.*

The Council on Foods and Nutrition expanded its educational activities. It continued to monitor the safety and quality of food products in a general way, but avoided anything as strenuous as the thrice yearly analysis of 2,400 brands of vitamin D milk. In a continuing program to improve nutritional knowledge among physicians, the council developed a series of twenty-five articles, published in *JAMA,* on the role of nutrition in the management of various medical conditions. The council also instituted symposia covering such topics as fats, cholesterol, and atherosclerosis; nutrition and pregnancy; and infant nutrition. The council developed frequent statements on nutritional questions for the AMA that were useful in the formation of public policies on artificial sweeteners, low sodium milk, the fluoridation of public water supplies, and so forth.

The Committee on Cosmetics widened its sphere of activities, a change reflected in its re-designation as the Committee on Cutaneous Health and Cosmetics in 1963. Through the accumulation, preparation, and dissemination of pertinent information, it continued to promote a better understanding of cosmetics and allied preparations among the medical profession and the public. It advocated a scientific approach to the formulation and manufacture of cosmetics through proper quality controls and through laboratory and clinical investigation of new products. The Council on Physical Medicine and Rehabilitation started to evaluate classes of apparatus and physical methods rather than individual brands of products. It prepared guides to the desirable performance and characteristics of apparatus and standard methods of testing, as well as consideration of the medical, diagnostic, and therapeutic aspects of rehabilitation.

Over the ten or fifteen years following the end of the Seal of Acceptance program, other councils and committees of the AMA also made significant scientific contributions. The Council on Mental Health convened a national congress on mental health and illness in 1962 that led to the formation of mental health committees by most of the state medical associations. It helped establish national priorities for mental health treatment, emphasizing community-based care. After community mental health centers were started in the early 1960s, the council monitored their progress and operation, making critical evaluations as to how well they were living up to their promises and mandate. The council continued its work on alcoholism and accomplished a great deal in helping the medical profession arrive at a better understanding of narcotics addiction.

Extending the interest of the Council on Industrial Health in occupational injuries, a Committee on Rating of Mental and Physical Impairment undertook an exhaustive study to establish scientific bases on which fair compensation could be made to the victims of injury and disease. The studies covered thirteen bodily systems—visual, cardiovascular, extremities and back, and so forth. They extended from 1958 to 1971, and afterwards were gathered in a book, *Guidelines for Evaluation of Permanent Impairment.*

The mid-1960s witnessed the high point of the AMA's long-established scientific programs conducted at the time of the two annual meetings of the House of Delegates. One of the AMA's earliest and possibly most valuable contibutions in the nineteenth century was to provide, through its annual convention, a forum before which physicians could present scientific papers for the edification of their colleagues. These were published in the annual *Transactions* (of the meetings), and one of the purposes in the founding of *JAMA* in 1883 was to speed up their publication.[12]

In terms of attendance, the June 1965 session in New York set the all-time record for AMA scientific meetings, with 70,000 people registered, 24,268 of them physicians. Organized by the Council on Scientific Assembly, the program consisted of six half-day symposia on such topics as adverse drug reactions, hearing disorders, and organ transplants. It took eighteen pages in *JAMA* to list the scientific exhibits and twenty-eight pages just to list the topics and authors of papers scheduled before the meetings of the twenty-one scientific sections of the AMA. Advance notices of the meeting included advice for physicians who would be arriving in their own airplanes; an exhibit of physicians' artworks was scheduled, even an eighteen-hole golf tournament. The scientific and educational events easily dominated the four days of the Scientific Assembly, however. The irrepressible *New York Daily News* gave reporter Richard D. Lyons' coverage of the convention the exuberant headline: "Biggest Doc Bash Ever."

The needs of medicine were changing, however. At one time, possibly about the end of World War II, the high technology of medicine was both comprehensible and interesting to virtually the whole of the profession. But by the 1970s the advances in drugs, surgical techniques, and the medical specialties had made the sum of scientific knowledge so complex that no one physician could even come close to understanding it all.[13] The trend, clearly evident in the growth of the medical specialty societies, was forcing the AMA to rethink its approach to scientific activities. Attendance at the AMA's scientific meetings started to decline after 1965, the interest siphoned away by programs put on by the specialty societies. After June 1978, in fact, the AMA gave up on scientific programs held simultaneously with the spring and fall meetings of the House of Delegates. It tried a series of smaller regional meetings for a while, but they were not successful either and were discontinued in 1980.

The growing specialization of medical knowledge was also having its effect on the work of the councils. It was becoming more and more frequently necessary for the councils to call in outside consultants to get authoritative answers to the questions that arose. The day was long gone when the expertise of the eight or ten members of a council could embrace all that was known in a given field. In response to such requirements, some councils elected to appoint special committees and subcommittees. Finally, the AMA concluded in the mid-1970s that its structure of councils and committees had outlived its usefulness and was no longer sufficiently productive to justify the costs. The association began developing new ways to conduct its scientific activities.

The reorganization adopted in 1975 merged the responsibilities of several councils into the new Council on Scientific Affairs. This was to be *the* AMA council on scientific matters, keeping the house and board informed on the important scientific developments in medicine and formulating strong policy positions in respect to them. The assignment given to the council at its first meeting, September 30, 1976, by the chairman of the board, Raymond T. Holden, M.D., was a broad one. "The council really had to decide for itself the direction in which it wanted to go," observed Richard J. Jones, M.D., a former associate professor of medicine at the University of Chicago who was brought in to serve as the first staff secretary to the council. "There was a certain amount of going back and forth at first. Some felt we should try to achieve immediate visibility by taking up some of the issues then in the headlines—laetrile [an unproven cancer cure], for example—but the consensus of the council was that we would not accomplish much by flag-waving; the members felt we should look for issues of substance."[14]

Following the first meeting, the council decided to set up committees to work under its direction on some of the more important scientific concerns. "When we went to the board to get authorization for these committees," says Jones, "they were all turned down." Reminded that the whole idea was to get rid of formally appointed committees, the council decided it would work through ad hoc advisory panels of consultants, which were given a specific task, a specific charge, and, implicitly, a time limit. The first panels—the council usually worked with fifteen or twenty at any given time— tended to focus on things that Jones considered "pretty well worked out," alcoholism, for example, and drug abuse. "We were not really tackling anything sharply controversial," he said. "I, for one, was eager to know if the council and the AMA could do that successfully."

The sort of issue the council had in mind presented itself in 1977 when the Veterans Administration released a report on its ten-year experience with aorto-coronary bypass graft surgery, or more simply, the coronary bypass operation. By replacing a narrowed section of coronary artery with a section of healthy vein, usually taken from the patient's leg, the operation relieved the painful symptoms of angina and corrected other manifestations of ischemic (constrictive or obstructive) heart disease, such as heart failure and myocardial infarction (a form of heart attack). The profession was sharply divided on the operation, then being done at the rate of about 75,000 a year. Cardiologists (specialists in heart disease) tended to think the operation did not prolong life as promised and was too often done without adequate justification; surgeons, taking a less conservative view, strongly disagreed.

Who was right? More to the point, could the AMA, through its new scientific council, settle an issue this divisive to the satisfaction of the whole profession?

After some initial hesitation, the council decided that it would try to establish the medical indications on which a decision to operate or not operate could properly be based. Proceeding slowly, the council appointed an eleven-physician advisory panel that included some highly respected cardiologists and some equally well regarded surgeons involved in the bypass technique. Meeting for the first time in early 1978 in a hotel near Chicago's O'Hare Field, the

panelists decided to base their findings on the peer-reviewed literature—the term refers to medical journal articles that, prior to publication, undergo a careful review by experts in the field. The re-
viewers evaluate both the methods used in the development of data
and the reasoning by which the author arrives at his conclusions.
They also protect against an author rendering judgments that are
not supported by the evidence.

A cardiologist himself, Jones served as the secretary to the advisory panel, and he got things underway by drafting a 2,500-word
working paper. This was mailed to the members of the panel to
stimulate reactions. When the comments came back, they were
incorporated in a second draft. This draft was mailed back to the
panelists to serve as the focus for discussion at a subsequent meeting. Meanwhile, news of what the AMA was doing had reached the
medical grapevine, stirring up expressions of doubt as to the merits
of the council's involvement. As the panel met for the second time,
the atmosphere had grown tense. One of the panelists, a bit huffily,
asked whether this AMA group was the proper forum for the discussion of such a specialized subject.

The other members of the advisory panel asked, in effect, "If this
is not the proper way to attack the problem, what do you suggest?"

After that, the panelists went through the paper line by line.
Another rewrite was circulated and, after the comments on that
were incorporated, the report of the panelists went to the council,
which gave its approval. The AMA Board of Trustees, receiving the
report next, recognized the controversial nature of what it was
reading but, deciding that it was a balanced report and that it was
the sort of thing it had created the council to handle, adopted it and
placed it on the agenda of the House of Delegates for its next meeting, in December 1978. The house also reacted to the controversial-
ity of the subject matter, but it adopted the report with changes so
minor that the sense of the findings remained intact.

Subsequent to this report, the house set new procedural rules for
reports of the Council on Scientific Affairs. No changes at all may be
made in the reports unless the council agrees to them; the house
itself may adopt or not adopt reports, but not alter them.

Published in *JAMA* in early 1979, the report did much to end
the wrangling between the cardiologists and the cardiac surgeons
over the circumstances under which the coronary bypass operation
should be done. Through an editorial in *Lancet*, the report was also
brought to the attention of a wide readership in Great Britain. Most

important of all, by working out the criteria for a commonly performed, controversial, difficult, and expensive procedure, the report helped to reduce the vehemence of the debate and, at the same time, to strengthen the credentials of the new council and reaffirm the AMA's role, nationally and internationally, in scientific policy-making.

The council generates fifteen to twenty reports a year, a few of them just as sensitive as the one on coronary bypass surgery. Because the reports represent the consensus of well-informed physicians, they are valuable in helping practitioners not closely linked to the research and teaching centers to evaluate new procedures and methods of treatment. They can have great influence, too, on the policy decisions made by federal and state health agencies.

In an extension of its work, the council in 1981 established a system of diagnostic and therapeutic technology assessment to determine whether certain medical procedures should be regarded as established, investigational, unacceptable, or indeterminate. Relying on a panel of about 500 physician-scientists in every field, to whom the council selectively refers questions, the technology assessment program allows the council to assess the value of technological advances rather than leaving such judgments to a governmental agency. It is a way for such questions to be resolved by the profession as matters of professional evaluation and consensus.

Closely allied with the work of the Council on Scientific Affairs, although functioning independently, are five related staff operations: programs on drugs, health and human behavior, environmental and occupational health, health education, and foods and nutrition. When the AMA pruned its council-committee structure in 1975, it did not intend to eliminate its traditional involvement in scientific activities. To preserve its role and insure continuity, the AMA shifted responsibility for much of its scientific work to the staff. Since that time, staff units have worked with the Council on Scientific Affairs, with ad hoc committees, task forces, and consultants, or independently, to accomplish specific objectives. The brief accounts that follow suggest, but are not intended to describe fully, the scope of activities pursued in these programs.

• The Division of Drugs, which published the first edition of *AMA Drug Evaluations* in 1971 when the Council on Drugs was in existence, has successfully produced updated editions, often relying—as it did in the first instance—on outside consultants for expert advice. Despite a high sale price, *AMA Drug Evaluations* has gained wide acceptance by the profession. In an expanded fifth edition (1984), it is the most complete accumulation of independent judgments on some 1,800 drugs that exists. The traditional compendium, the *Physicians' Desk Reference*, published by the magazine *Medical Economics* and sent free to high-prescribing doctors, does not attempt to evaluate products but simply repeats the package insert information on each drug required by the Food and Drug Administration.

In 1982 the information in *AMA Drug Evaluations* (which is the lineal descendent of the *New and Nonofficial Remedies* of 1905) was fed into the AMA's computerized medical information system, licensed to the General Telephone and Electronics Corporation for its Telenet Medical Information Network. Through this system, to which hospitals, medical groups, and individual physicians may subscribe, the information in *AMA Drug Evaluations* is electronically accessible through small terminals that can be tied into the system by telephone lines. Medical journal abstracts have been added to what is available through the Medical Information Network, and the assessments of diagnostic and therapeutic technology made by the Council on Scientific Affairs are also available.

In addition to informational programs conducted on its own, the Division of Drugs worked with the Council on Scientific Affairs to develop reports and statements on barbiturates, the use of amphetamines in the treatment of obesity, chymopapain (an enzyme used to treat slipped spinal discs), antidepressants, and estrogen replacement in menopause.

• Besides carrying on the work of the Council on Mental Health in alcoholism and drug abuse, the staff involved in the health and human behavior program has drawn public and professional attention to several other concerns. On the subject of violence on television and its possible effect on the behavior of young viewers, the AMA supported the exploratory work being done with substantial grants and pointed out to leading national advertisers, usually to their surprise, the amount of violence portrayed on the shows on which their commercials appeared. Aided by an advisory panel appointed by the Council on Scientific Affairs, a report on the prevention and treatment of child abuse was developed, reviewing the extent of the problem, possible legislative and administrative responses, the state of research, and other aspects of this complex problem. The report urged a greater response by physicians, pledged AMA support for programs at the state level, and recommended further educational and developmental efforts.

Problems within the profession have not escaped those involved in the AMA's human behavior program. Extending an earlier interest by the Council on Mental Health in physicians impaired by psychiatric disorders, including alcoholism and drug dependence, the AMA, in cooperation with the American Psychiatric Association, began a study of physician mortality, with particular attention to medical student and physician suicide. The purpose of the study was to improve detection, diagnosis, and treatment of those who are emotionally troubled.

With an eye still on problems within the profession, the AMA in 1982 brought together twenty interested groups to make a coordinated attack on the misuse and abuse of prescription drugs such as methaqualone ("ludes"). Of the drugs identified in drug-related emergency room episodes, at least 60 percent appear to be prescription drugs. The objective of this program, aside from serving as a focal point for organizations interested in the problem, is the development of a model by which the available statistics can be integrated so as to pinpoint the avenues in a given community by which prescription drugs find their way into the illegal market. Part of the problem is theft; part is illegal manufacture or import; part is the medical profession—prescribing physicians who are uninformed, dishonest, or mentally impaired.

• The environmental and occupational health program encompasses a wide span of activities, including those once grouped under the jurisdiction of the Council on Occupational Health. It deals with concerns related to the control of communicable diseases, clean air and safe drinking water, maternal and child health, chemicals, and health safety in the workplace. Working with the Council on Scientific Affairs and using panels of consultants, this staff unit helped generate reports dealing with environmental problems such as Agent Orange, dioxin, and ionizing radiation. In the interests of vehicular safety, it updated statements on airbags and seatbelts. The staff worked with the council in preparing reports in the field of sports medicine, one giving a definition of sports injuries, and others on the participation in athletics by asthmatics and diabetics. A popular booklet is *Travelers' Health Abroad—A Guide for Physicians*. The staff, under contract with the Federal Aviation Administration, produced an authoritative report on neurological and neurosurgical conditions associated with airplane crew members. An important undertaking updated the AMA's position on medical evaluations of healthy persons; that is, periodic physical examinations.

• Since 1923, when the Council on Health and Public Instruction was divided into several groups, one of which became the Bureau of Health Education, the AMA has conducted this activity primarily through staff. The broad objectives have remained relatively constant, though the programs have undergone changes to serve different needs.

At the present time, the AMA's health education program reaches in many directions. It acts as a clearinghouse to provide health information to both the public and the profession. For the public, it develops informational materials—both print and audio/visual—on common health and disease topics. To help answer the 2,000 or more inquiries it receives from the public in an average month, the AMA has stored in a data bank answers to 1,000 of the most commonly asked questions. A request to a computer results in an informational sheet that can easily be mailed to the person asking the question. References to other sources are listed in case more detailed information is desired.

For physicians and medical societies, the AMA offers descriptions of model health education programs suitable for presentation to patients, or at schools and in the workplace. Special consultation services are available to help local medical societies or other groups launch programs. Jointly with the radio/television department of the public relations office, health education is developing slide/tape presentations on such topics as how to quit smoking, home health care, and how patients can organize their thoughts so as to make a physician appointment more productive.

The health education staff is attempting to shift from a "retail" approach, in which the AMA does most of the educating, to a "wholesale" operation, which concentrates on generating materials, ideas, and programs that can be furnished to others whose cumulative efforts have the potential for reaching far more people than the AMA alone can. The staff actively explores new opportunities, such as those in the new telecommunications technology, and seeks answers to newly identified problems. Nearing completion is a study of the way cultural (not language) barriers often hamper the delivery of optimum care by an Anglo physician to a Hispanic family.

• In foods and nutrition, the staff continued the educational efforts that were emphasized by the Council on Foods and Nutrition, especially after the Seal of Acceptance program ended. In respect to the medical profession, there was expanded activity to stimulate further emphasis on the teaching of nutrition in medical schools. Conferences were sponsored on topics such as sodium-potassium in foods and the metabolic aspects of critically ill patients. As for the public, the AMA serves as an informational source for the media on food subjects and develops educational materials.

An outstanding achievement in nutrition during the 1970s was the development of new technology by which a person may receive intravenously *all* the proteins, minerals, and vitamins necessary to preserve life for a long period of time. This required development of a highly concentrated parenteral "food" to be introduced, not in the small veins of an arm or a leg, but into the fast-flowing, large-volume bloodstream in veins located close to the heart. The AMA's principal contributions were to establish the medical need for the highly concentrated intravenous "food," develop guidelines for its composition, and, finally, develop guidelines for clinical testing for safety and efficacy. Through position papers, reports, and symposia, the AMA has encouraged the rapid growth of this new technology.

In 1963, with expectations of financial support that were later to prove naive, the Board of Trustees led the AMA into a venture unique to its history: the Institute for Biomedical Research. Technically, the institute was the offspring of the AMA Education and Research Foundation,* but since the foundation's Board of Directors then consisted of five members of the AMA Board of Trustees, the actions of the two bodies are hard to disassociate. The institute occupied 40,000 square feet of space in the AMA headquarters building, operated with annual budgets of about $1.3 million, and was staffed by a complement of more than twenty scientists, two of whom were Nobel laureates. It was a scientific undertaking of considerable ambition.

The concept originated in the fertile mind of a young physician named Roy E. Ritts, M.D., who was a professor of microbiology at the Georgetown University School of Medicine. He came there in 1957 from the Rockefeller Institute of New York. Sometime in 1962 he discussed with his medical school dean (and friend) the idea

*See Chapter 14. Effective January 1, 1962, the AMA merged its educational and research foundations—separate organizations supported by voluntary contributions—into the AMA Education and Research Foundation.

that the AMA, with what he called "its vast resources," could sponsor something structured as the Rockefeller Institute had once been, a select center of scientific excellence with a group of noted scholars banded together for the broad study of a particular concept. The dean responded warmly during the several conversations they had and told him one night, "Write it all down."[15]

The dean happened to be Hugh H. Hussey, M.D., then chairman of the AMA Board of Trustees and president of the Board of Directors of the AMA Education and Research Foundation. He was also, as Ritts knew, on the point of resigning both of his AMA elected positions and his deanship to join the AMA staff as director of the Division of Scientific Activities.

Starting his new job on January 1, 1963, Hussey soon broached Ritts' idea to F.J.L. Blasingame, M.D., the executive vice president. A man who had more than an ordinary regard for the AMA's scientific traditions, Blasingame instinctively liked the idea. He could also see potential political advantages. The AMA was then in the middle of its strident opposition to the King-Anderson national health insurance bill; the press and, more importantly, parts of the medical profession, were critical of the AMA for overemphasizing legislative and political activities. The AMA had, in fact, recently launched the American Medical Political Action Committee, a decision that many of the traditionalists did not like. "We needed something on the other side of the ledger," Blasingame recalls. "The institute could be an asset. It could raise AMA prestige in the scientific community."[16] By May, Ritts had met with the foundation board; by April 15 he had written an eloquent, twelve-page prospectus for the institute.

"At this time," it read, "there is a beginning of a new biology... that of the intracellular molecular events that are life and the aberrations that are disease...There appears a need for an institute, representing and controlled by American physicians, to inquire into the disease process at the cellular level." What he envisioned specifically was a biomedical Camelot, "a prestige group of dedicated, imaginative and brilliant workers who, because of cross-fertilization of intellects, absolute freedom from external pressures and unmatched facilities, are capable of significant scientific achievements."

In addition to Ritts' proposal to study molecular biology in an unfettered environment and Blasingame's thought of political advantage, the idea of the institute aroused other feelings of support. Many physicians were uneasy about the way the federal government was fostering scientific exploration. The research grants so generously awarded to the medical schools often went for educational purposes instead; furthermore, the pursuit of grant money, or "grantsmanship," was thought by some to distort the basic purposes of research. Others felt that the disease orientation of the National Institutes of Health was wrong. Thus, the concept of a competing institute in the private sector, established by private practitioners, unrestricted by external direction, and dedicated to "pure" research, had a philosophical appeal.

Assembling in the Hotel Traymore in Atlantic City that June just before the 1963 annual meeting, the AMA Board of Trustees heard a presentation from Ritts, who had driven up from Georgetown to make it. Addressing the opening session of the House of Delegates a day or so later, on June 16, Raymond M. McKeown, M.D., who had succeeded Hussey as president of the Board of Directors of the AMA Education and Research Foundation, announced that it had authorized the Institute for Biomedical Research and that "the AMA board had reviewed this project and endorsed its early implementaton."[17]

Referred to a reference committee of the house (even though the delegates had no jurisdiction over foundation matters), the announcement drew a cool reception. The reference committee that received the report said that the delegates attending its hearing resented it as a *fait accompli*. Nevertheless, the committee expressed its opinion that the institute would be "valuable both in the terms of scientific research and enhancing the public's appreciation of the medical profession."[18]

The only explicit opposition came later from the Council on Medical Education. At its meeting in September 1963 the council "voiced its concern in regard to both the effectiveness of the proposed institute and that the board had developed its planning to the point of public announcement without providing the council an opportunity to express its views on a matter so closely related to the council's interest."[19] Though mild, the statement had an ominous ring.

Throughout the rest of 1963, all of 1964 and most of 1965, the preparatory work went forward, initially under Hussey's overall supervision. Hussey hired Ritts in November 1963 as assistant director of the Division of Scientific Activities. Ritts was appointed director of the institute in February 1964, responsible for its physical arrangements and the recruiting of staff. Additions were made to the east end of the headquarters building to house the laboratories and studies of the yet-to-be-engaged scientists. Plumbers working in the AMA building today are occasionally astonished to find the acid-proof piping that was installed at that time. Ritts helped design a ninth floor penthouse to shelter the large number of animals that would be needed in the cellular research that would be done.

The recruiting program was worldwide in scope. Ritts offered generous benefits: salaries generally higher than the prevailing rate, academic tenure, freedom from administrative and teaching requirements often attached to similar positions, allowances for travel to attend scientific conferences, few obligations regarding publication. Two of the first scientists to join came from the Rockefeller Institute, one of them as the director of the animal facility. Another recruit was Sir John Carew Eccles, an Australian who had won the 1963 Nobel prize for Physiology and Medicine. He was to continue his work in neurophysiology, concentrating on the structure of the cerebellum and its ability to process information and form thoughts. The institute opened to considerable fanfare in October 1965. An editorial in *JAMA* marked the event enthusiastically, saying, "The institute provides a prototype of the utopian research facility."

The work of the institute appeared to proceed productively. It was generally aimed at discovering more about the human cell— how different cell types discriminate among various chemical signals, how information is carried by chemical molecules, how viruses penetrate mammalian cells and make them malignant. Members of the institute contributed papers on their work to the scientific journals; they conducted symposia and published books, notably the 921-page *Neurobiology of Cerebellar Evolution and Development*, edited by Rodolfo Llinas, M.D., Ph.D., of the institute staff.

On the ninth floor the AMA boarded an extraordinary menagerie: alligators, electric fish, frogs, ferrets, gerbils, goats, hamsters, lobsters, guinea pigs, rabbits, rats, kangaroo rats, salamanders, sheep, squid, and squirrel monkeys. There were, in addition, cats suffering from virus-infection-induced ataxia (loss of coordination), and five strains of mice with recessive genes for different types of cerebellar lesions.[20] During the famous 1967 Chicago blizzard, which paralyzed the city for four days, the AMA furnaces ran dangerously low on oil, causing Blasingame genuine concern that if the oil trucks could not get through there could be a temperature drop in the building that would endanger "our $200,000 worth of mice." These were "gnotobiotic," according to an AMA report at the time, free of "ectoparasites, endoparasites and pathogenic microorganisms." (In other words, they harbored no disease-causing germs.)

By spring of 1967, the demands of the institute were beginning to stir questions among the delegates. The stream of front money that the foundation had received from industry, and which it had hoped would continue, began to dry up. The AMA itself was contributing $500,000 a year from its regular revenues. At the annual meeting in June the California delegation introduced a resolution that noted the recent increase in dues, the AMA's rising expenses, and a drop in the advertising revenues of AMA publications. The resolutions called for the appointment of a committee of the house to review the institute and "establish its relative priority among the objectives of the AMA."

The resolution was not adopted, but by the end of 1967 the institute was clearly in trouble. Ritts had announced his intention to accept an offer from the Mayo Foundation at the end of the year. A successor had been found, George W. Beadle, Ph.D., a distinguished biologist and a Nobel laureate in 1958. He had agreed to join the institute as director late in 1968 upon his retirement as president of the University of Chicago. Partly because of the needs for space in the AMA building, partly because of Beadle's conviction that the institute would function better in a university setting, it seemed that something close to $3 million for new quarters would soon be needed. This intensified the doubts about the whole idea of an AMA-supported research program. J. Alfred Fabro, M.D., a delegate from Connecticut, summarized a strong feeling in the house when he told the November 1967 meeting, "I seriously question that one of the purposes of the AMA is basic biomedical research."[21] But no action was taken.

A year later, at the December 1968 meeting, one of the reference committees, reporting to the house on its hearings, noted "the concern expressed on the allocation of ERF funds to biomedical research as compared to that for its educational effort. The point was made repeatedly that the need...of funds...in medical education is urgent...These observations were supported by a report of the Council on Medical Education which was made available to the committee."[22] Those close to medical education saw the annual contributions of the foundation to the medical schools being threatened by the growing financial demands of the institute. Working through the Council on Medical Education, they were trying to protect a source of income.

A special committee of the house was authorized at the meeting, not as suggested a year and a half earlier by California to "review" the institute, but to try to broaden the Education and Research Foundation's base of financial support. As it conducted its explorations, the liaison committee found the prospects dim, and, reporting back to the house in November-December 1969, noted the "vast" sums needed to construct a new home for the institute near the University of Chicago campus, the unpredictability of outside funds, and inevitably rising costs. It recommended that the institute be discontinued.[23] The house agreed.

The doors closed for good in July 1970, ending a serious, well-intentioned, $6.5 million experiment. As much as anything else, it was a victim of the AMA's inability to develop a reliable way to fund it.

Of all the scientific functions of the AMA, none has continued longer, served physicians better, or advanced scientific medicine farther than the publication of the journals. The oldest of these, *JAMA*, a publication of national and international stature, has appeared on a weekly or four-times-a-month schedule since 1883. With a 1982 circulation of 323,000 for its English language edition, it is the most widely read English-language medical journal in the world. In addition to *JAMA*, the AMA publishes nine monthly specialty journals, for which the editor of *JAMA* has traditionally had the overall editorial responsibility. Their titles, first year of publication, and 1982 circulation are listed in Table 1.

When Morris Fishbein, M.D., was forced out as the editor of *JAMA* in 1949, he left behind a publishing enterprise of unquestioned strength and vigor. The AMA's revenues from advertising* exceeded $2.4 million that year, then sufficient to finance a year's operation of the AMA under ordinary circumstances. Not only was the number of competing journals small, but *JAMA* also had an abundance of that ingredient so essential to any successful publication—a distinct character of its own, reflective of a strong personality in the editor's chair. Under Fishbein, *JAMA*'s pages crackled with his humor, his scholarship, his curiosity, his penchant for political broadside. The nation's top physician-scientists and researchers were eager to submit their most important papers to him for publication. His was a tough act to follow.

*The figure represents the revenues of all AMA publications. *JAMA* was, and is, by far the largest contributor.

TABLE 1
AMA Specialty Journals

	First year of Publication	1982 Circulation
American Journal of Diseases of Children	1911	25,000
The Archives of Dermatology[a]	1920	16,500
The Archives of General Psychiatry[b]	1919	19,700
The Archives of Internal Medicine	1908	67,700
The Archives of Neurology[b]	1919	14,000
The Archives of Ophthalmology	1929	15,300
The Archives of Otolaryngology	1925	11,200
The Archives of Pathology and Laboratory Medicine	1926	10,700
The Archives of Surgery	1920	43,900

(A tenth specialty journal, Occupational Medicine, started in 1946, became the Archives of Industrial Hygiene and Occupational Medicine in 1950 and the Archives of Environmental Health in 1960. Never able to establish a firm readership base, it was sold in 1976.)

[a]The Archives of Dermatology traces its ancestry to 1881 when it was published by the American Dermatological Association.

[b]The Archives of Neurology and Psychiatry began in 1919. By action of the Board of Trustees in 1959, it was split into separate journals.

Simultaneously with his departure, political events were forcing organizational change on the AMA. When the concept of Fellowship members gave way to regularly charged membership dues, *JAMA* became a benefit of membership. This boosted circulation from around 137,000 in 1949 to about 167,000 in 1951. Helped by a peak period for the introduction of new pharmaceutical products—particularly antibiotics—annual advertising revenues soared from $2.7 million in 1951 to more than $8 million in 1959. The size of the journal thickened to issues with as many as 300 pages, in contrast to a standard of 128 pages in the late 1940s. It had subscribers in 119 countries.

For nearly all of the 1950s, the new editor, Austin Smith, M.D., ran an operation quite different from Fishbein's. Promoted from his position as the staff secretary of the Council on Pharmacy and Chemistry, Smith had little editorial background.* Lacking Fishbein's flair, he methodically had readership studies done to identify the parts of the journal that were the best read and to help him decide how to allocate editorial space. He continued the humorous "Tonics and Sedatives" feature but toned it down and, of course, eliminated Fishbein's chatty "Dr. Pepys' Diary," which had often appeared in it. Unlike his predecessor, he kept the *JAMA* editorial page out of national politics. Smith reduced the size of the W.B. Saunders ad (for books and other publications) that had run across the bottom third of the front cover page for years. The change allowed for a more generous display of the table of contents above. He added new features, one on leisure activities and hobbies, one on the business aspects of medical practice, one called "Medicine at Work," which focused on how non-medical organizations worked with physicians on various problems.

Smith's major shift in editorial direction reflected his recognition of changes in the AMA. "I could see it," he recalled, "The AMA was changing from a scientific body to a partly politically-oriented organization...Some of this I supported; some I had reservations about...Anyway, my objective was to use the printed word to convey scientific information and organizational thinking. To this extent, my responsibilities were different from those of Morris."[24] Accordingly, Smith gave over about one article in ten to the reports and doings of the AMA councils and committees, hoping, as he stated in a 1951 report to the house, to draw "more attention to the activities of the various councils, bureaus and committees of the AMA so that their work may become better known and the information in their files more widely used."[25]

During the last of Smith's editorship and during the ten-month editorship of Johnson F. Hammond, M.D., in 1959, *JAMA* gave every outward appearance of robust health. The weekly issues were fat, allowing sometimes for the publication of 145 or more pages of editorial material. At nearly 180,000, circulation continued to climb. Helped by the introduction of the tranquilizers in the mid-1950s, advertising revenues proceeded on a steady upward path. But some of the former editorial vitality and spark was gone. A decade later, another *JAMA* editor had tart comments on the matter. "*The Journal* of the 1950s," wrote Hugh H. Hussey, M.D., "seems to have been

---

*After leaving *JAMA* at the end of 1958, he became, successively, president of the Pharmaceutical Manufacturers Association, chairman and chief executive officer of Parke, Davis & Co., and vice chairman of the board of Warner-Lambert Co.

guided by a conservatism common to behemoths and mammoths, doomed to a measure of inertia by size and lumbering movement."[26]

A slippage in editorial prestige is a factor of more than ordinary importance to a scientific journal. Unlike most regular magazines, the true scientific journal depends heavily on scientific papers that are voluntarily submitted for publication rather than on articles that are assigned or solicited. When leading physicians, scientists, and medical researchers think their work has progressed to the point where it should be published for the scientific community, they write a paper and submit it to what they consider the most respected journal in the field. Each hopes his manuscript will be accepted; if it is not, he sends it on to the less prestigious publications. When a scientific journal starts losing its editorial reputation, it thus loses first crack at the more desirable, news-making manuscripts. Forced to publish what has been rejected elsewhere, the journal suffers further loss of stature, causing even more slippage in the quality of material available to it. Over time, this turns into the classic vicious circle.

To reverse what it saw as a downward trend, the Board of Trustees in October 1959 appointed as editor John H. Talbott, M.D., a man with outstanding academic credentials and experience as a scientific journal editor. A graduate of the Harvard Medical School and a former member of the staff of the Massachusetts General Hospital, he had studied at Göttingen and Innsbruck. At the time of his appointment he was a professor of medicine at the University of Buffalo, a well-published author, a recognized authority on gout, and the editor of the respected quarterly, *Medicine*.

It took him little time to recognize what had to be done. To procure an increasingly high percentage of top quality manuscripts as early as possible, he wrote to the key department heads and the deans of all eighty-four medical schools, outlining his plans for an improved *JAMA*. His aim was "high quality medical information to both the non-specialist and (in the fields other than his own) the specialist."[27] In an early issue, April 23, 1960, he dropped the Saunders ad from the front cover, calling attention to the change in an editorial. He said it was "the initial presentation to the medical profession of the philosophy of the current regimen for improvement of the scientific publications of the AMA."[28]

Talbott had a number of changes to make. He reversed Smith's policy of using generous amounts of material supplied internally, telling the councils and committees that their reports would be considered along with other material but given no special priority. "The Council on Drugs is cooperating," he reported near the end of his first year, "by submitting brief reports instead of long and sometimes uninteresting material. The response of other councils and committees has not always been enthusiastic."[29] The House of Delegates backed him up in 1966 when he refused to accept for publication a paper presented by the chairman of one of the scientific sections at the Scientific Assembly. Talbott started a successful news section. He changed the binding of the journal from saddle-stitch (folded, then stapled) to perfect (squared off, like a book), enabling readers to tear out articles more easily for filing. Having dropped advertising from the cover, he first introduced a new, two-color logotype, then began using small, four-color photographs, and finally developed the basic cover format used from the later 1960s on—four-color reproductions of works of art.

At the end of the decade, Talbott retired, assuming a new title, Editor Emeritus. During his last two years, for reasons having to do more with marketing factors than his abilities as an editor, the advertising revenues of *JAMA* and other AMA publications turned sharply downward, sinking from $13.6 million in 1967 to $11.9 million in 1968 and to $10 million in 1969. The days of 300-page issues of *JAMA*, almost a standard in the early 1960s, vanished, and *JAMA*, like the AMA, entered a decade of leaner budgets and administrative tension.

As the AMA financial picture darkened, Hugh H. Hussey, M.D., the new editor, found his difficulties multiplied. He had to live with repeated economy drives, accepting cuts in the number of editorial pages as the number of advertising pages fell. Under pressure, he agreed to the interspersal of advertising, giving advertisers more favorable positions, instead of grouping all the ads together at the front and back of each issue. This, it was hoped, would increase sales. He did, however, deliver a firm "No" when it was suggested the *JAMA* might perform better financially on a fortnightly rather than a weekly publication schedule. Editorial space nevertheless stayed tight, and the backlog of accepted but unpublished manuscripts grew. In those straits, Hussey dropped the publication of council material in all but the most exceptional of circumstances. When he retired from the editorship near the end of 1973, not in the best of health, Hussey was respected as a scholarly and careful editor.

His successor, Robert H. Moser, M.D., was, by contrast, a wave-maker of formidable energy. A graduate of Georgetown, he had pursued his medical career in the United States Army, rising to chief of medicine at Walter Reed Hospital. When appointed to the editorship of *JAMA* in 1973, Moser came on like a medical version of General Patton. He knew exactly what he wanted to do: make *JAMA* an instrument for continuing medical education as well as a journal for reporting new advances and developments. In an interview at the time his apppointment was announced, he told *AMNews* "...I think some good can be accomplished in improving the general education of the American physician, and I feel *JAMA* may be the principal organ for achieving this."[30] Moser created an advisory board for *JAMA* consisting of some twenty-five top physicians in the major medical specialties and close to the major teaching centers. It was a much needed move. Scattered widely across the country, the advisors helped to recruit manuscripts, critique issues of the journal, pass on responsible comments from other physicians, and promote *JAMA* as a teaching medium for students and residents.

Convinced that a journal of *JAMA*'s stature should be doing more than it was internationally, Moser launched a Spanish language edition, working through a Barcelona-based physician-publisher.[31] The agreement called for the exchange of rights to publish *JAMA* material, under well-defined conditions, for royalties from the new *JAMA en Espanol*, circulated in Spain. If successful, the Spanish publisher would work with Moser in extending editions into Latin America. But Moser's aggressiveness led him into trouble with the fiscal restraints that were being applied. When he, along with the other AMA editors and division directors, was asked to cut costs further in early 1975, he threatened to resign rather than reduce the number of pages of *JAMA*. His resignation was accepted.

William R. Barclay, M.D., director of the Division of Scientific Activities since 1970 and before that a professor of medicine at the University of Chicago, succeeded him. As a senior staff executive, Barclay appreciated just how difficult the AMA's financial position was, which caused him to approach the editorship with restraint. "What the administration asked me to do," he said, "was to publish a respectable medical journal that would interest enough physicians to attract advertisers but require a minimum number of pages."

Though his background was teaching and research, Barclay edited *JAMA* with the practitioner in mind. He tended to emphasize what was established and known, "educational reminders of what good science was," he said. Highly technical articles, he thought, usually belonged in the specialty journals. "It was not practical to publish in a journal of 200,000 circulation information that might be understood and applied by only 3,000 or 4,000 physicians," he pointed out. "What *JAMA* tried to do was stay in the forefront of medical science in those areas that could be understood by the majority of physicians." More so than Hussey or Talbott, Barclay edited *JAMA* with a sure and unerring instinct for what the clinician needed to know.

Six months into Barclay's editorship, the staff reorganization that created the new position of publisher occurred. Under the publisher were grouped all of the business functions involved in getting out a journal—circulation fulfillment, printing, advertising sales, everything except the editorial operation. During Barclay's editorship and supported by his editorial efforts, the newly centralized management of the AMA made publishing decisions that expanded *JAMA's* role as an international journal. Starting in 1976, five additional Spanish language versions of *JAMA* were developed for Mexico, Central America, Colombia, Venezuela, and Argentina. Groundwork was laid for a Portuguese language edition in Portugal and Brazil. But the world wide economic troubles that spread in 1979 hit the Spanish-speaking areas with particular force, driving the AMA's Spanish publisher into bankruptcy and ending—temporarily, the AMA hoped—efforts to use *JAMA* in widening the availability of American medical knowledge.

In 1976 and 1977, as the additional Spanish language editions were getting underway, a broader outlook on international publishing was developing within the AMA, especially among several senior staff executives, notably James H. Sammons, M.D., the executive vice president, Joe D. Miller, his senior deputy, and Thomas F. Hannon, the new publisher. A trip to China in 1974 by a group of trustees and top staff executives opened a lot of eyes to American medical obligations—and opportunities—abroad. This was intensified a few years later when the AMA started having second thoughts about its resignation from the World Medical Association in 1972 because of an inequitable dues structure and overpermissive bylaws relating to participation and voting. In soliciting support from the Europeans and the Japanese for the bylaw changes it was preparing for that association, the AMA was further exposed to international medical concerns. At the time the World Medical Association adopted bylaw changes in 1978, satisfying the AMA's objections and paving the way for the AMA's re-entry the next year, the AMA made a deliberate long range commitment to an expanded international role for *JAMA*. The decision was neither a large financial risk nor an opportunity for immediate, sizeable financial returns; it was motivated more by the perception of an international societal obligation than anything else.

At the start of 1983, working through royalty arrangements with foreign medical publishers, *JAMA* had foreign language editions in French, German, Flemish, and Japanese appearing predominantly on a monthly basis in France, Germany, Switzerland, Belgium, and Japan. Making its own publishing arrangements through the Chinese Medical Association in Peking, the AMA was also producing a bimonthly Chinese language edition of *JAMA* in the People's Republic of China. Circulation of all the foreign language editions totaled 120,000.[32] In addition, an Italian edition was started in January 1984.

Following Barclay's retirement, George D. Lundberg, M.D., became the fourteenth editor of *JAMA* at the beginning of 1982. A medical graduate of the University of Alabama with a master's degree in science from Baylor, the forty-eight-year-old Lundberg had been professor of pathology at the University of Southern California and afterward Professor and Chief of the Department of Pathology at the University of California, Davis. A frequent contributor to medical journals, he had been a member of the *JAMA* advisory board.

Compared to what his three immediate predecessors had to work with, Lundberg inherited a *JAMA* in sturdy condition. Circulation stood at an alltime high, reflecting a wider AMA membership, a modest growth in paid subscriptions, and increased amounts of controlled circulation (that is, subscriptions sent free to physicians in some medical specialties considered particularly desirable by advertisers.) Under the new publisher, Thomas F. Hannon, and the new vice president for publishing, John T. Baker, AMA's overall advertising revenues slowly started to turn around after a low of $8.2 million in 1975. They rose to $10.8 million in 1977 and $12.1 million in 1980. In 1981, 1982, and 1983, however, income dramatically surged ahead, to $15.2 million in 1981, $20.8 million in 1982, and $23.8 million in 1983. Many factors contributed to the improvement: a better performance by all AMA publications; more products coming to market; the availability of new demographic advertising editions of *AMNews*. These permit an advertiser to place his ads only in the copies that go to the physicians likely to prescribe the advertised product. The advertiser thus does not have to pay for circulation that goes to readers outside of his targeted market. After *JAMA* initiated a demographic edition in 1983, it was able to compete far more successfully with what physicians often call throwaway publications (i.e. periodicals with totally controlled circulations) that had for years been able to tailor their distribution to maximize their appeal to advertisers.

Thanks to the improving revenues, Lundberg was soon editing 144-page issues of *JAMA* and working with seventy to ninety editorial pages each week. This was a decided improvement over the 100-page issues with fifty-five to sixty editorial pages that Hussey, Moser, and Barclay were often confined to.

As for operating philosophy, Lundberg quickly established himself as a man of definite ideas. From the beginning, he made it clear he would insist on a wider use of the peer review process than his predecessors. As a rule, the major articles in a peer review journal are subjected to review. But sometimes, when there is a staff authority present or in cases where the author is a widely known authority, exceptions are made. Lundberg, despite such circumstances, insisted on the review of many articles his predecessors might have exempted, on the theory that articles that have undergone the peer review process have more value than those that have not.

In a statement of guidelines developed with his editorial staff and the publisher's office, Lundberg spelled out some of his other editorial goals. *JAMA*, according to the statement, should be enjoyable to read as well as educational. Its scope should be international. Controversial issues should not be ducked but should be responsibly debated. As an official journal, *JAMA* should inform readers as to the AMA policy positions "as appropriate." Lundberg estimated, however, that only about 2 percent of *JAMA* would be taken up with internally generated material.

His overriding goal, he stated, was a well-informed reader. "We feel that a physician, if he reads only *JAMA* for a year but reads every issue cover to cover, should not, at the end of the year, be out of touch with anything in the general medical field. That is what we try to do."[33]

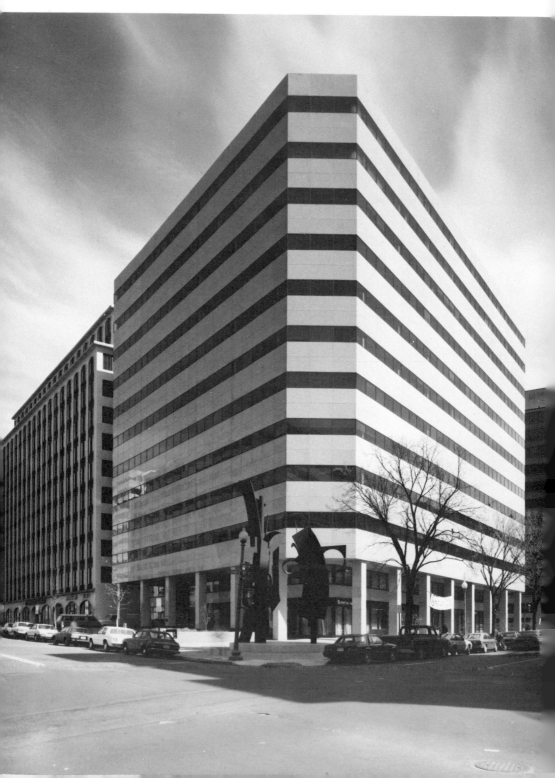

The AMA and Medical Care Today

Near the outset of this book, the statement was made that many forces have pushed and pulled at the United States medical care system during the last forty years and brought about substantial change. The pushing and the pulling and the changes having undergone an attentive examination in the intervening chapters, it may be instructive now to attempt some sort of retrospective appraisal—a weighing of the benefits achieved against the costs, an assessment of the new problems that have arisen to replace the old, and a final look at the role of the AMA in the whole process.

Without question, the American public has emerged a beneficiary, the health status of the nation having improved in remarkable ways. Life expectancy at birth for the American male is now more than seventy years, compared to sixty-one in 1940; for the American female, it is now more than seventy-seven years, versus sixty-five in 1940.[1] The infant mortality rate has plunged from forty-seven deaths per 1,000 live births to something under twelve, though the death rate for black infants approaches twice the rate of whites.[2] A number of common diseases about which medicine could once do little can now be prevented, cured, or managed. Tuberculosis, a crippling, chronic, and expensive disease in 1940, was also the fourth leading cause of death then; syphilis, with its devastating consequences, ranked as the eighth. Today, neither one appears as a significant item on the mortality tables.[3] Polio, once capable of sending waves of fear through whole communities, has all but disappeared, as has whooping cough. Measles and German measles, with their sometimes damaging after-effects, are well under control.[4] Heart disease, the number one killer, and stroke, the number three killer, have been reduced to the point where their death rates are approaching, respectively, two-thirds and a half of their former levels.[5]

Partly because people who might have succumbed to other diseases early in life now live to middle and old age, cancer, the number two killer, is a more common cause of death than it used to be. At the same time, however, treatment methods have become more effective. In 1940, according to the American Cancer Society, about 25 percent of cancer victims were alive five years after initial treatment; the 1982 figure is 38 percent.

Of the advances that have occurred, the ones having the sharpest impact are those affecting health at birth and soon thereafter. Life expectancy at age sixty-five has lengthened, but only from about fourteen additional years to just over sixteen.[6] What has shifted the demographics dramatically is the drop in the infant mortality rate. Many of the gains here are attributable to new medicines and more sophisticated medical care—new diagnostic techniques, including amniocentesis, which can sometimes identify disorders of the fetus, early identification and better management of high risk pregnancies, and advances in neonatal care. The main effect, however, is felt at the other end of the lifespan; in a significant way, it helps account for an over-sixty-five population of some twenty-six million Americans, more than double that of 1940.[7] Just in itself, this is a considerable population, equivalent roughly to that of Canada or of Norway and Sweden combined. Its financial strain on the Social Security system is well known; what has received less attention is its effect on medical care costs. As the risks of fatal disease among younger people decline, the risks of diseases associated with the later years increase. Unfortunately for the national health budget, the preponderance of these illnesses of the elderly, including heart disease and cancer, are often prolonged and expensive to treat. Thus, what success American medicine has had in making the nation healthier has raised, not lowered, the cost. If medical care continues to increase life expectancy, our national health bill will, presumably, continue to mount.

It is a mistake in logic to attribute better health statistics exclusively to better medicine. The truth is that good health results from many factors, of which medical care is only one. A person's genetic heritage affects health, as do nutrition, public sanitation, environment, living standards, education, and personal choices as to the use of tobacco, alcohol, and other drugs. Actually, to read what some scholars have written, you might conclude that medical care hardly makes any difference at all. The political scientist, Aaron Wildavsky, Ph.D., has even made an attempt to quantify medicine's role. "According to the Great Equation," he wrote, "Medical Care Equals Health. But the Great Equation is wrong. More available medical care does *not* equal better health. The best estimates are that the medical system (doctors, drugs, hospitals) affects only about 10% of the usual indices for measuring health."[8] Although Wildavsky may overstate his point, it is nonetheless valid. To attribute all progress in health to advances in medical science or to improvements in the medical care system is to oversimplify. Oversimplification, it might be noted, scarcely weakens political argument, and the Great Equation has been a well-used tool for those who have advocated sweeping changes in the medical care system over the decades, everyone from President Harry S. Truman to Senator Edward M. Kennedy.

Within the medical profession itself, possibly the greatest change in the last forty years, aside from the transformation wrought by specialization, has been a shift in practice patterns. Up until World War II, physicians were predominantly solo practitioners. Even today, Louis J. Goodman, Ph.D., director of the AMA Department of Health Care Financing and Organization, estimates that two-thirds of the 272,000 active, office-based physicians engaged in patient care are in solo practice or two-person partnerships. Yet there has been a pronounced trend toward group practice, defined as three or more physicians who deliver patient care, make joint use of equipment and personnel, and divide income by a prearranged formula.

A rarity in 1946, accounting for only 3,048 physicians, or 2.6 percent of the profession then,[9] group practice today attracts about a quarter of the active, office-based physicians engaged in patient care—88,290, according to the AMA's 1980 survey data. In one part of the United States, the West North Central states of North and South Dakota, Nebraska, Kansas, Missouri, Iowa, and Minnesota, over half of the office-based practitioners are in organized groups. And since the proportion of group physicians under thirty-five years of age has been increasing nationwide, it is not difficult to speculate that the trend will continue. Multispecialty groups have attracted a little over 61 percent of the physicians in group practice; single specialty groups, over 33 percent; and family practice groups, over 5 percent. Though there is one group with more than 1,400 physicians, most groups the AMA identified in its 1980 study have between eight and nine members. Of the 10,762 groups identified, 1,884 derived at least some revenue from care provided on a prepaid basis, that is, through a contract arrangement with a Health Maintenance Organization.[10]

In broad terms, the office-based, patient-care physician practices medicine in one of four ways. He may be a solo practitioner, charging his patients fees for each service rendered. He may practice in a fee-for-service group, in which the patient receives a bill for each service rendered, the physician group distributing overall revenues according to a prearranged formula. The other two modes of practice involve the physician with a Health Maintenance Organization.* Here, there are alternatives. One, the physician may be in prepaid group practice, meaning that the HMO has a closed panel of physicians (salaried, staff physicians in a clinic, for example) who provide the medical services for those enrolled. Or, two, the physician may be a member of an Independent Practice Association (IPA) with an open panel arrangement. In this case, the IPA (it can be a county medical society, for example) contracts with the HMO to provide services for so much per year per person enrolled. Patients may choose their physicians from among the membership of the IPA; the IPA reimburses the physician on a fee-for-service basis. It has become increasingly difficult to separate physicians exactly into those four compartments, however, for it is perfectly possible for an individual, office-based practitioner to derive income from more than one practice mode.

In the early 1980s, with the number of physicians growing and the competition for the health care dollar rising, more and more physicians entered new systems for the delivery and financing of care—preferred provider organizations (PPOs), which are prepaid groups offering low-cost contracts to deliver care to a specified population; surgicenters, which perform surgical services that do not require overnight hospitalization; and immediate care centers which are clinics to serve those who need to see a doctor "right now" but whose condition is not so serious as to merit a trip to a hospital emergency room.

Although the physician's office remains the most common place where medical care and consultation are given, the role of the hospital has grown to be far more important than it was forty years ago. In 1975, 13 percent of all physician visits took place in either a

---

*An HMO is an organization responsible for providing or arranging comprehensive health care services for a voluntarily enrolled population at so much per person per year. An enrollee's annual payment remains constant no matter how extensive the provided medical services may be.

hospital clinic or a hospital emergency room.[11] One reason for the new hospital role is its location for new medical technology; more and more, the patient with a serious complaint sees his doctor in a hospital. Another is that hospitals have expanded patient services; in addition to more than 60,000 resident physicians, there are now more than 40,000 full-time, hospital-based staff physicians providing patient care.[12] A third reason has to do with what has happened in the inner cities. Along with the flight of people to the suburbs, there has been a flight of some physician offices. Left in many places are the hospitals and, nearby, concentrations of low-income population, including many blacks. As a result, one out of every four physician visits by blacks is made in a hospital outpatient clinic or emergency room. The proportion for whites is one visit in eight.[13] House calls, which accounted for about 9 percent of visits in 1959, recently accounted for less than 1 percent of the total.[14]

As far as changes in the medical care system are concerned, the major shift since 1940 has been in the way medical treatment is financed. From overwhelming reliance on out-of-pocket payments in 1940, we now have a system that is basically insured. Medicaid, financed in part by federal appropriations and in part by contributions of individual states, covers about twenty-three million people—the welfare population and many (but by no means all) of the indigent. Medicare, financed largely by Social Security taxes and partly by contributions of the recipients, benefits about twenty-seven million retired people. As for the working population, the great majority of families that are self-supporting, health insurance is provided through private, voluntary programs, many of them financed entirely or in part by employers as a benefit of employment. Private health insurance, protecting only 12 million people in 1940, at the end of 1979 covered hospital charges for 183 million people, surgical charges for 174 million, and physician charges for 164 million; 148 million Americans had major medical coverage.[15]

Of all the money spent on physician services during 1982, direct payment by patients accounted for 37.7 percent; the rest was supplied either through government programs or by private insurance plans. Of all the money that went to cover hospital charges, direct payment by patients amounted to 10.8 percent; the rest was covered by government programs and private insurance.[16]

As in 1940, the American medical care system remains pluralistic—part private, part public. Since 1940, however, the government share of the total bill has grown from 20 percent to over 40 percent.[17] If those figures represent a fair measure, the long ideological struggle between those favoring private medicine and those advocating a publicly financed system may be said to have ended in something of a compromise. Though quiet, the conflict still exists, on one side the philosophical legatees of the New Deal, the Fair Deal, the Great Society; on the other, conservatives, many moderates, the AMA.

While solidly supporting private medicine and private medical insurance, physicians acknowledge a role for the government in the financing of medical care, though most of them ardently want the government role confined to help for those unable to finance their own care. They argue that mainstream Americans—those who support themselves in a basically private economy—should be served by a basically private medical care system. They believe that a patient should be free to choose among the various forms of medical care that are available; they value their own freedom to choose the type of practice they engage in.

Somewhere between the liberal and conservative viewpoints, and not very vocal, is a public that is not intensely committed either way. Poll after poll in the 1970s indicated wide public satisfaction with the quality of care received. According to a 1981 survey done by the Gallup Organization for the AMA, 90 percent of the respondents were either "fairly" or "well" satisfied with their last visit to a doctor. The public, however, is deeply concerned over the rising costs of care (as are physicians); 68 percent perceive a need for national health insurance. However, only 44 percent are in favor if it means an increase in taxes. Support for national health insurance runs most heavily among younger people, union members, and lower income and less educated groups. The ability to afford adequate health insurance coverage and the perception of others' ability to afford coverage also condition attitudes. Those who either cannot afford coverage themselves or assume that others cannot, tend to give responses favoring national health insurance.[18]

In the process of changing the way it finances medical care, the United States substantially reduced and in some cases even eliminated out-of-pocket cost for all but 10-15 percent of the population. What happened as a result is what usually happens when a desired service becomes easier to obtain: a surge in demand. Occurring in the presence of many technological improvements, a rise in living standards and a 71 percent population growth, the lowering of the economic barriers to medical care guaranteed an explosive increase in the use of the system. Some statistics:

- Hospital admissions rose from 13.6 million a year in 1940 to 36.2 million a year in 1980.[19]
- Physician visits per person, averaging something like two to three a year before 1940, now run to about five a year.[20]
- Between 1970 and 1979, total outpatient visits to hospitals increased 44 percent.[21]

The indices of utilization of the medical system rose especially rapidly following passage of Medicare and Medicaid in 1965. People in the lowest income brackets, for example, started seeing physicians more often than people in any other income category. Before 1965, those people, whose health statistics were also poor, saw physicians with the least frequency. At the same time, people in the more affluent brackets started seeing physicians less frequently. The reversal is apparent in Table 1.

TABLE 1
Physician Visits per Person per Year by Income

	$3,000 or less	$3-7,000	$7-10,000	$10-15,000	$15,000 or more
1963-4	4.3	4.5	4.7	4.8	5.8
1966-7	4.6	4.1	4.3	4.5	4.9
1973	6.0	5.2	4.8	4.9	5.1
1975	6.4	5.5 (est.)	5.0	4.8	4.9

Source: U.S. Department of Health, Education, and Welfare. *Vital and Health Statistics*, Series 10, Nos. 97, 128.

What about the differences in the utilization of medical services between whites and blacks? Table 2 shows two things; (1) blacks and whites both are seeing physicians more frequently than they used to; and (2) soon after Medicaid and Medicare, blacks started seeing physicians with nearly 50 percent more frequency than before.

TABLE 2
Physician Visits per Person per Year by Race

	White	Black
1963-4	4.7	3.3
1966-7	4.5	3.1
1975	5.1	4.7

Source: U.S. Department of Health, Education, and Welfare. *Vital and Health Statistics*, Series 10, Nos. 97, 128.

A federal government report that relies on later data states: "Minority groups are often assumed to have less access to or availability of medical care, but the data clearly do not indicate a pattern of differentials in the use of physician services. For example, black children showed less use than white children, but black young and middle-aged adults showed the same or more use as whites."[22]

Because of increasing demand, which actually began to grow before Medicare and Medicaid, the American medical care system has expanded five-fold to the point where it has become the employer of 5.1 million people, the third largest industry in the economy.[23] Medical schools now graduate more than three times the number of physicians they did in 1940. The ratio of physicians to population has grown from 135 to 205 per 100,000,[24] giving the United States a ratio that is higher than that of all but a few countries in the world. Thanks in large part to the Hill-Burton Act of 1946, the United States has modernized its hospitals, improved the distribution of medical facilities, and doubled the number of beds in short-term, general hospitals,[25] those that provide the bulk of care.

It scarcely needs to be said that the overall cost of the American medical care system has soared faster and higher than almost anything else—from annual expenditures of $4 billion in 1940 to something near $300 billion in 1982, from 4 percent of the annual Gross National Product to almost 10 percent.[26] The rate at which the dollars have poured into the system even causes wonder among those who witnessed it first-hand. Looking back in 1977, Lewis Thomas, M.D., the distinguished essayist and former chief executive of the Memorial Sloan-Kettering Cancer Center in New York, observed, "An alien historian would think, from a look at just the dollar figures for each of those years, that some sort of tremendous event must have been occurring since 1950. Either (1) the health of the nation had suddenly disintegrated, requiring the laying on of new resources to meet the crisis, or (2) the technology for handling health problems had undergone a major transformation, necessitating the installation of new effective resources to do things that could not be done before, or (3), another possibility, perhaps we had somehow been caught up in the momentum of a huge, collective, ponderous set of errors."[27]

What happened to costs can be explained in another way by the classic interplay among the three basic elements of a medical care system: access, quality, and cost.

Access means not only the geographical proximity to care, but also financial access—the ability to pay for services. Access is what the patient cares deeply about. "Can I get a doctor?" he or she asks. "Can I afford it?"

The doctors focus their attention on quality. They want the best training there is, for themselves, their colleagues, those who assist them. They want the best in hospitals and the latest equipment.

Those two elements affect cost. Low cost is, of course, what a person wants as a taxpayer or an insurance policy premium payer. It is also what he wants as a purchaser of consumer products, for he is aware that some part of the cost of his purchase pays the health insurance premiums of those who manufactured it. Nearly $500 of the price of a new car, for example, is accounted for by the premium cost of the health insurance for the autoworkers who built it.[28]

The extent to which these elements are emphasized determines the character of a nation's medical care system. Variations exist country by country, since national priorities vary. In the People's Republic of China, for example, the emphasis of the system is on access. "Barefoot doctors" minister to the needs of a vast and scattered population. But the Chinese also clamp a tight lid on cost, for they do not generate sufficient per capita income to do otherwise. The result is that Chinese medicine is, by and large, no match for Western medicine in terms of quality. In Peking and some other major cities, to be sure, medical capability does approach Western standards. But the quality of medicine that the average workman has available to him is not something the people of this country would accept.

Great Britain offers an example of a different sort. The British National Health Service, inaugurated in 1948 and climaxing nearly four decades of movement toward a nationalized service, started with the goal of free and universal access coupled with high standards of quality. Cost, it was argued, might be high initially. But once the existing medical conditions of the population were seen to, costs would ease downward to reasonable levels. That hope never materialized; the high costs persisted, and continued accessibility kept services in demand. To control costs, the British cut back on new facilities, new hospitals, and expenditures for modern equipment.

But the most intense pressure was applied to controlling access, which was eventually limited not by the imposition of fees but by the institution of waiting lists for non-emergency procedures—the queue. The effect has been the rationing of care, the queue serving as a control valve restraining patient use of the system. In the late 1970s in the industrial midlands of England, if you needed a total hip replacement, you had to endure a four- or five-year wait for the operation to be scheduled.[29] The queue has thrown some Englishmen back onto private medical care, and enrollment in private health insurance programs is growing. Nevertheless, the British remain loyal to their nationalized health system, tolerating delays, putting up with outdated facilities, and stoically accepting the denial of treatment under certain conditions.[30]

Not long after Medicare and Medicaid, the United States began to shift its priorities from the widening of access to the control of cost. The old, amiable impulses seemed to vanish, and the nation, like an expansive host once the party is over, began to grumble about paying the piper. But since no one was willing to revoke the earlier decisions on quality and access, what could be done to curb costs? As described in Chapter 18, the first response of Congress was a series of regulatory measures that accomplished almost nothing.

With the arrival of the Reagan administration, increasing attention turned to free market approaches to the cost problem. A number of so-called competition bills, some introduced by Democrats, some reintroduced from the previous Congress, gained a moderate amount of attention. One of them, bearing the name of Congressman Richard A. Gephardt of Missouri, encouraged employees to opt for low-cost, low-utilization insurance programs while discouraging employers from offering expensive, high-utilization plans. The bill won little support, however, many of those opposed to it (including the AMA) fearing it would favor the formation of company-dominated health provider groups.

Congress did pass legislation to change the way Medicare reimbursed hospitals, a major step since over 26 percent of total hospital revenues comes from Medicare. Replacing what was a cost-plus arrangement, the new prospective payment system (based on diagnosis-related groups) relies on flat rates—so much for every hip replacement, so much for every gallbladder removal, and so forth, regardless of length of stay, regardless of the number of services required.* Working against a predetermined reimbursement (based on the experience of a number of institutions), hospitals were thus given incentives to trim services and send patients home as quickly as possible. Some people regarded the change as the most revolutionary step in medical care reimbursement procedures to be made in several years. Others, like the AMA, feared it would lower the quality of needed care.

Private industries, which financed over 20 percent of the national health bill in 1982, also started to show a mounting concern over costs, especially as health insurance became a more significant factor in their own costs.[31] In 1980, shortly before his retirement as president of Blue Cross-Blue Shield, Walter J. McNerney noted:

> What industry senses is that the system can be pressurized to get some of the cost out without coming anywhere near damaging quality. When you look at the regional variations in length of hospital stay or compare the physician-to-population ratios in various sections of the country you can see tremendous variations. If the variations were small, that would be one thing. But they are not, and they do not seem to create a similar variation in the quality of care. We deal with eight of the ten biggest industries—Ford, U.S. Steel, AT & T, duPont, and so forth—and they have sophisticated unions and full-time people worrying about the costs of medical care for their employees. They are intelligent buyers of health insurance, and they are convinced that economy can be struck without compromise either to quality or access.[32]

Time and change have brought other problems to the fore in medical care, though none so urgent as the cost problem. After years of controversy about whether the United States had enough physicians, and after the decision in the 1960s to expand the medical schools, suddenly the question has changed to "Do we have too many physicians?" In a speech that must have given every preceding Democratic Secretary of Health, Education, and Welfare a turn, President Carter's Secretary, Joseph A. Califano, referred in 1978 to the "the

---

*Differentials were established, however, to recognize regional variations and the teaching function of many hospitals.

looming problem of physician oversupply."[33] One study, undertaken with the sponsorship of the Department of Health and Human Services, reported that the United States will have an oversupply of 70,000 physicians by 1990. Through 1983, the AMA had not taken a quantitative position, though it did extend and modify its 1951 stand (see Chapter 12) by recommending that free market processes determine the number of physicians.[34]

Two additional phenomena should be mentioned, both of them rare in 1940, but commonplace in the 1980s. For many years, medical liability was a matter of minor concern. What few malpractice awards were made in the 1960s, for example, were modest by later standards, averaging $100,000-125,000. Total physician premiums for malpractice insurance then came to something under $50 million a year. But in the early 1970s increasingly frequent claims and a sharp escalation in the size of awards to patients triggered a crisis. Premiums skyrocketed, many insurers abandoned the field, and liability insurance coverage simply became unavailable in some parts of the country. It was a temporary situation, however. Helped in places by the formation of physician-owned insurance companies and the start in 1975 of the American Medical Assurance Company, an AMA reinsurance subsidiary, physicians were again able to find insurance readily. Yet the problems worsened. A 1982 survey done by the AMA indicated that the average incidence of claims in recent years has doubled, increasing from 2.9 per 100 physicians per year prior to 1976 to 6.2 claims per year for the five following years.[35]

As the number of claims and the size of the awards grew, premiums rose, increasing at the rate of 14 percent a year after 1976. Many physicians in the high risk specialties—surgery, obstetrics/gynecology, and anesthesiology—paid $20,000 a year or more in 1982 for liability coverage. The total in premiums paid for medical liability insurance soared to more than twenty times what it was in the 1960s, $1.2 billion in 1982. This is a substantial new factor in medical care costs. No authority has identified the causes for the upsurge in claims and awards, though many factors clearly played a part: a more litigious society, new concepts of entitlement, greater public expectations from the well-publicized accomplishments of modern medicine.

The availability of more sophisticated technology also raised ethical dilemmas. Because the physician of 1940 was so limited as to what he could do for a patient on the edge of survival, the moral question of withholding treatment from a dying person seldom occurred. But surgical and biomedical progress changed that. Many heroic measures to save life, unknown forty years before, became widely available. But saving a life that could be useful and enjoyable was one thing. Extending the agonized days of the terminally ill, fighting to save a monstrously formed baby for a few weeks of misery, prolonging a life devoid of human quality—these dilemmas raised questions. More and more often in the 1970s and 1980s, physicians had to ask themselves not whether they could save a life but whether they should.

Before any sort of final view of the AMA's role in the formation of American medical care policy is attempted, a word should be said about how the AMA has itself changed in the process. It has obviously been one of the major participants in the evolutionary process that has affected the medical system, and rightly so. No matter what form a medical system takes, it is the physicians who provide and direct the care that the patient receives. Yet the AMA has been more than a participant in the process, more than an agent of change; it has been a recipient, changed itself in the interplay of forces.

The truth is that organized medicine has been transformed no less profoundly than the medical care system. By almost every yardstick—tempo, representation, program priorities, corporate personality—the AMA federation of the 1980s is far different from what it once was. Richard G. Layton, now the president of AMACO, the AMA reinsurance subsidiary, recalls what it was like to be the executive director of a county medical society years ago. "Multnomah county (Portland, Oregon) had a nice, quiet society," he remembers. "We took a lot of pride in the way we handled complaints. We weren't dealing with a whole bunch of regulations from a whole lot of government agencies. Malpractice was not even a problem then. Sometimes, it seems to me, our biggest worry was getting together with the Auxiliary each year and deciding on a theme for the annual dance."

Russell B. Roth, M.D., remembers the first county medical society meetings he went to in Erie, Pennsylvania, in the 1940s. They were, at first, almost completely educational. "They brought doctors together," he recalls, "to swap stories, discuss cases, trade experiences. For its time, it was continuing medical education at its best. But very soon," he adds, "we began to recognize that as a profession we had political problems, that people were going to start legislating at us."

Obviously that happened, and obviously the AMA had to respond. To highlight the change, it would be difficult to invent a sharper contrast than the one actually existing between the AMA Washington operation of 1940 and that of today. In 1940 the AMA had no representation in Washington. Only in 1944, after introduction of the first Wagner-Murray-Dingell proposal for national health insurance, did the AMA open an office there. It consisted of a solitary physician, who was not too clearly instructed as to his mission and was housed in a small rented office.

Symbolizing how organized medicine has changed since that time—or rather, has had to change to be effective in a different political climate—is the new $12 million office building the AMA built in Washington and opened in 1982. Sheathed in Spanish rose granite and bronze-tinted glass, the twelve-story structure at Vermont and L Streets houses a collection of contemporary American art with a modern sculpture by Louise Nevelson gracing a small plaza in front. The two upper stories provide quarters for the forty-person AMA Washington operation, headed by a vice president, Wayne W. Bradley. Responsible to him are three administrative divisions: The Washington staff (which includes six registered lobbyists), the Division of Political Education, and the Division of Legislation (based for the most part in the AMA's Chicago headquarters). Among its other assignments, the AMA monitors, tracks, and analyzes the approximately 2,500 pieces of legislation generated in each session of Congress that can have an effect on the health and medical care of the American people.

Although rent from the lower ten floors creates income, the AMA's Washington building was not undertaken as an investment. It was built, rather, as an assertion of the AMA presence in the nation's capital and the AMA's determination to take vigorous part in broad policy decisions affecting the future of American medicine.

Which brings up the final point: what is it, in the last analysis, that the AMA has been trying to accomplish all these years? It has clearly worked in the medical interests of the American people. But statements of that sort convey little more than what the AMA constitution says about its goals: "...to promote the science and art of medicine and the betterment of public health."[36] What may serve the purpose more aptly is an insight offered by the man who has known the AMA as well as any other, one who has certainly seen it at closer hand and for a longer time than any other during the period covered in this history. Ernest B. Howard, M.D., joined the AMA in the number two staff position in early 1948, before President Truman launched his major effort to obtain a national health insurance bill. He retired in 1974, voluntarily, at age 65, from the number one staff position, just as Senator Edward M. Kennedy was giving up on his efforts for a similar bill. In between, for twenty-six years, Howard sat in on all the meetings of the Board of Trustees, listened through all the sessions of the House of Delegates, and took part in all the major administrative decisions. His view of the organization and the profession is unique. His perception, a not entirely uncritical one, is of a group possessed by a strong dedication to high quality medicine and equal determination to protect it from external interference. He says,

> The major contribution has to be the development and maintenance of the high quality of physician performance in relation to the patient. That has to be first, no matter what the physician's type of practice—fee-for-service, HMO, hospital, government institution, whatever. The major preoccupation of the AMA—over all the years from the nineteenth century on—has been the creation of a high quality of physician performance.
>
> Now, coupled to that has been the feeling that high-quality physician performance is clearly related to the physician-government relationship, to the government role in medicine. I think this was the dominant feeling of my peers in American medicine for all the years that I was there. They were honestly feeling their way about government involvement, sometimes expressing their thoughts about this too violently, sometimes too dogmatically, other times quite reasonably.
>
> However they expressed it, there was a strong feeling that this excellent quality in the performance of the physician could not occur if the government harassed physicians, intervened too much in the practice of medicine.
>
> The two elements are related. That is why medicine has proceeded on two parallel courses over the years. One is clearly academic, clearly medical, clearly focused on the education of the physician. The other is clearly political, governmental, related to the prevention of the socializing or the nationalizing of medicine. The two courses are clearly related to each other.
>
> It isn't that the AMA is another National Association of Manufacturers or another conservative or even rightwing organization. It is the conviction of medical leaders that physicians in this country cannot provide the highest quality of medical care to patients in the context of a federalized system.[37]

The Physician Masterfile

When a medical student actually starts his or her formal training, the medical schools report each student's matriculation, and the student's name then enters the AMA's Physician Masterfile. A computerized data bank, this is the medical profession's official record of all United States physicians with an M.D. degree. (The American Osteopathic Association does much the same thing for those physicians who have a D.O. degree.) From that point on, whenever a medical school, a hospital, a state licensing board, or a medical specialty board takes an action relating to a physician's qualifications, the information is reported and recorded. Altogether, 2,100 organizations feed information on physicians into the Masterfile.

Periodically, the AMA sends a copy of the individual record to each physician so that he or she may check it for accuracy, give or update the office address, identify professional activity (teaching, research, administration, patient care, etc.), list specialty or specialties (surgery, pediatrics, family practice, etc.), and describe employment status (government-salaried, hospital-based, solo practice, group practice, partnership, etc.). Because the Masterfile gathers the essential statistical information about the profession, the AMA, in a sense, serves as the national medical census bureau.

Keeping the Masterfile current and extracting information from it takes three shifts of people a day and a large block of time on the AMA's computers. The Masterfile is used in the compilation of the *American Medical Directory*, published by the AMA since 1906 and periodically revised. It is a public document of four volumes, priced at over $300 but available in libraries, especially medical society libraries. If you want to look up a physician's educational qualifications, the *Directory* is where you will find them.

From the Masterfile come physician mailing lists that can be compiled by specialty and other population characteristics. The lists are used by the AMA publications and are available on a royalty basis to other organizations, *provided* that they have a legitimate informational or educational need to communicate with physicians. A physician may request that his or her name be carried on a do-not-contact basis, and about 5,000 do so.

In addition to the *Directory*, the Masterfile has served as the statistical base for many recent studies of physician distribution. The AMA actually began this work when it expanded its data-gathering activities in 1958, originally to develop information to help young physicians find places to practice. It launched a physician records service, information from which led to the publication of quarterly tables showing the distribution of physicians by professional activity ("private practice" or "not in private practice" were the only categories at that time), county and state. In 1959 the AMA first published *The Distribution of Physicians in the U.S.* With the increasing sophistication of the data gathered for the Masterfile, succeeding editions included more and more statistical information. A major program to improve and expand the file was undertaken in 1966, employing more exact and meaningful definitions of professional activity, specialty category, and employment status.

A recent version appearing in 1981, *Physician Characteristics and Distribution in the U.S.*, provides useful information on the geographic location of M.D.s by region, state and demographic county classification (i.e., urban, rural, etc.) with separate tabulations for women physicians and foreign medical graduate physicians. The book includes tables that show such characteristics as age, sex, board certification status, and country of medical school graduation. In addition, it contains population breakouts by professional activity and employment status. It is a must for anyone doing studies of physician manpower or wanting to identify the important demographic trends in American medicine.

U.S. Medical School Graduates by Year

These figures are those reported annually in the education issues of *JAMA*. See specifically: *JAMA* 75 (August 7, 1920): 382; 95 (August 16, 1930): 504; 186 (November 16, 1963): 661; 250 (September 23/30, 1983): 1512.

YEAR	GRADUATES	YEAR	GRADUATES
1900	5214	1922	2529
1901	5444	1923	3120
1902	5009	1924	3562
1903	5698	1925	3974
1904	5747	1926	3962
1905	5606	1927	4035
1906	5364	1928	4262
1907	4980	1929	4446
1908	4741	1930	4565
1909	4515	1931	4735
1910	4440	1932	4936
1911	4273	1933	4895
1912	4483	1934	5035
1913	3981	1935	5101
1914	3594	1936	5183
1915	3536	1937	5377
1916	3518	1938	5194
1917	3379	1939	5089
1918	2670	1940	5097
1919	2656	1941	5275
1920	3047	1942	5163
1921	3186	1943	5223

YEAR		GRADUATES	YEAR	GRADUATES
1944		5134	1964	7336
1944	(2nd Session)	5169	1965	7409
1945		5136	1966	7574
1946		5836	1967	7743
1947		6389	1968	7973
1948		5543	1969	8059
1949		5094	1970	8367
1950		5553	1971	8974
1951		6135	1972	9551
1952		6080	1973	10,391
1953		6668	1974	11,613
1954		6861	1975	12,714
1955		6977	1976	13,561
1956		6845	1977	13,607
1957		6796	1978	14,393
1958		6861	1979	14,966
1959		6860	1980	15,136
1960		7081	1981	15,667
1961		6994	1982	15,985
1962		7168	1983	15,728
1963		7264		

Response to COPE

Reprinted below is the AMA's rebuttal to charges made by COPE in 1960 alleging—without documentation—a number of obstructive and reactionary activities. The document appeared in the March 24, 1960, edition of the *Medical Legislative Digest*, published by the Council on Medical Service.

Quite the opposite of what labor said them to be, the AMA's basic and consistent views in favor of vaccination programs and other public health measures to control disease go back to the last century. See *JAMA* 32 (1899): 1276 and 1372.

On February 1, 1960, the AFL-CIO Committee on Political Education (COPE) published a political memorandum entitled "The Forand Bill and the Record of the AMA." The memorandum consists of sixteen charges purporting to show that the American Medical Association has opposed beneficial health measures. The memorandum suggests that the Association's opposition to the Forand Bill is another example of this so-called "reactionary" attitude.

Although the COPE statement cites no references, it is taken almost word for word from a campaign speech delivered on October 27, 1950, by former Congressman Eugene D. O'Sullivan from the Second Congressional District of Nebraska. After losing his campaign for re-election, Congressman O'Sullivan had the speech printed in the Congressional Record of December 8, 1950.

The memorandum contains so many falsehoods and distortions that AMA's President, Dr. Louis M. Orr has demanded a retraction of the statements. The demand for a retraction and a factual explanation of the Association's position on the health measures mentioned in the COPE memo were contained in a letter written by Dr. Orr on March 15, 1960, to George Meany, President of AFL-CIO. [There was no response.]

The following are the allegations and the facts:

Allegation

1. "A generation ago, the AMA opposed the requirement that all cases of tuberculosis be reported to a public authority—the foundation for all T.B. control methods."

Facts

The AMA has not opposed reporting cases of tuberculosis to a public authority.

The history of the Association's interest in the control of tuberculosis can be traced back to 1899, when the House of Delegates appointed a committee to report on the nature of tuberculosis, means of control, public education and the advisability of establishing national and state sanitariums.

The most recent AMA action on this subject was in 1944 when a resolution on the control of tuberculosis was approved. It stated in part "that it is necessary to extend procedures for careful, continuous supervision of the tuberculous by practicing physicians, who, in cooperation with duly constituted health authorities, federal, state and local, are in a position to deal with these problems by modern methods to prevent the spread of this communicable disease."

Allegation

2. "The AMA opposed the National Tuberculosis Act a week before Congress passed it unanimously."

Facts

Although the House of Delegates was in sympathy with the purposes of the proposed National Tuberculosis Act, it opposed the bill for the following reasons:

(1) Money could not be appropriated or expended for the purposes of the legislation without the approval of the Federal Security Agency;

(2) The objectives of the legislation could be obtained in other ways, as for example, direct aid to needy communities under the Lanham Act.

Allegation

3. "The AMA fought compulsory vaccination for smallpox."

Facts

This statement would be accurate if it said: The AMA fought *for* compulsory vaccination for smallpox, because in 1899, the House of Delegates adopted a resolution which urged local boards of health to adopt laws requiring compulsory vaccination for smallpox.

Allegation

4. "The AMA attacked provisions for immunization against diphtheria and other preventive measures against contagious diseases by public health agencies."

Facts

The AMA has not only cooperated with public health agencies for the prevention of contagious diseases, but also has made many recommendations for affirmative action in this field. The following are only a few examples of AMA activity:

(1) From 1875 to 1879 the AMA urged "that state boards of health be established in those states where such boards do not exist."

(2) In 1884 it recommended that Congress "make suitable appropriations for the prosecution of scientific research relating to the cause and prevention of the infectious diseases of the human race," and also in that year passed a resolution that "it is important that proper legislation be had at this session of the National Congress for the ultimate extermination...of pleuropneumonia."[6]

(3) In 1907 the Committee on Legislation was requested by the House of Delegates to take the necessary steps to secure national and state legislation for control of rabies.

(4) A report adopted by the House of Delegates in 1950 read, in part, as follows: "The basic services of the department of public health should be...prevention of disease and control of communicable diseases such as the diseases of childhood, venereal diseases and tuberculosis."

Allegation

5. "The AMA opposed the first bills to grant federal aid to the states to reduce infant and maternal deaths."

Facts

In 1922 the AMA opposed the Sheppard-Towner Maternity and Infancy Act, which authorized the payment of subsidies to the states over a fixed period of years because it believed that each state should be left free to formulate its own maternal-infant welfare programs with the cooperation of the United States Public Health Service and that any legislation involving cooperation *between the federal government and the states* should be jointly administered by the USPHS and state health authorities.

Allegation

6. "The AMA opposed the Social Security Act, passed in 1935."

Facts

The AMA has never taken a position on the retirement provisions of the Social Security Act.

Allegation

7. "In 1939, on behalf of the AMA board of trustees, Dr. Morris Fishbein condemned old-age and employment insurance as a 'definite step to either communism or totalitarianism'."

Facts

The quote attributed to Dr. Fishbein is taken out of context. In November of 1939, Dr. Fishbein, who was then Editor of the *Journal of the American Medical Association*, addressed the Annual Conference of Secretaries of Constituent Medical Associations on the AMA's position on health legislation. He said, "We are asking the government to go forward with the medical profession in attaining a wider distribution of medical and preventative services based on actually demonstrated needs of various communities..." He then went on to discuss medicine's plans for achieving this result and some problems which had resulted from the construction of facilities by the federal government where there was no demonstrated need. The only reference to social security occurred in the conclusion of the speech:

"The introduction into this nation of a federal security plan whereby the nation itself, as a federal agency, will step intimately into the sickness and life of every person in the country, will be the first step in the breakdown of American democracy. Indeed, all forms of security, compulsory security, even against old-age and unemployment, represent a beginning invasion by the state into the personal life of the individual, represent a taking away of individual responsibility, a weakening of national caliber, a definite step toward either communism or totalitarianism."

It is clear that the subject of Dr. Fishbein's remarks was health care, not social security. Even his one reference to social security showed more concern over the possible future consequences of compulsory programs than antagonism toward the old-age and unemployment insurance program. Since the AMA did not oppose old-age and unemployment insurance, it is difficult to see what this COPE allegation is trying to "prove."

Allegation

8. "The AMA opposed the creation of public venereal disease clinics."

Facts

The AMA has fought venereal disease as it has other diseases which have threatened the American public. In 1907 it resolved "that it should be the duty of the state boards of health to disseminate literature… to educate the people on the subject of venereal disease." Other actions have included:

(1) Cooperation of the American Medical Association with the United States Public Health Service for better control of venereal disease;

(2) Statements that the medical profession should cooperate with the official health agencies charged with the responsibility for and expanded program for the control of venereal diseases that has been made possible by federal grants-in-aid;

(3) A twelve point program for improved medical care which included "Establishment of local public health units and incorporation in health centers and local public health units of such services as …control of venereal diseases…"

(4) Approval of the treatment of nonindigents for venereal disease by public health clinics in instances when such treatment is not available through private sources.

Allegation

9. "The AMA opposed the creation of the free diagnostic centers for tuberculosis and cancer."

Facts

In 1948 the House of Delegates approved a resolution which authorized the
Association to cooperate with the American Cancer Society and other
agencies engaged in cancer detection "for the purpose of formulating
standards of procedure and conduct in the operation of cancer detection
and diagnostic centers and that the results of these studies be adequately
publicized to those concerned, including the medical profession and the
public."

As part of its program for improved medical care, the AMA approved
the diagnosis of tuberculosis by the treatment of indigents by public health
centers. In addition, it approved the treatment of nonindigents by these
centers if treatment is not available through private sources.

Allegation

10. "The AMA fought the American Red Cross plan to set up a nation-wide
reserve of civilian blood banks.

Facts

The AMA, instead of fighting the Red Cross plan for blood banks, actively
supported such a plan. This consistent approval is shown by the following
actions:

(1) 1947 — approval in principle of the American Red Cross Plan establishment of a national blood program;

(2) 1949 — the AMA statement that there was an urgent need for a
national blood program and that the Red Cross was the logical agency
to assume the responsiblity for such a program;

(3) 1953 — the House of Delegates urged the establishment of a coordinated national blood bank program to be organized by the AMA,
American National Red Cross, and other qualified organizations,

(4) 1954 — the AMA adopted a plan for a national blood program which was developed and unanimously approved by representatives of the American Red Cross, the American Hospital Association, the American Association of Blood Banks, the American Society of Clinical Pathologists and the Committee on Blood of the American Medical Association.

Allegation

11. "The AMA opposed federal aid to medical education even after AMA representatives had testified before Congress that the medical schools were in a dire financial emergency and that there was a serious shortage of doctors in the U.S."

Facts

The AMA would prefer to see necessary support for medical education received from private philanthropy or local public funds. However, it is recognized that until such support is provided, federal aid may be necessary if the legislation guarantees absolute freedom of medical education under government control.

In 1951, the Association endorsed the principle of one time grants-in-aid based on the Hill-Burton formula for the construction, equipment and renovation of the physical plants of medical schools. The funds were not to be used for operational expenses or salaries. This position has been reaffirmed by the House of Delegates several times.

The AMA has opposed bills for federal aid to medical education which did not guarantee freedom of medical education and which would have provided funds for salaries.

Allegation

12. "The AMA attacked voluntary health insurance plans as 'socialism, communism—inciting to revolution.' (Ho, hum.)" and

13. "It dismissed Blue Cross as 'a half-baked scheme'."

Facts

The first quotation is taken out of context. It is from an editorial in *JAMA*, December 3, 1932, concerning two reports of a Committee on the Cost of Medical Care. The majority report urged medical practice by organized groups of physicians associated with hospitals. Commenting on this, the *Journal* said: "The alignment is clear—on the one side, the forces representing the great foundations, public health officialdom, social theory— even socialism and communism—inciting revolution; on the other side, the organized medical profession of this country, urging an orderly evolution." It should be noted that this same editorial referred to health insurance as "foresighted, American, economical."

The second quotation does not even mention Blue Cross. It is from a *Journal* editorial of March 25, 1933, which criticized the attempts of some individuals to make large profits from health insurance. The AMA has never opposed the development of voluntary sickness insurance plans in this country as they exist today.

Allegation

14. "The AMA opposed school health service legislation."

Facts

This statement apparently refers to testimony given by the AMA on H.R. 3942, 81st Congress. Our witness stated that the Association was in agreement with the general purpose of the bill and considered it so worthwhile that we would not oppose it if we did not feel that, in its present form, it would fail to accomplish its purpose. It should be remembered that there is a great deal of difference between opposing the principles of a particular type of legislation and opposing an ineffectual bill.

Allegation

15. "The AMA fought federal aid to public health units."

Facts

The following statement, which reflects the AMA's position in regard to this subject, is taken from testimony given before the House Interstate and Foreign Commerce Committee on July 6, 1949: "We, the American Medical

Association, have long believed that the existence of...public health units is basic to the maintenance of and improvement of the health of our people. Recognition of this conviction was reflected in action taken by the Association as early as 1883, when a report was made at our annual meeting for that year covering a survey conducted to ascertain what states and counties had at that time health departments." The AMA has not opposed aid to public health units, but has suggested amendments which would define the term "public health" as used in the proposed laws and which would exclude care of the sick.

Allegation

16. "The AMA blasted a Defense Department request to Congress to give government medical care to dependents of men in the Armed Forces, with particular reference to the men then fighting in Korea as 'unpractical and harmful to National Defense'."

Facts

The AMA testified on H.R. 7994, 84th Congress, which became the Dependent Medical Care Act and in this testimony stated:

"As you know, on the basis of our previous testimony, the American Medical Association has taken no position on the question of whether it is the responsibility of the government to provide medical care for the dependents of military personnel. In our opinion this is a question for Congress to decide. We do strongly urge, however, in the event such care is to be provided, that increased emphasis be placed on the utilization of civilian facilities and the services of civilian physicians."

The quote in the allegation does not appear in the testimony or in any statement of AMA policy. In fact, the House of Delegates, when expounding its policy on medicare [the term used in the 1950s to describe federally sponsored medical care for dependents of U.S. military personnel], specifically stated: "The policy advocated should not in any way be construed as one of opposition by the American Medical Association to dependent medical care;...."

Interviews

In developing this history, the author interviewed several AMA employees, retirees, elected officers and officials, plus a number of people with no connection to the AMA. The interviews, conducted between 1979 and 1983, were recorded on 8 mm. tape cassettes, and these have been turned over to the AMA archive library. The author is indebted to those listed below for the time they generously contributed.

Annis, Edward R.; AMA president, 1963; trustee, 1967-69.

Baker, John T.; joined AMA in 1972 as advertising sales executive; vice president for publishing 1978-.

Baldwin, David G.: communications director of AMPAC 1961-69; director of communications, AMA Washington Office, 1969-81.

Balfe, Bruce; director of the AMA Office of Planning during 1970s; vice president for policy development and planning 1981-.

Ballantine, H. Thomas, Jr.; delegate from Massachusetts; AMA trustee 1977-80.

Ballin, John C.; a member of the AMA Department of Drugs since 1955; director of the department (later the Division of Drugs and Technology) 1969-.

Barclay, William R.; director of scientific activities 1970-75; editor of *JAMA* from 1976 until retirement in 1981.

Blasingame, Francis J. L.; AMA trustee 1949-57, vice chairman of the board 1955-57; executive vice president 1958-68.

Boston, Larry; writer in AMA science news department 1965; later Washington correspondent for *American Medical News*; editor of *AMNews* from 1975 until resignation in 1982.

Bradley, Wayne W.; joined AMA as Washington lobbyist in 1970; director, Division of Public Affairs, 1974-78; in Washington as vice president for public affairs since 1979.

Brown, Leo E.; AMA director of communications 1951-60; assistant to the executive vice president 1961 until retirement in 1975.

Budde, Norbert W.; director, Division of Survey and Data Resources.

Carden, Terrence; editor of the *New Physician*, journal of the Student American Medical Association in the early 1970s. An editor of *JAMA* briefly in the late 1970s.

Chilcoat, Theodore R., Jr.; joined AMA Field Service Division 1965; director, Department of Specialty Society Relations; senior vice president for health services and public affairs; assistant executive vice president 1981-.

Clousson, J. Paige; labor relations consultant, director of the AMA Division of Negotiations in mid-1970s.

Cohan, William M.; joined AMA Division of Medical Service in 1970; associate director, director of Division of Health Program Development 1982-.

Cohen, Wilbur J.; U.S. government official; Secretary of Department of Health, Education, and Welfare 1968. Professor of Public Affairs, University of Texas in early 1980s.

Coleman, Frank C.; member, first board of directors, AMPAC; AMPAC chairman 1965; alternate delegate from Florida from 1964.

Coursey, James; director, AMA Division of Membership since 1978.

Crawford, Susan; AMA librarian during the late 1950s; director of library and archive services 1975-81.

Crawshaw, Ralph C.; Portland, Oregon, psychiatrist; a former president of Multnomah County Medical Society.

Egan, Richard L.; joined AMA Division of Medical Education in 1971; director since 1976.

Erfert, Jan W.; joined AMA as Director of Finance 1975; vice president for Real Estate and New Product Development 1983-.

Fauser, John J.; director, AMA Department of Allied Health Education and Evaluation.

Fenninger, Leonard D.; joined the AMA in 1973 after service with the Bureau of Health Manpower, U.S. Department of Health, Education, and Welfare; group vice president for medical education after 1976; vice president for medical education and scientific policy 1982-84.

Finkel, Asher; joined AMA in 1970; director of environmental, public and occupational health; group vice president for scientific affairs 1975-80.

Gienapp, John C.; director, AMA Department of Graduate Medical Education.

Golin, Carol Brierly; assistant executive editor, *AMNews*.

Hannon, Thomas F.; joined AMA in 1975 as group vice president for publishing; senior vice president for business services 1978; deputy executive vice president for business affairs 1981-84.

Harrison, Bernard P.; joined AMA as secretary to AMA Council on Legislative Activities in 1963; director, Division of Medical Practice 1970-75; then group vice president for external affairs; retired in 1981.

Henningsgaard, Blair; director and then chairman of the Board of Directors of AMPAC 1968; member of AMA Judicial Council 1975-80.

Hinton, Harry R.; joined AMA field staff in 1961; director of Washington office 1969-75; director, Division of Professional Relations 1975-.

Hirsh, Bernard; joined AMA as member of the law division in 1954; general counsel from 1965 until retirement in 1983.

Howard, Ernest B.; joined AMA as assistant secretary-general manager 1948; assistant executive vice president 1958- 68; executive vice president 1968-74.

Hunter, Robert B.; delegate 1965-71; trustee 1971-79; chairman of the board 1977-79; president 1980.

Jensen, Lynn E.; director, AMA Center for Health Policy Research 1975-.

Jones, Richard J.; joined AMA as director, Division of Scientific Activities in 1976; secretary to Council on Scientific Activities 1976-83.

Kernodle, John R.; trustee 1968-73; chairman of the board 1972-73.

Lauer, Peter; director, Division of Political Education/AMPAC 1980-.

Layton, Richard G.; joined AMPAC field staff 1963; joined AMA field staff 1968, director, 1970-75; vice president of American Medical Assurance Company 1976-.

Lewis, Ted, Jr.; Washington correspondent and columnist for *AMNews* 1959-82.

Lundberg, George D.; editor of *JAMA*, 1982-.

McNerney, Walter J.; appointed president of Blue Cross Association 1961; president of Blue Cross-Blue Shield at the time of retirement in 1981.

Miller, Joe D.; joined AMA as research assistant, Division of Medical Service 1957; executive director of AMPAC 1961- 68; director, AMA Division of Public Affairs 1968-70; assistant executive vice president 1970-74; deputy executive vice president (and senior vice president for socioeconomic affairs until 1978); senior deputy executive vice president at time of retirement in 1982.

Monroe, Kenneth E.; joined AMA research center in 1971; group vice president for health service policy 1980-.

Nesbitt, Tom E.; vice speaker of the House of Delegates 1972-73; speaker 1973-77; president 1978.

Parrott, Max H.; delegate 1962-66; trustee 1966-74; chairman of the board 1970-72; president 1975.

Peterson, Harry N.; joined AMA legislative department in 1965; director, Department (later Division) of Legislative Activities, 1979-.

Ramsey, William R.; joined AMA field staff in 1960s; executive director of the American Society of Internal Medicine 1969-83.

Rappel, James F.; joined AMA as assistant director of corporate services 1976; vice president for information systems 1980-.

Renshaw, Charles C.; editor of *Prism* 1972-76; vice president, AMA Consumer Book Program 1977-.

Ritts, Roy E.; director, AMA-ERF Institute for Biomedical Research 1963-67.

Roth, Russell B.; member of the Council on Medical Service in early 1960s, later vice chairman; delegate, vice speaker and speaker of the House of Delegates 1969-72; president 1973; delegate from American Association of Clinical Urologists in early 1980s.

Ruhe, C.H. William; joined AMA Department of Medical Education 1960; director, Division of Medical Education 1967-78; senior vice president for scientific affairs and medical education at time of retirement in 1982.

Sammons, James H.; delegate 1964-70; chairman, Board of Directors of AMPAC 1969; AMA trustee 1970-74; chairman of the AMA board 1973-74; AMA executive vice president 1974-.

Seekins, Steven V.; director then vice president, for AMA public and federation relations 1978-.

Stetler, C. Joseph; director, AMA Law Department (later) Legal and Socioeconomic Division in 1950s till 1963; president, Pharmaceutical Manufacturers Association 1963-80.

Strobhar, Whalen M.; joined AMA in 1965; director, Division of Public Affairs 1970-73; assistant executive vice president 1974; senior vice president in 1977; and deputy executive vice president for public, scientific and health service policy 1981-.

Theodore, Chris N.; joined AMA research operation 1962; director of AMA Center for Health Service Research and Development in 1970s; vice president for human resources 1981-.

Watson, William L.; joined AMPAC staff in early 1960s; staff director AMPAC 1968-80.

White, Philip L.; secretary to AMA Council on Foods and Nutrition 1956-72; director of AMA food and nutrition program 1973-82; director of Division of Personal and Public Health Policy 1982-.

Wolman, Walter; joined AMA chemical laboratory in 1945; director, Department of Mental Health 1962-75.

Wood, Donald E.; member of Board of Directors AMPAC 1961-63, chairman 1964; AMA trustee 1971-74.

Zapp, John S.; joined AMA Washington office in 1975; director of the Washington office 1979-.

Chairmen and Presidents of the AMA since 1940

The term of office for both the president and the chairman is for one year. Elections take place at the annual meeting. Since these usually occur in June, the term of office extends from one June to the next. Presidents serve for one year; in recent times, the chairman has usually been elected for a second, one-year term.

YEAR	CHAIRMAN	PRESIDENT
1940-41	Arthur W. Booth	Nathan B. Van Etten
1941-42	Arthur W. Booth	Frank H. Lahey
1942-43	Roger I. Lee	Fred W. Rankin
1943-44	Roger I. Lee	James E. Paullin
1944-45[a]	James R. Bloss	Herman L. Kretschmer
1945-46	Roscoe L. Sensenich	Roger I. Lee
1946-47	Roscoe L. Sensenich	Harrison H. Shoulders
1947-48	Elmer L. Henderson	Edward L. Bortz
1948-49	Elmer L. Henderson	Roscoe L. Sensenich
1949-50	Louis H. Bauer	Ernest E. Irons
1950-51	Louis H. Bauer	Elmer L. Henderson
1951-52	Dwight H. Murray	John W. Cline
1952-53	Dwight H. Murray	Louis H. Bauer
1953-54	Dwight H. Murray	Edward J. McCormick
1954-55	Dwight H. Murray	Walter B. Martin
1955-56	Gunnar Gundersen	Elmer Hess
1956-57	Gunnar Gundersen	Dwight H. Murray
1957-58	Edwin S. Hamilton	David B. Allman
1958-59	Leonard W. Larson	Gunnar Gundersen
1959-60	Leonard W. Larson	Louis M. Orr
1960-61	Julian P. Price	E. Vincent Askey

YEAR	CHAIRMAN	PRESIDENT
1961-62	Hugh H. Hussey	Leonard W. Larson
1962-63[b]	Hugh H. Hussey	George M. Fister
	Percy E. Hopkins	
1963-64	Percy E. Hopkins	Edward R. Annis
1964-65	Percy E. Hopkins	Norman A. Welch, (d.),
		Donovan F. Ward
1965-66	Percy E. Hopkins	James Z. Appel
1966-67	Wesley W. Hall	Charles L. Hudson
1967-68	Wesley W. Hall	Milford O. Rouse
1968-69	Burtis E. Montgomery	Dwight L. Wilbur
1969-70	Burtis E. Montgomery	Gerald D. Dorman
1970-71	Max H. Parrott	Walter C. Bornemeier
1971-72	Max H. Parrott	Wesley W. Hall
1972-73[c]	John R. Kernodle	Carl A. Hoffman
1973-74	James H. Sammons,	Russell B. Roth
	Richard E. Palmer	
1974-75	Richard E. Palmer	Malcolm C. Todd
1975-76	Raymond T. Holden	Max H. Parrott
1976-77	Raymond T. Holden	Richard E. Palmer
1977-78	Robert B. Hunter	John H. Budd
1978-79	Robert B. Hunter	Tom E. Nesbitt
1979-80	Lowell H. Steen	Hoyt D. Gardner
1980-81	Lowell H. Steen	Robert B. Hunter
1981-82	Joseph F. Boyle	Daniel T. Cloud
1982-83	Joseph F. Boyle	William Y. Rial
1983-84	John J. Coury, Jr.	Frank J. Jirka, Jr.
1984-85	John J. Coury, Jr.	Joseph F. Boyle

[a]Because the annual meeting of 1945 was held in December that year, Bloss served from June 1944 to December 1945, when Sensenich succeeded him. Kretschmer's term as president was similarly short, from December 1945 to June 1946.

[b]Hussey, after being re-elected to a second year as chairman in June 1962, resigned in November of that year to join the AMA staff. Hopkins succeeded him at that point.

[c]Kernodle, after being elected to a second year term in June 1973, resigned in October of that year, to be succeeded by Sammons. Sammons upon being elected executive vice president resigned in March 1974 to be succeeded by Palmer for the remainder of the term. Palmer was re-elected chairman in June 1974 for a full year term.

REFERENCE NOTES

Many of the citations in this history refer to the *Proceedings of the AMA House of Delegates* or to *JAMA*, the *Journal of the American Medical Association*. The published *Proceedings* are not generally available in regular libraries. However, they can be found in the libraries maintained by major county, state, and specialty medical societies, medical school libraries, and of course, the AMA library in Chicago. *JAMA* is more generally available in libraries, and it actually published the annual proceedings through the June 1950 meeting. Many cited documents, such as congressional testimony, speeches, and the like are available in the archives or departmental files of the AMA. The *Transcripts*, which are frequently cited, are also in the archive library.

Chapter 1. The Elements of Change.

1. Odin W. Anderson, *Blue Cross Since 1929* (Cambridge, Massachusetts: Ballinger, 1975): 16-17.

2. Victor Fuchs, "The Political Economy of Health Care," *New England Journal of Medicine* 300 (1979): 1485.

3. Arthur D. Bevan, "Report of the Council on Medical Education," *JAMA* 72 (1919): 1751-61, 1832; Arthur D. Bevan, "Cooperation in Medical Education and Medical Service," *JAMA* 90 (1928): 1173-77.

4. "State Board Examinations in 1904," *JAMA* 44 (1905): 1454, insert at 1477.

5. Council on Medical Education, "Report of Second Annual Conference," *JAMA* 46 (1906): 1853-58.

6. Council on Medical Education, "Report of Third Annual Conference," *JAMA* 48 (1907): 1701-1703.

7. Bevan, "Cooperation in Medical Education," 1175.

8. Ibid.

9. Bevan, "Report of the Council," 1753.

10. David Halberstam, *The Powers That Be* (New York: Alfred A. Knopf, 1979): 12.

11. Morris Fishbein, *A History of the American Medical Association* (Philadelphia: W.B. Saunders, 1947): 413.

12. Wilbur J. Cohen, interview with author, February 22, 1980.

13. Monte M. Poen, *Harry S. Truman Versus the Medical Lobby* (Columbia, Missouri: University of Missouri Press, 1979): 22-36.

14. James MacGregor Burns, *Leadership* (New York: Harper and Row, 1978): 67.

15. AMA House of Delegates, *Proceedings* December 1945: 59, 71. (Subsequent references to these records of the AMA House of Delegates' actions will be cited simply as *Proceedings*.)

16. *Proceedings*, July 1946: 3.

Chapter 2. "Overnight We Became Optimists..."

1. John C. Ballin, interviews with author, April 13, 14, 1979.

2. *Prescription Drug Industry Factbook* (Washington: Pharmaceutical Manufacturers Association, 1976): 1.

3. Lewis Thomas, "Medical Lessons from History," in *The Medusa and the Snail* (New York: Bantam Books, 1980): 136.

4. David Schwartzman, *Innovation in the Pharmaceutical Industry* (Baltimore: Johns Hopkins University Press, 1976): 38.

5. *Our Smallest Servants* (Brooklyn: Charles Pfizer and Company, Inc., 1955): 14, 15.

6. Michael J. Halberstam, *The Pills in Your Life* (New York: Grosset and Dunlap, 1972): 76.

7. Julius D. Richmond, "Why Americans are Healthiest Ever," *U.S. News and World Report* 87 (October 29, 1979): 63-66.

8. Frank H. Clarke, *How Modern Medicines are Discovered* (Mount Kisco, New York: Futura, 1973): 64.

9. Bernard Dixon, *Beyond the Magic Bullet* (New York: Harper and Row, 1978): 51.

10. William R. Barclay, interview with author, November 8, 1979.

Chapter 3. The Breakthroughs in Surgery

1. H. Thomas Ballantine, interview with author, October 18, 1979. Subsequent quotations from Ballantine in this chapter come from the same interview.

2. Owen H. Wangensteen and Sarah D. Wangensteen, *The Rise of Surgery* (Minneapolis: University of Minnesota Press, 1978): 36.

3. Rosemary Stevens, *American Medicine and the Public Interest* (New Haven: Yale University Press, 1971): 543.

4. William R. Barclay, interview with author, November 8, 1979.

5. Julius H. Comroe, "The Heart and Lungs," in *Advances in American Medicine: Essays at the Bicentennial*, Vol. 2, ed. J.Z. Bowers and E.P. Purcell (New York: Josiah Macy, Jr. Foundation, 1976): 484-526.

6. Frances D. Moore, "Surgery," in *Advances in American Medicine: Essays at the Bicentennial*, Vol.2, ed. J.Z. Bowers and E.P. Purcell (New York: Josiah Macy, Jr. Foundation, 1976): 614-76.

7. "Kidney Transplantation and Cancer," *JAMA* 235 (1976): 1195-99.

8. *Surgery in the U.S.*, Vol. 2 (Chicago: American College of Surgeons/American Surgical Association, 1975): 1547-55.

9. Ibid.

10. George W. Pickering, "The View from the United Kingdom," in *Advances in American Medicine: Essays at the Bicentennial*, Vol. 2, ed. J.Z. Bowers and E.P. Purcell (New York: Josiah Macy Jr. Foundation, 1976): 774.

Chapter 4. The Move to Specialization

1. Rosemary Stevens, *American Medicine and the Public Interest* (New Haven: Yale University Press, 1971): 181.

2. Harold C. Lueth, "Postgraduate Wishes of Medical Officers," *JAMA* 127 (1945): 759.

3. "Residency Training of Physician Veterans," *JAMA* 131 (1946): 1356.

4. American Medical Association, *Directory of Approved Residency Training Programs* (Chicago: AMA, 1950, 1960, 1980).

5. American Medical Association, *Profile of Medical Practice* (Chicago: AMA, 1978): 152.

6. Edithe J. Levit and William D. Holden, "Specialty Board Certification Rates," *JAMA* 239 (1978): 407-12.

7. American Medical Association, *Physician Manpower and Medical Education II* (Chicago: AMA, June 1978): 9-10.

8. Richard L. Egan, interview with author, September 20, 1979. Subsequent quotations from Egan in this chapter come from the same interview.

9. Stevens, *American Medicine*: 300. Stressing the impact of the GI bill, Stevens notes the increase in the number of surgeons between 1945 and 1950, surgery being a popular choice of residency training during the immediate postwar period. She attributes the high proportion of surgeons in the United States medical profession to the opportunities offered by the GI Bill.

10. Donald S. Fredrickson, "The National Institutes of Health: Yesterday, Today and Tomorrow," *Public Health Reports* 93 (1978): 642-47.

11. Russell A. Nelson, "Medical Care, " in *Advances in American Medicine: Essays at the Bicentennial*, Vol. 1, ed. J.Z. Bowers and E.P. Purcell (New York: Josiah Macy, Jr. Foundation, 1976): 348; also, *NIH Data Book* (Washington: National Institutes of Health, 1983): 21.

12. John A.D. Cooper, "Undergraduate Medical Education," in *Advances in American Medicine: Essays at the Bicentennial*, Vol. 1, ed. J.Z. Bowers and E.P. Purcell (New York: Josiah Macy, Jr. Foundation, 1976): 277.

13. Hugh H. Hussey, interview with author, May 30, 1979. Subsequent quotations and information in this chapter attributed to Hussey come from the same interview.

14. *Journal of Medical Education* 37 (1962): 1066-68, gives 3,933 as the number of full-time medical school faculty in 1951. *JAMA* 238 (1977): 2767, lists 41,394 full-time faculty positions in United States medical schools for 1976-77.

15. Paul Jolly, Division of Operational Studies, Association of American Medical Colleges.

16. Blair Henningsgaard, interview with author, July 24, 1979.

Chapter 5. The AMA: What Does It Do?

1. Michael J. Halberstam, "Why I'm Finally Joining the AMA," *Medical Economics* 49 (1972): 117-28.

2. American Medical Association, *Budget*, 1982, 1983.

3. American Medical Association, *AMA Membership Department Report* (Chicago: AMA, 1979).

4. David R. Hyde, et al. "The AMA: Power, Purpose and Politics in Organized Medicine," *Yale Law Journal* 63 (1954): 938-1022.

5. John G. Freymann, "Leadership in American Medicine: A Matter of Personal Responsibility," *New England Journal of Medicine* 270 (1964): 710-19.

6. "Undergraduate Medical Education," *JAMA* 243 (1980): 851.

7. American Medical Association, "Committee on Organization: Preliminary Report," *JAMA* 36 (1901): 1435-37.

8. William H. Welch, "Fields of Usefulness of the American Medical Association," *JAMA* 54 (1910): 2015.

9. F.D. Sturdivant, J.D. Kirby, and M.J. Hobor, "Comparative Analysis of the AMA Versus Other Organizations," unpublished report prepared for the AMA by Management Analysis Inc., Columbus, Ohio, December 1, 1977.

10. American Medical Association, "1972 Membership Opinion Poll," *Proceedings*, June 1972: 188-220.

11. American Medical Association, *Opinions of AMA Members* (Chicago: AMA, 1975): 14-16, 56-58.

12. "Public Opinion Survey About Doctors," *JAMA* 160 (1956): 471- 72.

13. "Public Attitudes Toward Health Care and Health Care Issues," unpublished reports prepared for the AMA by the Gallup Organization, Inc., Princeton, New Jersey, 1976 and 1979.

Chapter 6. The Making of a Physician

1. "Undergraduate Medical Education," *JAMA* 244 (1980): 2816.

2. Ralph Crawshaw, interview with author, May 12, 1980. Subsequent quotations from Crawshaw in this chapter are from the same interview.

3. Hugh H. Hussey, correspondence with author, June 5, 1979. Subsequent quotations from Hussey in this chapter come from that correspondence and an interview with the author on May 30, 1979.

4. John W. Tarnasky, interview with author, May 13, 1980.

5. H.S. Becker, *Boys in White* (Chicago: University of Chicago Press, 1961): 77.

6. C.H. William Ruhe, interview with author, March 10, 1980. Subsequent quotations from Ruhe in this chapter are from the same interview.

7. Russel V. Lee and Sarel Eimerl, *The Physician* (New York: Time-Life Books, 1967): 57.

8. Ann Landers, *The Ann Landers Encyclopedia* (Garden City, New York: Doubleday, 1978): ix.

9. Article in *Medical/Mrs.* quoted in the *New York Times*, May 7, 1979.

10. Carol Brierly Golin, "The Health Hazards of Being a Physician," *AMNews*, (June 23, 1978); Impact section: 7.

11. Ralph Crawshaw, et al., "An Epidemic of Suicide Among Physicians on Probation," *JAMA* 243 (1980): 1915-17.

12. William R. Barclay, interview with author, November 8, 1979.

13. J. Paige Clousson, interview with author, February 13, 1980.

14. Jacques Barzun, "The Professions Under Siege," *Harper's* (October, 1978): 61-68.

Chapter 7. The House of Delegates

1. American Medical Association, *Socioeconomic Monitoring System*, Vol. 2, No. 4, July 1983.

2. Figure developed by cross-referencing delegates' names (1980) with listings in *Directory of Medical Specialists*.

3. "The AMA House of Delegates," *Medical World News* 12 (June 18, 1971): 37-48.

4. Ibid.

5. "AMA Committee on Reorganization: Preliminary Report," *JAMA* 36 (1901): 1435-51; A. L. Reed, "President's Address," *JAMA* 36: 1605-1606; "Reorganization Committee on Revision of Constitution and By-laws," *JAMA* 36: 1643-48.

6. N.S. Davis, "Report of the Special Committee on Changes in the Plan of Organization," *JAMA* 8 (1887): 711-16.

7. "The House of Delegates," *JAMA* 38 (1902): 1443.

8. Terrence S. Carden, interview with author, May 19, 1980. Subsequent quotations from Carden in this chapter come from the same interview.

9. Gerald D. Dorman, "Address of the President," *Proceedings*, November-December 1969: 47-50.

10. *Proceedings*, November December 1969: 257-58.

11. Theodore R. Chilcoat, Jr., interview with author, September 24, 1980.

12. Rather than cite all the actions by the house on this subject, the author has referenced only the major turning-points. *Proceedings*, June 1962: 96-97; November 1962: 102-13 (Appel Report); June 1968: 135-48; July 1969: 242-49 (Quinn Report); November-December 1975: 125-27; December 1977: 112-16.

13. William R. Barclay, interviews with author, October 8 and 10, 1980.

14. *Proceedings*, November 1962: 103.

15. *Proceedings*, June 1977: 125-6.

16. "Specialty Society Representation Plan Turned Down," *AMNews* 20 (July 4, 1977): 8.

17. "Specialty Societies Get AMA House Seats," *AMNews* 20 (December 12, 1977): 1.

Chapter 8. Moving Through the Chairs

1. Alexis de Tocqueville, *Democracy in America* (New York: Mentor, New American Library, 1956): 198.

2. Ibid., 201.

3. American Medical Association, *The American Health Care System 1982* (Chicago: AMA, 1982): 70.

4. Robert B. Hunter, interview with author, May 9, 1980. Subsequent quotations from Hunter in this chapter are from the same interview.

5. Hugh H. Hussey, interview with author, May 30, 1980.

6. Donald E. Wood, interview with author, April 22, 1980.

7. Lester S. King, "The Founding of *JAMA*, 1883," *JAMA* 250 (1983): 177-180.

8. *Transactions* 33 (1882): 38-40.

9. "The Report of the Special Committee on Changes in the Plan and Organization and Bylaws of the Association," *JAMA* 8 (1887): 711-16.

10. *Proceedings*, June 1975: 35.

11. Max H. Parrott, interview with author, May 11, 1980.

12. Actions relating to the role of the AMA president are to be found in *Proceedings*, December 1976: 181, 211; June 1977: 127-30; December 1977: 66, 232.

Chapter 9. The End of an Institution

1. "Angry Voice," *Time* 49 (June 16, 1947): 61.

2. Ibid.

3. "Reports of Officers," *JAMA* 131 (1946): 406, 431, 432; *Proceedings*, December 1945: 8; July 1946: 6.

4. Morris Fishbein, *A History of the American Medical Association* (Philadelphia: W.B. Saunders, 1947): 349, 493, 494.

5. Morris Fishbein, *Morris Fishbein, M.D., An Autobiography* (Garden City, New York: Doubleday, 1969): 265.

6. Milton Mayer, "The Rise and Fall of Dr. Fishbein," *Harper's* 199 (November, 1949): 76-85.

7. John C. Ballin, interview with author, April 4, 1981.

8. Bernard D. Hirsh, interview with author, May 24, 1979.

9. Ernest B. Howard, interview with author, April 7, 1979.

10. F.J.L. Blasingame, interview with author, October 23, 1980.

11. Morris Fishbein, "The Committee on the Costs of Medical Care," *JAMA* 99 (1932): 1950-52.

12. Wilbur J. Cohen, interview with author, February 2, 1980.

13. Howard Hassard, letter to author, March 9, 1981. This letter is source for the information regarding Fishbein's difficulties with the California Medical Association.

14. *Proceedings*, June 1944: 83.

15. *Transcript*, June 1944: 6-18.

16. American Medical Association, *Digest of Official Actions 1846-1948* (Chicago: AMA, 1959): 321, 324.

17. Morris Fishbein, "Health Insurance Legislation in California," *JAMA* 127 (1945): 398.

18. *Proceedings*, December 1945: 62, 74.

19. *Transcript*, December 1945: 103, 104.

20. Ibid., 117.

21. Ibid., 119, 120.

22. *Proceedings*, 1945: 68, 70, 73, 74, 83.

23. Milton D. Krueger, letter to author, February 23, 1979. The letter describes the contents of the resolution adopted by the California Medical Association.

24. *Proceedings*, July 1946: 67-69.

25. "Remedy for Fishbein," *Time* 48 (July 15, 1946): 92.

26. Mayer, "The Rise and Fall:" 79, 80.

27. Fishbein, *Autobiography*: 308.

28. William L. Laurence, "AMA to Retire Dr. Fishbein," *New York Times*, June 7, 1949: 1, 14: "AMA Glosses over the Fishbein Case," *New York Times*, June 8, 1949: 31,53.

Chapter Ten. Political Challenge and Response

1. American Medical Association, *Digest of Official Actions 1846-1958*, (Chicago: AMA, 1959): 321.

2. John M. Glasgow, "The Compulsory Health Insurance Movement in the United States" (unpublished Ph.D. thesis, Department of Economics, University of Colorado, 1965): 154-56.

3. Morris Fishbein, "Wagner-Murray-Dingell Bill," *JAMA* 122 (1943): 609-611.

4. *Proceedings*, June 1943: 68-71.

5. United States versus the American Medical Association, 371 U.S. 519 (1943).

6. *Transcript*, June 1943: 31-34.

7. Joe D. Miller, interview with author, April 19, 1979.

8. Board of Trustees, minutes, June 1943.

9. Key actions establishing the Council on Medical Service are to be found in *Proceedings*, June 1943: 68-71, 84, 85.

10. *Proceedings*, June 1944: 55-61.

11. Board of Trustees, minutes, September 22-23, 1944.

12. *Proceedings*, June 1944: 58, 61.

13. Board of Trustees, minutes, July 1946: 216; *Proceedings*, July 1946: 43.

14. *Transcript*, December 1945: 187.

15. *Proceedings*, July 1946: 48, 67, 70; *Transcript*, July 1946: 3.

16. *Transcript*, June 1944: 23-24.

17. *Transcript*, December 1945: 185-86.

18. Board of Trustees, minutes, June 1945: 219.

19. *Transcript*, December 1945: 185-86.

20. *Transcript*, July 1946: 15-16.

21. "National Physicians' Committee for the Extension of Medical Service," *JAMA* 113 (1939): 2062-63.

22. U.S. Senate, Committee on Education and Labor, hearings, April 19, 1946.

23. "The Dan Gilbert Letter," *JAMA* 139 (1949): 588.

24. "A National Health Program," *JAMA* 130 (1945): 1021-23.

25. Monte M. Poen, *Harry S. Truman Versus the Medical Lobby* (Columbia: University of Missouri Press, 1979): 73.

26. "The President's National Health Program and the New Wagner Bill," *JAMA* 129 (1945): 950-53.

27. "Compulsory Sickness Insurance," *JAMA* 129 (1945): 632.

28. "The Wagner-Murray-Dingell Bill," *JAMA* 130 (1945): 1021-23.

29. Odin W. Anderson, *Blue Cross Since 1929* (Cambridge, Massachusetts: Ballinger, 1975): 62.

30. *Proceedings*, December 1945: 74-83.

31. "Hearings on S. 1606—To Provide for a National Health Program," *JAMA* 131 (1946): 225-35.

32. Raymond T. Rich, unpublished report prepared for the AMA, 1946.

33. Board of Trustees, minutes, June 29-July 4, 1946; *Proceedings*, July 1946: 67-69.

34. *Transcript*, July 1946: 122-23.

35. *Proceedings*, July 1947: 39, 73-74.

36. Board of Trustees, minutes, February 1946: 75-85.

37. *Transcript*, July 1946: 24-25.

38. *Proceedings*, December 1946: 18.

39. "Prepaid Medical Care," *JAMA* 128 (1945): 1173-77.

Chapter Eleven. The Nation Makes a Choice

1. Robert T. Elson, *The World of Time Inc.* (New York: Atheneum, 1973): 245.

2. *Proceedings*, November-December 1948: 2.

3. Ibid., 55, 62-65, 72-74.

4. Ernest B. Howard, interview with author, March 28, 1979.

5. "Hearings on Health Insurance," *JAMA* 140 (1949): 893.

6. "Hearings on S. 1606—To Provide for a National Health Program," *JAMA* 131 (1946): 1439-40.

7. Monte M. Poen, *Harry S. Truman Versus the Medical Lobby* (Columbia: University of Missouri Press, 1979): 114, 115.

8. "Hearings on Health Insurance," *JAMA* 140 (1949): 817-18.

9. James G. Burrow, *AMA: Voice of American Medicine* (Baltimore: Johns Hopkins University Press, 1963): 355.

10. American Medical Association, *Secretary's Letter*, No. 85, November 29, 1948.

11. "The Assessment and Public Opinion," *JAMA* 138 (1948): 1230-31.

12. Clem Whitaker, speech to House of Delegates, *Proceedings*, June 1949: 36. His estimate of "45,000 full-time and part-time press agents and propagandists in Washington supported by taxpayers at a cost of $75 million" is not documented. While Whitaker's numbers are to be questioned, the fact of a strong press capability within government is not.

13. Al Weisman, "The Campaign Against Compulsory Health Insurance," *St. Louis Post-Dispatch*, May 1, 1949.

14. Theodore H. White, *Breach of Faith* (Garden City, New York: Doubleday, 1976): 14, 15; Carey McWilliams, "Government by Whitaker and Baxter," *The Nation* 172 (April 14, 21; May 5, 1951); 346-48; 366-69; 419-21.

15. *Proceedings*, June 1951: 15.

16. "Doctors at War," *Time* 56 (July 10, 1950): 30, 33, 34.

17. Elmer L. Henderson, "The Responsibilities of American Medicine," *JAMA* 143 (1950): 783-85.

18. "Which Medicine?" *Time* 53 (June 21, 1949): 48.

19. *Source Book of Health Insurance Data* (Washington: Health Insurance Institute, 1980): 13.

20. *Proceedings*, June 1949: 35.

21. Ernest B. Howard, interview with author, April 7, 1980.

22. Poen, *Truman Versus the Medical Lobby*: 167.

23. Ibid., 165-67.

24. "Statement by the Board of Trustees on Investigations of Medical Organizations," *JAMA* 141 (1949): 465; "Report of the Bureau of Legal Medicine and Legislation," *JAMA* 144 (1950): 645.

25. Poen, *Truman Versus the Medical Lobby*: 164, 177.

26. John B. Martin, *Adlai E. Stevenson of Illinois*, Vol. 1 (Garden City, New York: Doubleday, 1976): 610.

27. *Proceedings*, December 1945: 45, 49, 71.

28. Frank G. Dickinson, "An Analysis of the Ewing Report," *Bulletin 69*, Bureau of Medical Economic Research, American Medical Association (Chicago: AMA, August 1949).

29. "Hearings on S. 1606—To Provide a National Health Program," *JAMA* 131 (1946): 1023-29

30. Ibid., 151-162.

31. "Hearings on National Health Insurance, *JAMA* 140 (July 2, 1949): 817-19.

32. Dickinson, "An Analysis of the Ewing Report."

33. American Medical Association, *Digest of Official Actions 1846-1958* (Chicago: AMA, 1959): 198-201.

34. Bernard DeVoto, "Letter to A Family Doctor," *Harper's Magazine* 202 (January 1951): 56-59.

35. Carol Brierly Golin, interview with author, April 25, 1980.

36. *Proceedings*, June 1950: 5, 6, 10-12; June 1951: 6, 10-12.

Chapter Twelve. The Not-So-Quiet 1950s

1. John A.D. Cooper, "Undergraduate Medical Education" in *Advances in American Medicine: Essays at the Bicentennial*, Vol. 1, ed. J.Z. Bowers and E.P. Purcell (New York: Josiah Macy, Jr. Foundation, 1976): 274.

2. *Proceedings*, December 1949: 52-53.

3. Richard Carter, *The Doctor Business* (Garden City, New York: Doubleday, 1958), 91-92.

4. *Proceedings*, June 1951: 41.

5. "Commission on Financing Higher Educaton," *JAMA* 146 (1951): 376.

6. "New Support for Medical Education," *JAMA* 144 (1951): 1378-79.

7. *Proceedings*, June 1951: 41.

8. The final debate on this issue is recorded in *Transcript*, June 1956: 124-43; previous discussions may be found in *Proceedings*, June 1955: 123, 139: June 1956: 55, 67; see also June 1960: 95.

9. American Medical Association, *Money and Medical Students*, (Chicago: AMA, 1963): 18.

10. American Medical Association, *The American Health Care System 1982* (Chicago: AMA, 1982): 46.

11. *Proceedings*, June 1951: 16-17.

12. "Medical Education in the United States and Canada," *JAMA* 77 (1921): 530-31.

13. Frank Billings, "Medical Education in the U.S.," *JAMA* 40 (1903): 1272.

14. George H. Simmons, "Medical Education and Preliminary Requirements," *JAMA* 42 (1904): 1205.

15. "Medical Education in the United States and Canada," *JAMA* 144 (1950): 115.)

16. Herman G. Weiskotten, *A History of the Council on Medical Education* (Chicago: AMA, 1959): 13.

17. U.S. Bureau of the Census, *Historical Statistics of the U.S.: Colonial Times to 1970*, Part I (Washington: U.S. Government Printing Office, 1975): 176.

18. *Proceedings*, June 1933: 28.

19. Walter L. Bierring, "The Family Doctor," *JAMA* 102 (1934): 1997-98.

20. "Medical Education in the United States," *JAMA* 144 (1950).

21. Leonard W. Larson, *Report of the Commission on Medical Care Plans*, *JAMA* (Special Issue, January 17, 1959): 89-90.

22. M.I. Roemer and J.W. Friedman, *Doctors in Hospitals* (Baltimore: Johns Hopkins University Press, 1971): 5.

23. L. Powers, J.F. Whiting, and K.C. Opperman, "Trends in Medical School Faculties," *Journal of Medical Education* 37 (1962): 1068-70.

24. *Proceedings*, June 1955: 110-11.

25. *Transcript*, June 1955: 73.

26. *Proceedings*, June 1957: 26.

27. Morris Fishbein, "The Committee on the Costs of Medical Care," *JAMA* 99 (1932): 1950-52.

28. *Proceedings*, June 1959: 65.

29. Louis M. Orr, "The President's Page," *JAMA* 170 (1959): 1554.

30. *Transcript*, June 1951: 82-85; *Proceedings*, June 1952: 34; June 1954: 29-30; 38, *Transcript*, June 1954: 114-16; *Proceedings*, November-December 1955: 111-16, 134; June 1956: 53-55; November 1956: 103, 107-108.

31. *Proceedings*, November-December 1955: 134.

32. *Proceedings*, June 1957: 25.

33. *Proceedings*, June 1952: 4-5.

34. *Proceedings*, June 1955: 16-21.

35. Ibid., 167-83, 209.

36. *Proceedings*, June 1959: 58-60.

37. Unpublished report for AMA Board of Trustees, Robert Heller and Associates, Cleveland, Ohio, 1957.

38. Ernest B. Howard, interview with author, April 7, 1980.

39. Ibid.

40. "Public Opinion Survey About Doctors," *JAMA*: 160 (1956): 471-73.

41. *Proceedings*, December 1957: 106.

42. *Proceedings*, December 1958: 60-61.

43. Joe D. Miller, interview with author, March 25, 1980.

44. F.J.L. Blasingame, notes prepared for presentation, August 1, 1958.

45. *Proceedings*, December 1958: 111-16.

46. Frank C. Coleman, interview with author, June 8, 1981.

47. F.J.L. Blasingame, interview with author, October 23, 1980.

Chapter Thirteen. A Careful Plunge into Political Action

1. Frank C. Coleman, interview with author, June 8, 1981. Subsequent quotations from Coleman in this chapter are from the same interview.

2. C. Joseph Stetler, memo to F.J.L. Blasingame, March 24, 1959.

3. Joe D. Miller, interview with author, April 19, 1979.

4. Ernest B. Howard, interview with author, April 7, 1980.

5. C. Joseph Stetler, interview with author, June 15, 1979. Subsequent quotations from Stetler in this chapter are from the same interview.

6. William L. Watson, interview with author, October 13, 1981. Subsequent quotations from Watson in this chapter are from the same interview.

7. AMA Council on Legislative Activities, minutes, October 22, 1960.

8. David G. Baldwin, interview with author, June 14, 1979. Subsequent quotations from Baldwin in this chapter are from the same interview.

9. AMA Board of Trustees, minutes, May 27-28, 1961.

10. *Transcript*, November 1961: 118, 121, 123.

11. Joe D. Miller, interview with author, April 25, 1979. Subsequent quotations from Miller in this chapter are from the same interview.

12. Ibid.

13. *Proceedings*, June 1965: 23.

14. Donald E. Wood, "Remarks to the House of Delegates," *Proceedings*, November 1962: 12-13.

15. Blair Henningsgaard, interview with author, July 24, 1979.

16. Alfred Balitzer, *A Nation of Associations* (Washington: American Society of Association Executives, 1981): 84.

17. As quoted in *The Washington Lobby*, second edition (Washington: Congressional Quarterly Inc., 1974): 1-2.

18. Theodore H. White, *Breach of Faith* (Garden City, New York: Doubleday, 1976): 69.

19. A good example is the presidential address of George M. Fister, M.D., at the November 1962 meeting of the House of Delegates. One paragraph reads, "We will not compromise the fundamental principles in which we believe and for which we have fought in the past with courage and good judgment. We will not jeopardize our position either by indicating a willingness to consider a compromise which would damage our basic principles, or by hasty action which might be misinterpreted."

Chapter Fourteen. A Liberalized Policy on Education

1. Edward L. Turner, "Looking Ahead," *JAMA* 165 (1957): 1460.

2. U.S. Bureau of the Census, *Historical Statistics of the U.S., Colonial Times to 1970*, Part I (Washington: U.S. Government Printing Office, 1975): 49.

3. Landon Y. Jones, *Great Expectations* (New York: Ballantine Books, 1980): 2-3.

4. Frank G. Dickinson, "Supply of Physician Services," *JAMA* 145 (1951): 1260-64.

5. "Undergraduate Medical Education," *JAMA* 248 (1982): 3245.

6. John A.D. Cooper, "Undergraduate Medical Education," in *Advances in American Medicine: Essays at the Bicentennial*, Vol. 1, ed. J.Z. Bowers and E.P. Purcell (New York: The Josiah Macy Jr. Foundation, 1976): 277.

7. F.J.L. Blasingame, letter to Kenneth A. Roberts, Chairman, Subcommittee on Health and Safety, Interstate and Foreign Commerce Committee, U.S. House of Representatives, June 6, 1960.

8. C.H. William Ruhe, interview with author, December 7, 1981. Subsequent quotations from Ruhe in this chapter come from the same interview.

9. *Proceedings*, November 1960: 128.

10. *Proceedings*, December 1963: 79.

11. Christopher C. Fordham, "The Bane Report Revisited," *JAMA* 244 (1980): 354-57.

12. Frank G. Dickinson, "An Analysis of the Ewing Report," *Bulletin* 69, Bureau of Medical Economic Research, American Medical Association (Chicago: AMA, August 1949): 8-11.

13. *Costs of Education in the Health Professions: Report of a Study*, Part I (Bethesda, Maryland: Institute of Medicine, 1974): 2.

14. *Proceedings*, November-December 1964: 29, 30.

15. Gerald D. Dorman, testimony before the U.S. House of Representatives, Interstate and Foreign Commerce Committee, February 7, 1963.

16. *Proceedings*, June 1963: 36.

17. Ibid

18. AMA statement to the Subcommittee on Health, Committee on Labor and Public Welfare, U.S. Senate. Submitted by mail, September 8, 1965.

19. *Proceedings*, June 1965: 68.

20. *Proceedings*, June 1966: 65, 85, 86, 101.

21. *JAMA* 244 (1980): 2813, 2845-49.

22. American Medical Association, *Socioeconomic Issues of Health* (Chicago: AMA, 1980): 151.

23. Statement to the health subcommittee, U.S. Senate, September 8, 1965.

23. Statement to the health subcommittee, U.S. Senate, September 8, 1965.

24. *Proceedings*, June 1966: 65, 66.

25. *Proceedings*, November 1967: 113, 248.

26. *Proceedings*, June 1968: 93-94.

27. "Undergraduate Medical Education," *JAMA* 246 (1981): 2917.

28. *The American Health Care System 1982* (Chicago: AMA, 1982): 46-47.

29. *Proceedings*, November 1967: 113, 248.

Chapter Fifteen. Medicare and Medicaid

1. Odin W. Anderson, *Blue Cross Since 1929* (Cambridge, Massachusetts: Ballinger, 1975): 85-86.

2. Theodore R. Marmor, *The Politics of Medicare* (Chicago: Aldine, 1973): 14-15.

3. Richard Harris, "Annals of Legislation: Medicare, All Very Hegelian," *New Yorker*, July 2, 1966.

4. Martha Derthick, *Policymaking for Social Security* (Washington: The Brookings Institute, 1979): 130-131.

5. Ibid., 122.

6. Ibid., 116.

7. Ibid., 321.

8. *Proceedings*, June 1961: 163.

9. *Proceedings*, November 1961: 2-6.

10. Leonard W. Larson, testimony before the Committee on Finance, U.S. Senate, June 30, 1960; *Proceedings*, June 1960: 4, 89.

11. David G. Baldwin, interview with author, June 14, 1979. Subsequent quotations from Baldwin in this chapter are from the same interview.

12. "The Big Push," *New England Journal of Medicine* 265 (1961): 1317.

13. Everett R. Spencer, *A Society of Physicians* (Boston: Massachusetts Medical Society, 1981): 342.

14. William R. Ramsey, interview with author, June 15, 1979. Subsequent material attributed to Ramsey in this chapter is from the same interview.

15. Richard Reinauer, interview with author, April 1979. Subsequent quotations from Reinauer in this chapter are from the same interview.

16. Richard Harris, "Annals of Legislation: Medicare, We Do Not Compromise," *New Yorker*, July 16, 1966.

17. Edward R. Annis, interview with author, July 24, 1979.

18. "Hardship Case Still a Mystery," *AMNews* 5 (June 11, 1962): 4.

19. "The Moment of Truth," *AMNews* 5 (June 11, 1962): 5.

20. Harris, "Annals of Legislation: We Do Not Compromise."

21. "Rallies Fail to Draw Crowds," *AMNews* 5 (May 28, 1962): 1. Accompanying the *AMNews* story is a photograph by the *Charleston Mail* showing the sparsely occupied auditorium.

22. Spencer, *A Society of Physicians*, 344.

23. *Proceedings*, June 1963: 152-53.

24. Wilbur J. Cohen, interview with author, February 22, 1980.

25. "The Moment of Truth," *AMNews*.

26. Max H. Parrott, interview with author, May 11, 1980.

27. Bernard P. Harrison, interview with author, March 2, 1979.

28. Harris, "Annals of Legislation: We Do Not Compromise."

29. Wayne W. Bradley, interview with author, April 13, 1979.

30. Marmor, *The Politics of Medicare*: 56.

31. *Proceedings*, February 6-7, 1965: 3.

32. *Proceedings*, November-December, 1964: 153.

33. *Transcript*, February 6-7, 1965: 46-47.

34. *Proceedings*, February 6-7, 1965: 19.

35. Robert J. Myers, *Medicare* (Bryn Mawr, Pennsylvania: McCahan Foundation, 1970): 54-63.

36. Donovan Ward, testimony before the Committee on Finance, U.S. Senate, May 11, 1965.

37. Minority Report of the Committee on Finance, U.S. Senate, reprinted in *AMNews* 8 (July 5, 1965): 1, 7.

38. *Proceedings*, June 1965: 115-16.

39. Memoranda from the Lyndon B. Johnson Library, Austin, Texas: Wilbur Cohen to Douglass Cater of the White House staff; Cater to the President, July 28, 1965.

40. This account of the meeting was constructed with the help of interviews with Russell B. Roth on August 22, 1979, and Wilbur J. Cohen on February 22, 1980. Further quotations from Roth and Cohen in this chapter are from these interviews.

41. The Cohen and Roth interviews plus a memorandum from Ernest B. Howard to F.J.L. Blasingame, August 31, 1965.

42. *Transcript*, October 2-3, 1965: 75-76.

43. *Proceedings*, October 2-3, 1965: 6-7.

44. Charles E. Phelps, "Public Sector Medicine: History and Analysis," in *New Directions in Public Health Care* (San Francisco: the Institute for Contemporary Studies, 1976): 135-36.

Chapter Sixteen. The Pragmatists Come to Power

1. *Proceedings*, June 1965: 75; October 1965: 9, 30; November-December 1965: 103-104, 179-80.

2. F.J.L. Blasingame, interview with author, October 23, 1980.

3. Ted Lewis, Jr., interview with author, June 14, 1979.

4. Max H. Parrott, interviews with author, July 23 and 29, 1979. Subsequent quotations from Parrott in this chapter come from the same interviews.

5. Ernest B. Howard, interview with author, April 7, 1980.

6. William R. Ramsey, interview with author, June 15, 1979.

7. Joe D. Miller, interview with author, April 25, 1979. Subsequent quotations from Miller in this chapter come from the same interview.

8. Blair Henningsgaard, interview with author, July 24, 1979.

9. This account of the actions that culminated in Dr. Blasingame's dismissal is based on interviews with Max H. Parrott, James H. Sammons, and Joe D. Miller. It also relies on the minutes of the September 5-8, 1968, meeting of the Board of Trustees and a letter written by Montgomery quoted in the next paragraph.

10. Board of Trustees, minutes, September 17-18, 1968.

11. *Proceedings*, December 1968: 186-87; *Transcript*, December 1968: 141-64.

12. Excerpts taken from the annual addresses of the Student American Medical Association presidents, given at the AMA annual meetings. They may be found in the appropriate *Proceedings*.

13. Ernest B. Howard, "Organized Medicine: The AMA," *Scope*, November-December 1970, publication of Boston University Medical Center.

Chapter Seventeen. NHI: The High-Water Mark

1. "Lobby Planned to Push National Health Insurance," *AMNews* 11 (November 25, 1968): 1, 8.

2. Bernard P. Harrison, interview with author, April 2, 1979.

3. Russell B. Roth, interview with author, April 11, 1980. Subsequent quotations from Roth in this chapter are from the same interview.

4. *Proceedings*, November 1962: 199.

5. Ibid., 113-16, 200.

6. *Proceedings*, June 1968: 76-85, 126-27, 193, 216-17.

7. *Proceedings*, December 1968: 111-15, 217.

8. Russell B. Roth, testimony before Ways and Means Committee, U.S. House of Representatives, November 3, 1969.

9. This opinion was expressed by Russell B. Roth (see note 3) and also by Ernest B. Howard in an interview with the author, March 28, 1979.

10. "National Health Insurance Proposals," *Legislative Analysis* No. 19 (Washington: American Enterprise Institute, 1974): 37-54.

11. Louis Harris, "Confidence in Major Institutions Slips Sharply," news release by the Harris Survey, *Chicago Tribune-New York News* Syndicate Inc., October 25, 1971.

12. Before 1968 the *Proceedings* did not carry the text of the president's inaugural address. The quotation here is taken from the copy of President Rouse's speech in the AMA archive library.

13. Daniel Bell, *The Cultural Contradictions of Capitalism* (New York: Basic Books, 1976): 41.

14. Edward M. Kennedy, "Introduction of the Health Security Act," *Congressional Record* 116 (August 27, 1970): 30142-45.

15. "It's Time to Operate," *Fortune* 81 (January 1970): 79.

16. Ernest B. Howard, letter to Julian Goodman, president of NBC- TV, January 10, 1973; Frank D. Campion, "Point of Contact," *Canadian Medical Association Journal* 111 (1973): 232, 238-39.

17. *National Health Insurance, Hearings before the Committee on Labor and Public Welfare, U.S. Senate*, Part I (Washington: U.S. Government Printing Office, 1970): 208.

18. Max H. Parrott and Russell B. Roth, testimony before the Subcommittee on Health, U.S. Senate, March 15, 1971, and before the Ways and Means Committee, U.S. House of Representatives, November 10, 1971.

19. For further discussion of the difficulty in comparing international vital statistics see: *Handbook of Vital Statistics Methods* (New York: Statistical Office of the United Nations, 1955): 8-9.

20. "What America Thinks of Itself." *Newsweek* 82 (December 10, 1983): 40.

21. *Proceedings*, June 1977: 11.

22. Wayne W. Bradley, interview with author, April 13, 1979.

23. This account of the high-water mark of national health insurance legislation is based upon and borrows heavily from articles in *AMNews* August 26, 1974, by Ted Lewis Jr. It also relies on the interview with Bradley, see note 22.

24. Wilbur J. Cohen, "Observations Regarding National Health Insurance," in *National Commission on the Cost of Medical Care*, Vol. 2 (Chicago: AMA, 1977): 208.

25. Stephan P. Strickland, *U.S. Health Care: What's Wrong and What's Right?* (New York: Universe Books, 1972): 26-30. In the early 1970s, polls done by *LIFE* magazine, the *Washington Post*, the Continental Illinois Bank of Chicago, Black Opinion Survey of Washington, D.C., Roper Reports and the University of Michigan Institute for Social Research indicated that from 70-85 percent of the publics sampled were "satisfied" or "well satisfied" with the health care they received.

Chapter Eighteen. The Politics of Rising Costs

1. Lynn E. Jensen, "Trends in Health Care Costs and Prices," *National Commission on the Cost of Medical Care 1976-1977*, Vol. 2 (Chicago: AMA, 1978): 3-4.

2. U.S Bureau of the Census, *Historical Statistics of the U.S.: Colonial Times to 1970*, Vol. 1 (Washington: U.S. Government Printing Office, 1975): 82.

3. Marjorie Smith Mueller and Robert M. Gibson, "National Health Expenditures, Fiscal Year 1975," *Social Security Bulletin*, (February, 1976): 3, table.

4. C.R. Fisher, "Differences by Age Groups in Health Care Spending," *Health Care Financing Review* 1 (Spring 1980): 81-83.

5. Walter J. McNerney, interview with author April 4, 1980.

6. Mueller and Gibson, "National Health Expenditures:" 3.

7. Committee on Finance, U.S. Senate, *Medicare and Medicaid* (Washington: U.S. Government Printing Office, 1970): 1.

8. *Proceedings*, June 1970: 63-65.

9. William O. LaMotte, testimony before the Committee on Finance, U.S. Senate, September 23, 1970.

10. "AMA Clarifies the Record on PSRO," *AMNews* 16 (November 19, 1973): 1, 5, 14-15.

11. "MDs' Doubts Demonstrated at Conference," *AMNews* 16 (December 10, 1973): 12.

12. *Proceedings*, December 1973: 26.

13. "AMA Expands PSRO Policy to Seek Repeal," *AMNews* 16 (December 10, 1973): 1, 3, 4, 14.

14. "Delegates Refuse to Seek PSRO Repeal," *Proceedings*, June 1974: 323, 378-80.

15. Helen L. Smits, "The PSRO in Perspective," *New England Journal of Medicine* 303 (1981): 258.

16. *Proceedings*, December 1978: 12.

17. "HEW Agrees to Issue Revised Medicare List," *AMNews* 20 (March 20, 1977): 1, 4, 10.

18. Smits, "PSRO in Perspective:" 258.

19. *Proceedings*, June 1971: 232-45.

20. *Proceedings*, July 1980: 128-33; also, *Health Maintenance Organizations* (Chicago: AMA, 1980).

21. Harold S. Luft, *Health Maintenance Organizations* (New York: John Wiley & Sons, 1981): 1, 36, 39.

22. *Proceedings*, July 1980: 133.

23. *Proceedings*, June 1981: 153-54.

24. *Proceedings*, December 1981: 145-46.

25. *The National Health Maintenance Organization Census of 1980* (Washington: Office of Health Maintenance Organizations, U.S. Department of Health and Human Services, 1981).

26. Russell B. Roth, testimony before the Subcommittee on Health, Committee on Labor and Public Welfare, U.S. Senate, March 20, 1974.

27. *Proceedings*, December 1978: 54.

28. "HSA Failures: The Most Damning Report to Date," *Medical Economics* 58 (1981): 251-60.

29. Karen Garloch, "CORVA Using Kid Gloves with Funds, Plans," *Cincinnati Enquirer* (August 11, 1981): D-1.

30. *Proceedings*, December 1978: 12-18.

31. American Medical Association, *Opinions and Reports of the Judicial Council* (Chicago: AMA, 1977): 41.

32. *Proceedings*, December 1978: 13.

33. *Proceedings*, June 1978: 30.

34. Lynn E. Jensen, interview with author, June 24, 1982.

35. *Proceedings*, June 1978: 31-49.

36. Victor M. Zink, "The Public's Expectations," in *National Commission on the Cost of Medical Care*, Vol. 2 (Chicago: AMA, 1978): 192.

37. Walter J. McNerney, "Consumer Demand for Services: Health Insurer's View," in *National Commission on the Cost of Medical Care*, Vol. 2 (Chicago: AMA, 1978): 127.

38. Dan Rostenkowski, "Hospital Cost Containment," *Congressional Record* 123 (November 2, 1977): H12086.

39. Max H. Parrott, "Medical Care Costs," *National Journal* June 26, 1976.

Chapter Nineteen. A Gathering of Troubles

1. *Proceedings*, June 1968: 46; July 1969: 52; June 1970: 36.

2. James H. Sammons, "Report to the Special Committee," April 20, 1975, *Proceedings*, June 1975: 344.

3. *Proceedings*, June 1970: 37-44.

4. Ibid., 42, 80-84.

5. Ibid., 317-19.

6. *Transcript*, June 1970: 543-44, 555, 568.

7. Ibid., 555-59.

8. Max H. Parrott, letter to Joseph T. Painter, April 17, 1975.

9. *Proceedings*, June 1971: 43-45.

10. *Proceedings*, November-December 1971: 138-40, 282-84; Board of Trustees, minutes, November 29, 1971: 26-27.

11. Robert B. Hunter, interview with author, May 9, 1980.

12. Parrott, letter to Painter.

13. *Proceedings*, November-December 1970: 3-5.

14. *Proceedings*, November 1972: 69-72.

15. *Proceedings*, July 1969: 260.

16. "Turmoil at the AMA," *Medical World News* 15 (May 10, 1974): 12, 51-55, 60-62.

17. "Showdown at the AMA—Delegates Take Charge." *Medical World News* 15 (July 19, 1974): 15-18.

18. James H. Sammons, interview with author, May 16, 1980. Subsequent quotations from Sammons in this chapter are from the same interview.

19. Joe D. Miller, interview with author, March 27, 1980. Subsequent quotations from Miller in this chapter are from the same interview.

20. *Proceedings*, December 1974: 105-15.

21. The number of AMA employees varies in the reports made at this time. The figures used here are taken from a report Sammons made to the House of Delegates. See *Proceedings*, June 1975: 364.

22. *Proceedings*, December 1974: 130-31.

23. "A 10-Hour Shootout in Portland," *AMNews* 17 (December 9, 1974): 1, 8.

24. *Proceedings*, December 1974: 105-12, 375-77.

25. *Transcript*, December 1974; 258, 272.

26. *Proceedings*, December 1974: 130-31.

27. Theodore R. Chilcoat, Jr., interview with author, August 10, 1982.

28. *Proceedings*, June 1975: 105.

Chapter Twenty. The Turnaround

1. *Proceedings*, June 1975: 106-107, 326-30, 341-52, 358-59, 365.

2. *Proceedings*, December 1979: 85.

3. *Proceedings*, June 1975: 282-361

4. *AMNews* 18 (June 23-30, 1975): 1, 19; *Transcript*, June 1975: 477-92.

5. *Proceedings*, June 1975: 365-66.

6. James W. Coursey, interview with author, August 17, 1982.

7. *Proceedings*, June 1975: 344.

8. Larry Boston, interview with author, January 20, 1981.

9. Edward W. Barrett, letter to author, January 27, 1979.

10. *Proceedings*, June 1975: 359.

11. *Transcript*, June 1975: 539-96.

12. Joe D. Miller, interview with author, August 5, 1982.

13. Thomas F. Hannon, interview with author, December 18, 1980.

14. Board of Trustees, minutes, March 11-13, 1976.

15. *Proceedings*, November-December 1969: 156.

16. Ibid., 316.

17. Bruce Balfe, interview with author, March 9, 1981. Subsequent quotations from Balfe in this chapter are from this same interview.

18. Ibid.

19. Ibid.

20. *Proceedings*, June 1973: 47.

21. James H. Sammons, memorandum to the Board of Trustees, August 28, 1975.

22. Jan W. Erfert, interview with author, February 25, 1981.

23. *Proceedings*, December 1976: 175.

24. AMA Staff Task Force, "Report on Council and Committee Structure," May 1975.

25. *Proceedings*, June 1968: 158.

26. *Proceedings*, July 1969: 53-77.

27. Ernest B. Howard, "Critique of the Two Reports by Cresap, McCormick, and Paget," memorandum to the Board of Trustees, March 14, 1969.

28. *Proceedings*, July 1969: 58.

29. Ibid.

30. *Proceedings*, November 1972: 69-72.

31. Max H. Parrott, interview with author, July 25, 1979.

32. John C. Ballin, interview with author, May 15, 1979.

33. *Proceedings*, June 1973: 451.

34. Board of Trustees, minutes, October 1974.

35. *Proceedings*, June 1975: 3, 6-25.

36. Ibid., 358

37. Ibid., 349-50.

38. *Proceedings*, November-December 1975: 139-65.

39. *Transcript*, November-December 1975: 624-30.

40. *Proceedings*, June 1975: 352.

41. Joe D. Miller, interview with author, March 26, 1981. Subsequent quotations from Miller in this chapter are from the same interview.

42. James H. Sammons, interview with author, May 16, 1980. Subsequent quotations from Sammons in this chapter are from the same interview.

Chapter Twenty-One. The AMA and Medical Education

1. "Report of the Council on Medical Education," JAMA 45 (1905): 269; Arthur D. Bevan, "Report of the Council on Medical Education," JAMA 72 (1919): 1751-61; Arthur D. Bevan, "Cooperation in Medical Education and Medical Service," JAMA 90 (1928): 1173-77; Victor Johnson, "The Council on Medical Education and Hospitals," in Morris Fishbein, A History of the American Medical Association (Philadelphia: W.B. Saunders, 1947): 893-903.

2. JAMA 244 (1980): 2816.

3. Leonard D. Fenninger, interview with the author, November 22, 1982. Subsequent quotations from Fenninger in this chapter come from the same interview.

4. American Medical Association, Future Directions in Medical Education (Chicago: AMA, 1982): 53.

5. Rosemary V. Stevens, American Medicine and the Public Interest (New Haven: Yale University Press, 1971): 55. A statement of the economic rationale is to be found here though Stevens believes that the reform was "partly educational, partly restrictionist."

6. C.H. William Ruhe, interview with author, December 10, 1982. Subsequent quotations from Ruhe in this chapter are from the same interview.

7. Johnson, "A History of the Council on Medical Education," 899.

8. Stevens, Medicine and the Public Interest, 75-115, and AMA, Future Directions, 66-72, are the author's main sources of information on the specialization of American medicine.

9. Proceedings, April 1920: 31-32.

10. George A. Silver, "Family Practice," JAMA 185 (1963): 188.

11. The Citizens Commission on Graduate Medical Education, The Graduate Education of Physicians (Chicago: American Medical Association, 1966): 38.

12. Ibid., vi.

13. Ibid., 5-7.

14. Proceedings, November 1966: 134.

15. Citizens Commission, Graduate Education, 98.

16. *Proceedings*, December 1968: 101-103

17. C.H. William Ruhe, memo filed with the minutes of the March 12-14, 1970, meeting of the Council on Medical Education.

18. Council on Medical Education, minutes, June 18-20, 1971: 30.

19. *Proceedings*, June 1972: 72-76.

20. John C. Gienapp, interview with author, November 19, 1982.

21. Douglas D. Vollan, *Postgraduate Medical Education in the U.S.* (Chicago: American Medical Association, 1955): 28.

22. Jerome D. Freedman, "Explanation of the CME Advisory Committee Draft of Guidelines to the Essentials," *AMA Continuing Medical Education Newsletter* 12 No. 2 (1983): 2-7.

23. *Proceedings*, December 1979: 17.

24. *JAMA* 159 (1955): 600; 202 (1967): 796; 244 (1980): 2837.

25. *Allied Health Education Directory*, tenth edition (Chicago: American Medical Association, 1981): 1-2.

26. *Proceedings*, November-December 1969: 179-82.

27. AMA, *Future Directions*: 91.

28. American Medical Association, *U.S. Medical Licensure and Statistics* (Chicago: AMA, 1980): 4-5.

29. James J. Haug and Rosemary V. Stevens, "Foreign Medical Graduates in the U.S. in 1963 and 1971: A Cohort Study," *Inquiry* 10 (March 1973): 26-32.

30. Thomas D. Dublin, *The Changing Role of the FMG* (Philadelphia: Educational Commission for Foreign Medical Graduates, 1981): 4. Dublin gives 22.9 percent as the total at the end of 1979.

31. *Proceedings*, June 1954: 57-58.

32. AMA, *Future Directions*: 79-80.

33. AMA, *Future Directions*: 80; *Proceedings*, June 1975: 125-79.

34. AMA, *Future Directions*: 81.

35. *JAMA* 246 (1981): 2917, 2939.

36. Thomas D. Dublin, "Foreign Physicians: Their Impact on U.S. Health Care," *Science* 185 (August 2, 1974): 407-14.

37. *Proceedings*, June 1975: 127.

38. Dublin, "Foreign Physicians," 411.

39. Stephen S. Mick, "The Foreign Medical Graduate," *Scientific American* 232 (February 1975): 17.

Chapter Twenty-Two. The AMA and Science

1. American Medical Association, *1983 Budget*: 13, 15. The figure is arrived at by adding the entire $28,952,000 for Mission B (provide scientific information) to the $12,584,000 for scientific policy and information under Mission A (represent the profession).

2. John Duffy, *The Healers: The Rise of the Medical Establishment* (New York: McGraw-Hill, 1976): 109-28.

3. Frank Billings, "Address of the President," *JAMA* 45 (1905): 1901.

4. Austin Smith, "The Council on Pharmacy and Chemistry," in Morris Fishbein, *A History of the American Medical Association* (Philadelphia: W.B. Saunders Company, 1947): 870-75.

5. Bliss O. Halling, "The Bureau of Investigation," in Morris Fishbein, *A History of the American Medical Association* (Philadelphia: W.B. Saunders, 1947): 1034-38.

6. Philip L. White, "A Brief History of the AMA's Council on Foods and Nutrition," *Nutrition Today* (January-February 1975): 10-14.

7. *Proceedings*, November-December 1955: 26-35.

8. Board of Trustees, minutes, June 18, 1954: 199.

9. White, "History of the Council on Foods and Nutrition:" 11.

10. Board of Trustees, minutes, February 4, 1955: 109-110.

11. Bernard D. Hirsh, interview with author, May 24, 1979.

12. Lester S. King, "The Founding of *JAMA*," *JAMA* 250 (1983): 177.

13. William R. Barclay, interview with author, February 9, 1983. Subsequent quotations from Barclay in this chapter come from the same interview.

14. Richard J. Jones, interview with author, February 25, 1983. Subsequent quotations from Jones in this chapter are from the same interview.

15. Roy E. Ritts, interview with author, May 20, 1980.

16. Francis J.L. Blasingame, interview with author, March 10, 1983.

17. *Proceedings*, June 1963: 7.

18. Ibid., 9.

19. Walter S. Wiggins, memorandum to F.J.L. Blasingame, M.D., September 20, 1963.

20. *Proceedings*, December 1968: 90.

21. *Transcript*, November 1967: 214.

22. *Transcript*, December 1968: 210.

23. *Proceedings*, November-December 1969: 220-22, 304.

24. Austin Smith, letter to the author, February 4, 1983.

25. *Proceedings*, December 1951: 9.

26. Hugh H. Hussey, editorial, *JAMA* 211 (1970): 113.

27. *Proceedings*, November 1962: 6.

28. John H. Talbott, "Cover—1960 Design," *JAMA* 173 (1960): 1030.

29. *Proceedings*, November-December 1960: 74.

30. "Dr. Moser New Editor of AMA Journal," *AMNews* (July 16, 1973): 12.

31. J.H. Sammons, J.D. Miller, and T.F. Hannon,"The Journal and Publications in Other Languages and Countries," *JAMA* 250 (1983): 236-41.

32. Ibid.

33. George D. Lundberg, interview with author, March 14, 1983.

Chapter Twenty-Three. The AMA and Medical Care Today

1. National Center for Health Statistics, *Health—United States, 1981.* (Washington: U.S. Government Printing Office, 1981): 111; U.S. Bureau of Census, *Statistical Abstract of the United States, 1982-83* (Washington: U.S. Government Printing Office, 1983): 71.

2. Bureau of Census, *Statistical Abstract, 1982-83*: 75.

3. U.S. Department of the Census, *Historical Statistics of the United States, Colonial Times to 1 970*, Part I (Washington: U.S. Government Printing Office, 1975): 58; Bureau of the Census, *Statistical Abstract, 1982-83::* 76.

4. Bureau of Census, *Historical Statistics to 1970*: 58.

5. Center for Health Statistics, *Health—United States, 1981*: 120, 135.

6. Ibid., 111.

7. Bureau of the Census, *Statistical Abstract, 1982-93*: 30; Bureau of the Census, *Historical Statistics to 1970*, Part I: 10.

8. Aaron Wildavsky, "Doing Better and Feeling Worse," *Daedalus*, (Winter, 1977).

9. G.H. Hunt and M. Goldstein, "Medical Group Practice in the United States," *United States Public Health Service Publications* 77 (1951): 49.

10. Sharon R. Henderson, Richard J. Odem, and Karen M. Ginsberg, *Medical Groups in the United States, 1980* (Chicago: AMA, 1982): 6, 13, 14, 88.

11. Augustine Gentile, "Physician Visits: Volume and Interval Since Last Visit," *Vital and Health Statistics*, Series 10, No. 128 (1975): 1.

12. American Medical Association, *The American Health Care System 1982* (Chicago: AMA, 1982): 53.

13. National Center for Health Statistics, *Health—United States, 1979* (Washington: U.S. Government Printing Office, 1979): 13.

14. Gentile, "Physician Visits," 9.

15. Health Insurance Institute, *Source Book of Health Insurance Data, 1980-81* (Washington: Health Insurance Association of America, 1981): 8-9.

16. Robert M. Gibson and Daniel R. Waldo, "National Health Expenditures, 1981," *Health Care Financing Review*, 4, No. 1 (1982): 25.

17. Ibid., 19, 20.

18. AMA, *The American Health Care System 1982*: 2-4.

19. American Hospital Association, *Hospital Statistics* (Chicago: AHA, 1981): 5.

20. AMA, *The American Health Care System 1982*: 24.

21. Ibid., 21.

22. Center for Health Statistics, *Health—United States, 1979*: 13.

23. AMA, *The American Health Care System 1982*: 1.

24. Ibid., 19.

25. AHA, *Hospital Statistics*, (1981): 5.

26. Gibson and Waldo, "National Health Expenditures," 25.

27. Lewis Thomas, "On the Science and Technology of Medicine," in *Doing Better and Feeling Worse*, ed. John N. Knowles (New York: W.W. Norton, 1977): 35.

28. "Business Aims to Trim Health Costs," *AMNews* (November 18, 1983): 7. Article quotes William Winters, a spokesman for General Motors.

29. Cotton M. Lindsay and Arthur Seldon, "More Evidence on Britain and Canada," in *New Directions in Public Health Care*, ed. Cotton M. Lindsay (San Francisco: Institute for Contemporary Studies, 1980): 85.

30. William B. Schwartz and Henry J. Aaron, "Rationing Hospital Care, Lessons from Britain," *New England Journal of Medicine* 310 (1984): 54.

31. L.S. Richman, "Health Benefits Come under the Knife," *Fortune* 107 (1983): 95-110.

32. Walter J. McNerney, interview with author, April 8, 1980.

33. Joseph A. Califano, speech to the American Association of Medical Colleges, New Orleans, Louisiana, October 24, 1978.

34. *Proceedings*, December 1981: 25-31.

35. "Recent Trends in Physician Liability Claims and Insurance Expenses," *SMS Reports* (Chicago: AMA, October 1982): 1.

36. AMA Constitution, Article II.

37. Ernest B. Howard, interview with author, April 7, 1980.

Picture Credits

Chapter 5. Pages 1 and 2: Joseph F. Fletcher, AMA staff photographer; Disney characters, © Walt Disney Productions. Page 3: AMA Archive Library. Pages 4 and 5: Fletcher.

Chapter 9. Page 1: *Chicago Daily News* photograph, from the Morris Fishbein Collection, the Regenstein Library, University of Chicago; Carl Mydans, copyright 1937, Time Inc. Pages 2 and 3: AMA Archive Library.

Chapter 11. Pages 1 and 2: courtesy Wyeth Laboratories, Philadelphia, Pa. Pages 3 and 4: Fletcher, AMA Archive Library. Page 5: courtesy John M. Goin; AMA Archive Library.

Chapter 13. Pages 1 and 2: Fletcher.

Chapter 15. Page 1: Lang, *The Daily Oklahoman.* Page 2: Crawford, Newspaper Enterprise Association. Pages 3 and 4: Fletcher. Page 5: Wide World Photos. Page 6: Troy/Beaumont.

Chapter 16. Page 1: Fletcher, AMA Archive Library.

Chapter 17. Pages 1 and 2: Fletcher. Page 3: Fletcher, AMA photographic file.

Chapter 19. Pages 1 and 2: Fletcher.

Chapter 23. Page 1: Maxwell MacKenzie.